Comparative Effectiveness Review
Number 112

Local Nonsurgical Therapies for Stage I and Symptomatic Obstructive Non–Small-Cell Lung Cancer

Prepared for:
Agency for Healthcare Research and Quality
U.S. Department of Health and Human Services
540 Gaither Road
Rockville, MD 20850
www.ahrq.gov

Contract No. 290-2007-10058-I

Prepared by:
Blue Cross and Blue Shield Association Technology Evaluation Center
Evidence-based Practice Center
Chicago, IL

Investigators:
Thomas A. Ratko, Ph.D.
Vikrant Vats, Ph.D.
Jennifer Brock, M.P.H.
B W. Ruffner, Jr., M.D.
Naomi Aronson, Ph.D.

AHRQ Publication No. 13-EHC071-EF
June 2013

This report is based on research conducted by the Blue Cross and Blue Shield Association Technology Evaluation Center Evidence-based Practice Center (EPC) under contract to the Agency for Healthcare Research and Quality (AHRQ), Rockville, MD (Contract No. 290-2007-10058-I). The findings and conclusions in this document are those of the authors, who are responsible for its contents; the findings and conclusions do not necessarily represent the views of AHRQ. Therefore, no statement in this report should be construed as an official position of AHRQ or of the U.S. Department of Health and Human Services.

The information in this report is intended to help health care decisionmakers—patients and clinicians, health system leaders, and policymakers, among others—make well-informed decisions and thereby improve the quality of health care services. This report is not intended to be a substitute for the application of clinical judgment. Anyone who makes decisions concerning the provision of clinical care should consider this report in the same way as any medical reference and in conjunction with all other pertinent information, i.e., in the context of available resources and circumstances presented by individual patients.

This report may be used, in whole or in part, as the basis for development of clinical practice guidelines and other quality enhancement tools, or as a basis for reimbursement and coverage policies. AHRQ or U.S. Department of Health and Human Services endorsement of such derivative products may not be stated or implied.

This document is in the public domain and may be used and reprinted without permission. Citation of the source is appreciated.

Persons using assistive technology may not be able to fully access information in this report. For assistance contact EffectiveHealthCare@ahrq.hhs.gov.

Suggested citation: Ratko TA, Vats V, Brock J, Ruffner BW Jr, Aronson N. Local Nonsurgical Therapies for Stage I and Symptomatic Obstructive Non–Small-Cell Lung Cancer. Comparative Effectiveness Review No. 112. (Prepared by Blue Cross and Blue Shield Association Technology Evaluation Center Evidence-based Practice Center under Contract No. 290-2007-10058-I.) AHRQ Publication No. 13-EHC071-EF. Rockville, MD: Agency for Healthcare Research and Quality; June 2013. www.effectivehealthcare.ahrq.gov/reports/final.cfm.

Preface

The Agency for Healthcare Research and Quality (AHRQ), through its Evidence-based Practice Centers (EPCs), sponsors the development of systematic reviews to assist public- and private-sector organizations in their efforts to improve the quality of health care in the United States. These reviews provide comprehensive, science-based information on common, costly medical conditions, and new health care technologies and strategies.

Systematic reviews are the building blocks underlying evidence-based practice; they focus attention on the strength and limits of evidence from research studies about the effectiveness and safety of a clinical intervention. In the context of developing recommendations for practice, systematic reviews can help clarify whether assertions about the value of the intervention are based on strong evidence from clinical studies. For more information about AHRQ EPC systematic reviews, see www.effectivehealthcare.ahrq.gov/reference/purpose.cfm.

AHRQ expects that these systematic reviews will be helpful to health plans, providers, purchasers, government programs, and the health care system as a whole. Transparency and stakeholder input are essential to the Effective Health Care Program. Please visit the Web site (www.effectivehealthcare.ahrq.gov) to see draft research questions and reports or to join an email list to learn about new program products and opportunities for input.

We welcome comments on this systematic review. They may be sent by mail to the Task Order Officer named below at: Agency for Healthcare Research and Quality, 540 Gaither Road, Rockville, MD 20850, or by email to epc@ahrq.hhs.gov.

Carolyn M. Clancy, M.D.
Director
Agency for Healthcare Research and Quality

Stephanie Chang, M.D., M.P.H.
Director, EPC Program
Center for Outcomes and Evidence
Agency for Healthcare Research and Quality

Jean Slutsky, P.A., M.S.P.H.
Director, Center for Outcomes and Evidence
Agency for Healthcare Research and Quality

Supriya Janakiraman, M.D., M.P.H.
Task Order Officer
Center for Outcomes and Evidence
Agency for Healthcare Research and Quality

Acknowledgments

The authors gratefully acknowledge the following individuals for their contributions to this project: Claudia Bonnell, R.N., M.L.S.; Lisa Garofalo, B.A.; Sarah Godfrey, M.P.H.; David Samson, M.S.; Lisa Sarsany, M.A.; Kathleen Ziegler, Pharm.D.

Key Informants

In designing the study questions, the EPC consulted several Key Informants who represent the end-users of research. The EPC sought the Key Informant input on the priority areas for research and synthesis. Key Informants are not involved in the analysis of the evidence or the writing of the report. Therefore, in the end, study questions, design, methodological approaches, and/or conclusions do not necessarily represent the views of individual Key Informants.

Key Informants must disclose any financial conflicts of interest greater than $10,000 and any other relevant business or professional conflicts of interest. Because of their role as end-users, individuals with potential conflicts may be retained. The TOO and the EPC work to balance, manage, or mitigate any conflicts of interest.

The list of Key Informants who participated in developing this report follows:

James Adamson, M.D.
Vice President and Medical Officer for
  National Accounts
Arkansas Blue Cross and Blue Shield
Little Rock, AR

James D. Cox, M.D.
Professor
Department of Radiation Oncology
Stringer Distinguished Chair in Oncology
University of Texas M.D. Anderson Cancer
  Center
Houston, TX

David Sturges
Patient Advocate
Lung Cancer Foundation of America
New Ulm, MN

Lynn Tanoue, M.D.
Professor of Medicine
Co-Director, Yale Cancer Center Thoracic
  Oncology Program
Yale School of Medicine
New Haven, CT

Robert D. Timmerman, M.D.
Professor of Radiation Oncology and
  Neurosurgery
University of Texas Southwestern Medical
  Center
Dallas, TX

Technical Expert Panel

In designing the study questions and methodology at the outset of this report, the EPC consulted several technical and content experts. Broad expertise and perspectives were sought. Divergent and conflicted opinions are common and perceived as healthy scientific discourse that results in a thoughtful, relevant systematic review. Therefore, in the end, study questions, design, methodologic approaches, and/or conclusions do not necessarily represent the views of individual technical and content experts.

Technical Experts must disclose any financial conflicts of interest greater than $10,000 and any other relevant business or professional conflicts of interest. Because of their unique clinical or content expertise, individuals with potential conflicts may be retained. The TOO and the EPC work to balance, manage, or mitigate any potential conflicts of interest identified.

The list of Technical Experts who participated in developing this report follows:

James Adamson, M.D.
Vice President and Medical Officer for
    National Accounts
Arkansas Blue Cross and Blue Shield
Little Rock, AR

Damian Dupuy, M.D.
Professor, Diagnostic Imaging
Warren Alpert Medical School
Brown University
Director of Tumor Ablation
Rhode Island Hospital
Providence, RI

Mark Ferguson, M.D.
Professor of Surgery
Head, Thoracic Surgery Service
University of Chicago Cancer Research
    Center
Chicago, IL

Brian Funaki, M.D.
Section Chief, Vascular/Interventional
    Radiology
University of Chicago Medical Center
Chicago, IL

Renuka Malik, M.D.
Instructor, Radiation/Cellular Oncology
University of Chicago Hospitals
Chicago, IL

Jyoti Patel, M.D.
Associate Professor, Hematology/Oncology
Feinberg School of Medicine
Northwestern University
Chicago, IL

Douglas Wood, M.D.
Chief, Cardiothoracic Surgery
University of Washington
Seattle, WA

Peer Reviewers

Prior to publication of the final evidence report, EPCs sought input from independent Peer Reviewers without financial conflicts of interest. However, the conclusions and synthesis of the scientific literature presented in this report does not necessarily represent the views of individual reviewers.

Peer Reviewers must disclose any financial conflicts of interest greater than $10,000 and any other relevant business or professional conflicts of interest. Because of their unique clinical or content expertise, individuals with potential nonfinancial conflicts may be retained. The TOO and the EPC work to balance, manage, or mitigate any potential nonfinancial conflicts of interest identified.

The list of Peer Reviewers follows:

Jessica Donington, M.D.
Assistant Professor of Cardiothoracic
   Surgery
New York University School of Medicine
New York, NY

Stephen M. Hahn, M.D.
Chair, Department of Radiation Oncology
Director, Photodynamic Therapy Program
Perelman Center for Advanced Medicine
Philadelphia, PA

Michael Lanuti, M.D.
Director, Thoracic Oncology
Division of Thoracic Surgery
Massachusetts General Hospital
Boston, MA

William Moore, M.D.
Chief of Thoracic Imaging
Stony Brook Cancer Center
Stony Brook, NY

Local Nonsurgical Therapies for Stage I and Symptomatic Obstructive Non–Small-Cell Lung Cancer

Structured Abstract

Objectives. We prepared this report on the comparative effectiveness and harms of lung-directed nonsurgical therapies for non–small-cell lung cancer (NSCLC) in three distinct patient populations: (1) patients with stage I NSCLC who are not surgical candidates (Key Question 1), (2) patients with stage I NSCLC who are deemed operable but decline surgery (Key Question 2), and (3) patients with endoluminal NSCLC causing obstruction (Key Question 3). For stage I NSCLC, the local nonsurgical interventions could include conformal radiotherapy modalities and radiofrequency ablation (RFA). For patients with airway obstruction due to an endoluminal NSCLC, local nonsurgical interventions could include those for the stage I setting, as well as conventional wide-field radiotherapy, brachytherapy, laser and mechanical debridement, endoluminal stents, cryoablation, and photodynamic therapy. Surgical resection of any type is not considered as a comparator for any of the Key Questions.

Data sources. MEDLINE®, Embase®, and the Cochrane Controlled Trials Registry were searched from January 1, 1995, to July 25, 2012. A search of the gray literature included databases with regulatory information, clinical trial registries, abstracts and conference papers, and information from manufacturers.

Review methods. We sought studies reporting overall survival, cancer-specific survival, local control, symptom relief, adverse events, and quality of life among our populations of interest. Data were abstracted for each Key Question by a team of reviewers, with independent data verification. Study quality and the risk of bias of randomized controlled trials (RCTs) were assessed using the United States Preventive Services Task Force criteria. The quality and risk of bias of single-arm studies were assessed using the Carey and Boden criteria. The strength of the body of evidence was assessed according to the Agency for Healthcare Research and Quality Methods Guide.

Results. In our searches, we identified 4,648 unique titles and screened 1,178 in full text. Of the latter, 55 met the inclusion criteria. Thirty-five studies were relevant to Key Question 1, considering medically inoperable patients with stage I NSCLC; 6 were relevant to Key Question 2, considering medically operable patients with stage I NSCLC who decline surgery; and 17 were relevant to Key Question 3, considering patients with inoperable endoluminal NSCLC causing symptoms of obstruction. Three studies addressed both Key Questions 1 and 2. All studies relevant to Key Questions 1 and 2 were single-arm design, prospective (n=15), retrospective (n=21), or not specified (n=2). Among 17 papers included for Key Question 3, 5 were RCTs, 1 was a nonrandomized comparative study, and 11 were single-arm studies. Because comparative study evidence on RFA and debridement and stenting was unavailable for Key Question 3, we included evidence from two single-arm studies involving stents and one on RFA. All RCTs were of poor quality. Only one comparison was available per study, with no two studies examining the same set of interventions. Outcomes of therapy for all Key Questions included overall survival, adverse effects, and quality of life.

Conclusions. Evidence on localized nonsurgical therapies for patients with stage I NSCLC who are not surgical candidates or who decline surgery consists only of single-arm studies, with no direct comparisons among interventions. The best evidence for NSCLC patients with endoluminal obstruction consists of poor-quality single RCTs for each comparison; we did not identify evidence that permitted us to draw conclusions based on indirect comparisons. Overall, evidence is insufficient to permit conclusions on the comparative effectiveness of local nonsurgical therapies for inoperable or operable patients with stage I NSCLC or inoperable NSCLC patients with endoluminal tumor causing pulmonary symptoms.

Contents

Tables

Figures

Appendixes

Executive Summary

Background

Non–small-cell lung cancer (NSCLC) refers to any type of epithelial lung cancer other than small-cell lung cancer.[1] The disease arises from epithelial cells of the lung, from the central bronchi to terminal alveoli. The histological type correlates with site of origin, reflecting the variation in respiratory tract epithelium by location. The most common types of NSCLC are adenocarcinoma, squamous cell carcinoma, and large cell carcinoma. Several other types occur less frequently; all can occur in unusual histological variants. Squamous cell carcinoma typically originates near a central bronchus. Adenocarcinoma and adenocarcinoma in situ (formerly called bronchioalveolar carcinoma) usually arise in peripheral lung tissue. Adenocarcinomas are frequently associated with cigarette smoke but may also occur in patients who have never smoked.

More than 1 million deaths are attributed per year to NSCLC, making it the leading cause of cancer-related mortality worldwide.[2] In the United States, lung cancer is the leading cause of cancer death, and an estimated 222,520 cases were expected to be diagnosed in 2010, with 157,300 deaths due to the disease.[2]

NSCLC may be symptomatic at presentation or it may be incidentally discovered at a routine chest imaging examination. The most common symptoms at presentation are progressive cough or chest pain. Other presenting symptoms include hemoptysis, malaise, weight loss, dyspnea, and hoarseness. Symptoms may result from local invasion or compression of adjacent thoracic structures, such as compression of the esophagus causing dysphagia, compression of the laryngeal nerves causing hoarseness, or compression involving the superior vena cava causing facial edema and distension of the superficial veins of the head and neck. Symptoms from distant metastases may also be present and include neurological defect or personality change from brain metastases or pain from bone metastases. Physical examination may identify enlarged supraclavicular lymphadenopathy, pleural effusion or lobar collapse, unresolved pneumonia, or signs of associated disease, such as chronic obstructive pulmonary disease or pulmonary fibrosis.

The prognosis of an NSCLC patient and the subsequent treatment plan are a function of disease stage.[3] NSCLC stage is defined by the TNM system, which was initially developed by the Union Internationale Contre le Cancer (UICC) and the American Joint Committee for Cancer Staging (AJCC). The TNM system takes into account the size of the primary tumor (T), the extent of regional lymph node involvement (N), and the presence or absence of distant metastases (M).[4] The UICC and AJCC have adopted the current Revised International System for Staging Lung Cancer, which is based on information from a clinical database of nearly 70,000 patients.[4] Imaging methods used to stage NSCLC patients may include 18F-fluorodeoxyglucose positron emission tomography (FDG PET), computed tomography (CT), or magnetic resonance imaging (MRI).[5] The presence of symptoms, physical signs, or laboratory findings, or perceived risk of distant metastasis ultimately drive evaluation for nodal and distant metastatic disease. Bone scans, FDG PET, CT, or MRI may be performed if initial assessments suggest nodal or more distant metastases, or if a patient with more advanced disease is under consideration for aggressive local and combined-modality treatments. Surgical staging of the mediastinum is considered the standard to evaluate local nodal status.

Treatment Options for NSCLC

NSCLC patients can be divided into three general groups that reflect the extent of disease, which in turn dictates the initial treatment approach, not considering systemic therapies:

- Surgically resectable disease (generally stage I, stage II, and selected stage III tumors)
- Potentially operable or inoperable locally (T3–T4) or regionally (N2–N3) advanced disease, including endoluminal lesions
- Inoperable distant metastatic disease, including distant metastases (M1) that are found at the time of diagnosis

Surgery is the standard of care for patients with resectable stage I NSCLC. However, alternative treatments are needed for two subsets of stage I NSCLC patients. First is a subset that comprises about 20–30 percent of stage I patients: those who have resectable tumors but are deemed medically inoperable, primarily because of preexisting diminished cardiac reserve, poor pulmonary function, and poor performance status.[6-9] A second, much less common subset comprises patients who are deemed operable but decline surgery. It is assumed that medically inoperable patients are more likely to die from intercurrent illness than from lung cancer; however, evidence exists to question this assumption.[9] For example, among a group of 128 patients with stage I or II NSCLC treated between 1994 and 1999, 49 did not receive any surgical treatment, as they were deemed medically inoperable, and yet 53 percent of them died due to lung cancer.[10] Among 1,432 untreated medically inoperable stage I NSCLC patients reported to a registry in California, the lung cancer–specific survival rate at 5 years was 16 percent, suggesting the need for alternative interventions in such patients.[11]

This report aims to compare the effectiveness and harms of local nonsurgical therapies for medically inoperable NSCLC stage I patients, medically operable NSCLC stage I patients who refuse surgery, or patients with inoperable NSCLC who have symptoms secondary to the presence of an endoluminal lesion. Comparisons of ablation versus surgery or systemic chemotherapy versus local nonsurgical therapy are outside the scope of this report.

Local Nonsurgical Treatment Options for Stage I NSCLC

Radiotherapy has a role in the definitive treatment of patients with stage I NSCLC who are deemed medically inoperable or those who decline surgery.[7,9] Ideally, radiotherapy balances delivery of a cytotoxic dose of ionizing radiation to the tumor volume, attempting to minimize adverse effects of radiation on adjacent normal lung tissue and thoracic structures. Several radiotherapy modalities have been used to treat patients with stage I NSCLC. Conventional wide-field two-dimensional radiation therapy (2DRT) has been used extensively to treat medically inoperable patients with stage I NSCLC. Delivery of radiation to a total dose that ranged from 31 to 103 Gray (Gy), in daily fractions of 1.8-2 Gy, has been reported to produce overall survival rates of 17 percent to 42 percent among patients with early-stage disease.[8] However, conventional 2DRT is no longer in routine use in modern radiation oncology practice in this setting and thus was not considered in this comparative effectiveness review (CER).

A quest to improve on survival rates achieved with 2DRT has led to development of conformal radiotherapy methods for definitive (curative) treatment of inoperable patients with stage I NSCLC. Conformal radiotherapy refers to modalities in which cytotoxic radiation beams are "shaped" to cover the tumor volume plus a surrounding tissue margin to treat microscopic disease that may reside there. Photon-based modalities include three-dimensional conformal radiation therapy (3DRT); intensity-modulated radiation therapy (IMRT); and stereotactic body radiation therapy (SBRT), which is also known as stereotactic ablative radiotherapy.[12-14] For purposes of this report, we use the term "SBRT." Charged particle–based therapy such as proton beam radiotherapy (PBRT) is also available.[15]

The optimal definitive external radiotherapy modality is not defined for patients with medical contraindications (medically inoperable patients) or for those with stage I NSCLC who elect nonsurgical treatment.[14] All radiotherapy procedures listed above are time intensive, require significant training, and necessitate substantial advance planning.[13,16] Institutional quality control processes are required to assure their safe and effective use, in particular IMRT.[17] Analysis of the application of PBRT to NSCLC presents challenges because of the small number of institutions that have experience with this technique and small reported patient numbers.[15]

Interventional treatment options for stage I NSCLC include radiofrequency ablation (RFA).[18,19] Percutaneous RFA is a minimally invasive technique that uses high-frequency electric currents to heat and destroy tumors and is typically performed in a single session.[20] The most frequent complication of RFA is pneumothorax.[21] Analysis of the application of RFA to NSCLC presents challenges because of the small number of institutions that have experience with this technique and small number of patients.[15,20,22]

Local Nonsurgical Treatment Options for Symptomatic Endobronchial NSCLC

Patients with airway obstruction from nonresectable primary or recurrent endoluminal lung tumors comprise 20–30 percent of NSCLC cases and manifest symptoms of disabling dyspnea, cough, and hemoptysis.[23,24] Up to 40 percent of lung cancer deaths may be attributed to such locoregional disease. Management of these patients is a significant challenge. For example, the ability to promptly alleviate airway distress may be lifesaving, as some patients may succumb to suffocation within hours of presentation.[24-26] Patients with such advanced disease often require emergency treatment to relieve airway obstruction or stop bleeding. These interventions are palliative but are performed in some patients with curative intent.

Patients with good performance status may benefit from external-beam radiotherapy (EBRT), which comprises conventional 2DRT or conformal methods, outlined above, to ameliorate symptoms (hemoptysis, cough, chest pain, dyspnea, obstructive pneumonia, dysphagia, etc.) associated with an airway obstructive tumor.[26] However, if they have already been heavily pretreated or the tumor is located too close to radiosensitive organs or other anatomic structures, interventional options may become necessary.

Brachytherapy is another option for relieving airway obstruction and can be used alone or with EBRT to boost the total dose of irradiation used.[26,27] Brachytherapy has been used in combination with high-dose EBRT as a potentially curative primary treatment in selected cases. Serious complications have been described with brachytherapy, including massive hemoptysis, tracheoesophageal fistulas, bronchial stenosis, and radiation bronchitis.[27]

The role of brachytherapy for the palliative treatment of symptomatic patients with airway obstruction is unclear. Brachytherapy has been used as a palliative treatment in case of endobronchial tumor recurrence after EBRT. Brachytherapy also may be an option for patients in whom EBRT fails to relieve symptoms or those with an obstructive endobronchial lesion who require lung reexpansion before or in conjunction with EBRT.[26]

Several interventional methods involve tumor debulking to palliate symptoms in patients with advanced endobronchial NSCLC.[19,25,26,28] Interventional bronchoscopy with mechanical tumor debridement and stent placement can rapidly reestablish airway patency and relieve dyspnea and respiratory distress in patients with airway obstruction due to a malignant endoluminal tumor.[25,28] Debridement and stent placement may be complemented by subsequent application of radiotherapy to extend the durability of palliation and may offer definitive therapy for local tumors.

Laser resection involving the neodymium-doped yttrium aluminum garnet (Nd-YAG) laser and photodynamic therapy (PDT) using porfimer sodium have been investigated in this setting, with suggestion of symptomatic improvement in some cases.[19] RFA also has been used in cryosurgery.

Objectives

This CER is intended to be a comprehensive systematic review of the relative benefits and harms of lung-directed nonsurgical therapies in two disease settings encompassing three distinct patient populations. The disease setting and patient populations are defined in the Key Questions section. Available therapies include conformal radiation modalities (3DRT, IMRT, SBRT, PBRT) and interventional methods such as RFA. Likewise, numerous methods are used to treat patients with symptomatic malignant airway obstruction: EBRT methods, brachytherapy, surgical debridement and stent placement, and others (e.g., Nd-YAG laser, cryoablation).

Surgery is the standard of care for eligible patients with stage I NSCLC. However, a substantial subset of stage I NSCLC patients exists for whom surgery is contraindicated due to the existence of underlying comorbidities. Alternatives also are needed for another smaller proportion of stage I patients who are medically operable but decline surgery. Comparison of outcomes with alternative procedures to those achieved with surgery is outside the scope of this CER. Instead, the CER is focused on comparison of local nonsurgical modalities for inoperable patients in Key Question 1 and for operable patients in Key Question 2.

Key Question 3 addresses the comparative benefits and harms of local nonsurgical therapies in patients with inoperable NSCLC who have symptoms secondary to the presence of an endoluminal lesion. The optimal approach in these patients is not established. These patients often require urgent care; typically, they have a short expected lifespan and interventions are often palliative.

All of the alternative modalities under consideration are clinically relevant and merit comparative evaluation due to uncertainty surrounding their optimal use in these settings. Alternatives to surgery are important to health care providers, patients, and policymakers, given the substantial disease burden of NSCLC, especially in the elderly population.

Key Questions and Analytical Framework

The Key Questions and CER analytical frameworks (Figures A and B) are structured to be consistent with the populations, interventions, comparisons, outcomes, timing, and settings (PICOTS) framework (Table A), as laid out in the Agency for Healthcare Research and Quality (AHRQ) Evidence-based Practice Center (EPC) "Methods Guide for Effectiveness and Comparative Effectiveness Reviews" (Methods Guide).[29]

The Key Questions are:

Key Question 1. What are the comparative benefits and harms of local nonsurgical definitive therapies for documented (clinical or biopsy) stage I (T1N0M0, T2N0M0) NSCLC in adult patients (age 18 years or older) who are not surgical candidates because of the presence of contraindications to major surgery—for example, cardiac insufficiency, poor pulmonary function, presence of severe intercurrent illness, or poor performance status?

Key Question 2. What are the comparative benefits and harms of local nonsurgical definitive therapies for documented (clinical or biopsy) stage I (T1N0M0, T2N0M0) NSCLC in adult patients (age 18 years or older) who are deemed operable but decline surgery?

Key Question 3. What are the comparative short- and long-term benefits and harms of local nonsurgical therapies given with palliative or curative intent to patients with endoluminal NSCLC causing obstruction of the trachea, main stem, or lobar bronchi and recurrent or persistent thoracic symptoms such as hemoptysis, cough, dyspnea, and postobstructive pneumonitis?

Figure A. Analytical framework for comparative effectiveness of local nonsurgical definitive therapies for adult patients (age 18 years or older) with documented (clinical or biopsy) stage I (T1N0M0 or T2N0M0) medically inoperable NSCLC or those with documented stage I NSCLC who are deemed operable but decline surgery

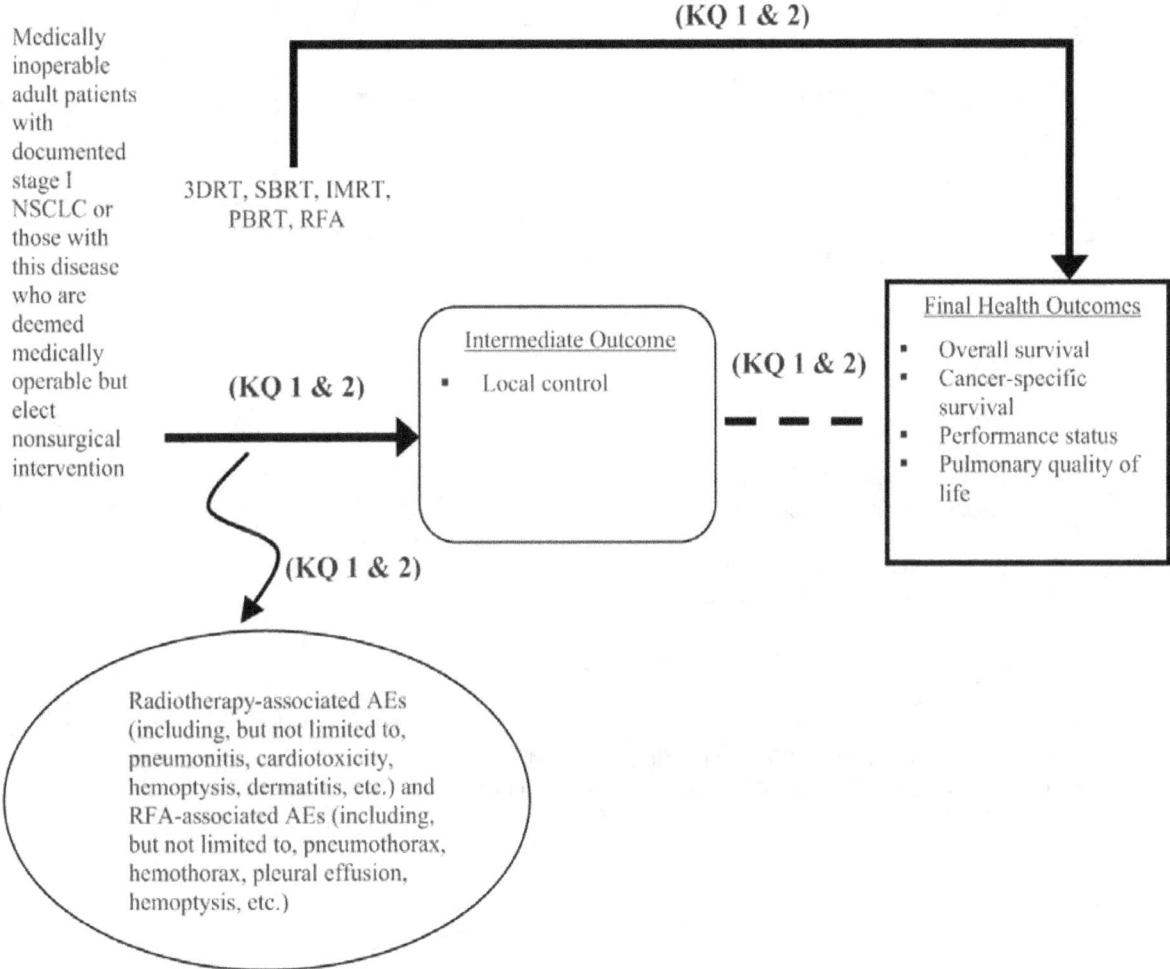

3DRT = three-dimensional radiotherapy; AE = adverse event; IMRT = intensity-modulated radiotherapy; KQ = Key Question; NSCLC = non–small-cell lung cancer; PBRT = proton beam radiotherapy; RFA = radiofrequency ablation; SBRT = stereotactic body radiotherapy
Note: T, N, and M refer to tumor, lymph node involvement, and metastasis in the TNM staging system.

Figure B. Analytical framework for comparative effectiveness of local nonsurgical curative or palliative therapies for adult patients (age 18 years or older) with symptomatic inoperable airway obstruction due to NSCLC

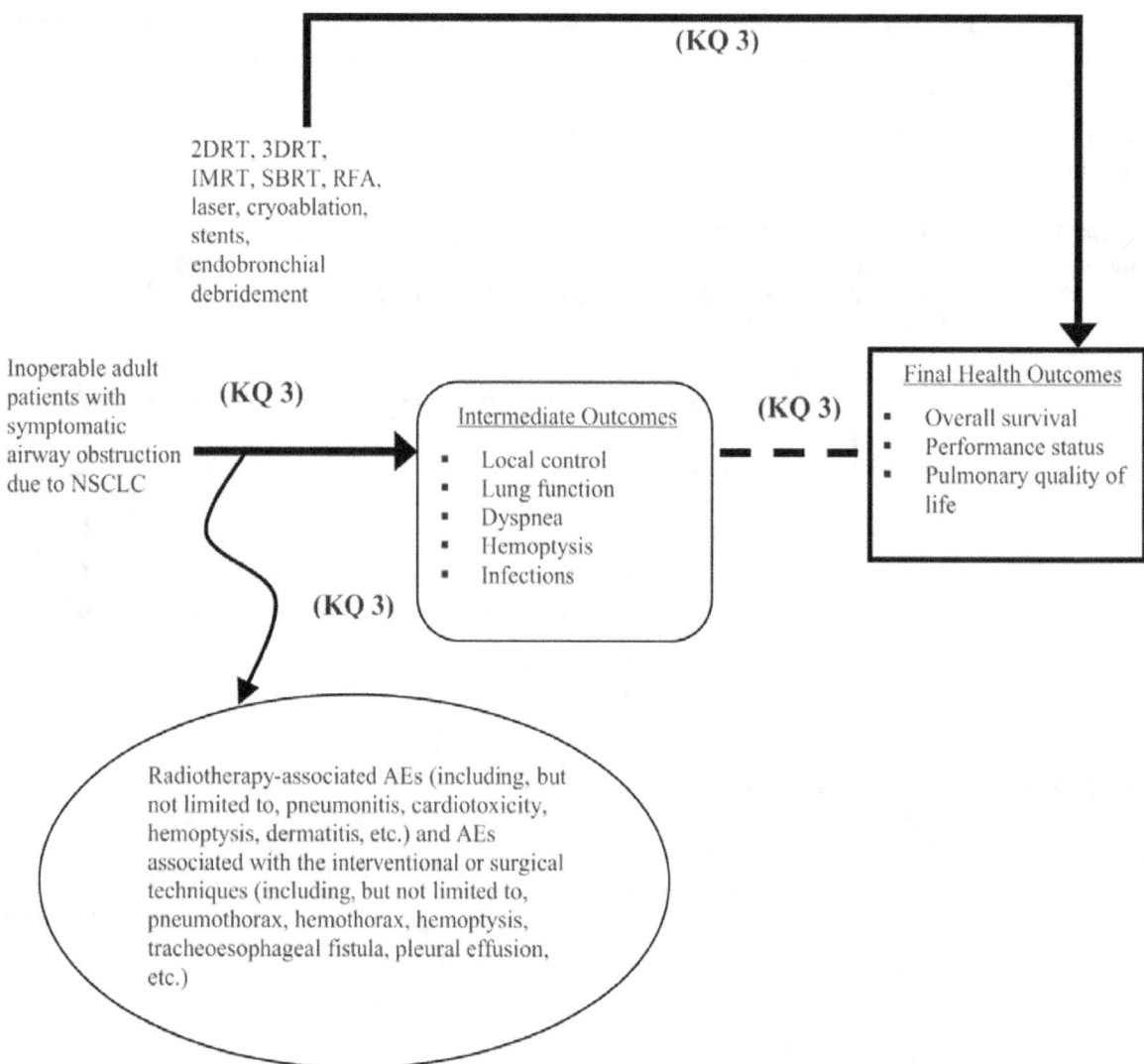

2DRT = two-dimensional radiotherapy; 3DRT = three-dimensional radiotherapy; AE = adverse event; IMRT = intensity-modulated radiotherapy; KQ = Key Question; NSCLC = non–small-cell lung cancer; RFA = radiofrequency ablation; SBRT = stereotactic body radiotherapy

Table A. PICOTS for the Key Questions

PICOTS	Key Questions 1 and 2	Key Question 3
Population	**Key Question 1:** Adult patients (age 18 years or older) with documented (clinical or biopsy) stage I (T1N0M0 and T2N0M0) NSCLC not deemed surgical candidates because of the documented presence of contraindications to major surgery—for example, cardiac insufficiency, poor pulmonary function, severe intercurrent illness, or poor performance status **Key Question 2:** Adult patients (age 18 years or older) with documented (clinical or biopsy) stage I (T1N0M0 and T2N0M0) NSCLC who would be deemed surgical candidates according to current clinical criteria but decline surgery	Adult patients (age 18 years or older) with endoluminal NSCLC causing obstruction of the trachea, main stem, or lobar bronchi and recurrent or persistent thoracic symptoms such as hemoptysis, cough, dyspnea, and postobstructive pneumonitis who were treated with curative or palliative intent
Intervention	All interventions are first-line (definitive), nonsurgical therapies: • Conformal external-beam radiotherapy methods (including SBRT, 3DRT, and IMRT) • PBRT • RFA	• Conventional 2DRT • Conformal PBRT methods (including SBRT, 3DRT, and IMRT) • Brachytherapy • RFA • Cryoablation • Laser therapy • Endobronchial debridement and stents • PDT • Electrocautery • Combinations—for example, endobronchial debridement plus a stent compared with debridement alone or combination of 2DRT with brachytherapy compared with radiotherapy alone • Because systemic therapy (chemotherapy) is used with radiotherapy or local nonsurgical interventional methods in stage III or greater patients, we collected information on chemotherapy to use in categorizing and assessing outcomes to ensure that relevant and appropriate comparisons are made, particularly as they relate to possible harms. Such comparisons may be segregated and reported accordingly if it is not possible to discern interventional therapeutic effects
Comparator	• Comparators comprise the interventions noted above	• Comparators comprise the interventions noted above
Outcome	• **Final health outcomes:** OS, CSS, performance status, pulmonary QOL • **Intermediate outcomes:** LCT • **Adverse outcomes:** Radiotherapy-associated AEs (including, but not limited to, pneumonitis, cardiotoxicity, hemoptysis, dermatitis, etc.) and RFA-associated AEs (including, but not limited to, pneumothorax, hemothorax, hemoptysis, pleural effusion, etc.)	• **Final health outcomes:** OS, performance status, pulmonary QOL • **Intermediate outcomes:** LCT, lung function, pulmonary symptoms (e.g., dyspnea, hemoptysis), respiratory tract infection • **Adverse outcomes:** Radiotherapy-associated AEs (including, but not limited to, pneumonitis, cardiotoxicity, hemoptysis, dermatitis, etc.) and AEs associated with the interventional or surgical techniques (including, but not limited to, pneumothorax, pleural effusion, hemoptysis, transesophageal fistula, pericardial effusion)

Table A. PICOTS for the Key Questions (continued)

PICOTS	Key Questions 1 and 2	Key Question 3
Timing	• The relevant periods occur from the time of treatment through followup over months (palliation) or years (OS)	• The relevant periods occur from the time of treatment through followup over months (palliation) or years (OS)
Setting	• Inpatient and outpatient	• Inpatient and outpatient

2DRT = two-dimensional radiotherapy; 3DRT = three-dimensional radiotherapy; AE = adverse event; CSS = cancer-specific survival; IMRT = intensity-modulated radiotherapy; LCT = local control; NSCLC = non–small-cell lung cancer; OS = overall survival; PBRT = proton beam radiotherapy; PDT = photodynamic therapy; PICOTS = population, intervention, comparator, outcome, timing, and setting; QOL = quality of life; RFA = radiofrequency ablation; SBRT = stereotactic body radiotherapy
Note: T, N, and M refer to tumor, lymph node involvement, and metastasis in the TNM staging system.

Methods

Input From Stakeholders

The topic for this report came via the Effective Health Care Program Web site. Initially, a panel of Key Informants recruited by the Evidence-based Practice Center (EPC) gave input on draft Key Questions. The draft Key Questions were posted on AHRQ's Web site for public comment on October 5, 2011, for 4 weeks. During this period, the EPC drafted a protocol for the CER and recruited a Technical Expert Panel (TEP) that comprised individuals with clinical expertise in radiation oncology, thoracic surgery and surgical oncology, pulmonology, and general oncology. In response to the comments received and with TEP input, we eliminated a Key Question aimed at "technically inoperable" patients, and expanded the list of adverse events (AEs) we would attempt to capture for each intervention. These changes were documented in the final protocol for this report, which was posted on AHRQ's Web site on February 22, 2012.

The TEP provided input throughout the development of the review but was not involved in subsequent evidence analysis or drafting the report.

Data Sources and Selection

A medical librarian conducted electronic searches of MEDLINE®, Embase®, and the Cochrane Controlled Trials Registry, seeking randomized, nonrandomized comparative, and observational studies published between January 1, 1995, and July 25, 2012. We truncated the search at 1995 to ensure comparability of procedures and technologies. The search was limited to English-language studies based on the following rationale. First, evidence suggests that language restrictions do not change results of systematic review for conventional medical interventions.[30] Second, input from the TEP suggested that most if not all of the pivotal studies in this area would be captured in the English-language evidence base and that restriction to English would not introduce bias. Our search strategy used the National Library of Medicine's Medical Subject Headings (MeSH®) keyword nomenclature developed for MEDLINE® and adapted for use in other databases. The full search strings and strategies are listed in Appendix A of the full report.

We reviewed scientific information packets from the Scientific Resource Center and gray literature from the U.S. Food and Drug Administration Web site, ClinicalTrials.gov, and conference abstracts (American Society of Clinical Oncology and American Society for Radiation Oncology). We limited the gray literature to include only phase 3 randomized controlled trials (RCTs) through 2010. We did not contact study authors for unpublished results.

Inclusion Criteria

Studies of any design were included if they fulfilled all of the following inclusion criteria.

Key Questions 1 and 2

- Study included medically inoperable NSCLC stage I patients (T1N0M0 and T2N0M0) or medically operable NSCLC stage I patients (T1N0M0 and T2N0M0) who refuse surgery
- Such patients received only one of the following local nonsurgical interventions as first-line (definitive) treatment:
  - Conformal radiotherapy methods (including SBRT, 3DRT, IMRT)
  - PBRT
  - RFA
- Study reported ≥ 1 of the following types of outcome data for such patients:
  - Survival outcome (overall survival or cancer-specific survival)
  - Local control (an outcome defined as the arrest of cancer growth at the site of origin)
  - Pulmonary quality of life (QOL)
  - AEs specific to radiotherapy techniques or to RFA

Key Question 3

- Study included NSCLC patients of any stage with a symptomatic endoluminal obstruction
- Such patients received ≥ 1 of the following local nonsurgical interventions:
  - Conformal radiotherapy methods (including SBRT, 3DRT, IMRT)
  - Conventional 2DRT
  - PBRT
  - RFA
  - Brachytherapy
  - Cryoablation
  - Laser therapy, including PDT
  - Electrocautery
  - Endobronchial debridement and stents
- Study reported data ≥ 1 of the following types of outcome data for such patients:
  - Survival outcome (overall survival or cancer-specific survival)
  - Local control (an outcome defined as the arrest of cancer growth at the site of origin)
  - Symptom relief
  - Pulmonary QOL
  - AEs specific to radiotherapy or interventional techniques (e.g., RFA, cryoablation, electrocautery) or to surgical techniques (laser or mechanical debridement and stents)

Exclusion Criteria

- Editorials, commentaries, abstracts, animal studies, case reports, non–English-language, and diagnostic accuracy studies were excluded.
- Primary studies published prior to January 1, 1995, were excluded.

- If we identified more than one article that included the same patients, interventions, and outcomes, we included the article with the longest followup, excluding the earlier paper(s). The latter were cross-indexed in the abstraction tables.
- For Key Questions 1 and 2, we compared single interventions—for example, two different conformal radiotherapy methods, or RFA compared with a conformal radiotherapy method. We excluded studies that used any postintervention systemic (e.g., chemotherapy) or local nonsurgical therapy but did not define the therapy or disaggregate the clinical outcomes of such patients. Failure to stratify or disaggregate outcome data according to the treatment received—for example, a local nonsurgical intervention with subsequent chemotherapy at progression—precludes determining whether an outcome such as overall survival could be attributed to the local intervention, the chemotherapy, or the combined effect of both therapies.

The list of excluded studies and reason for exclusion are provided in Appendix B of the full report.

Data Abstraction and Quality Assessment

Electronic search results were transferred to EndNote® and subsequently into DistillerSR® for study screening and selection. Using the study selection criteria outlined above for screening titles and abstracts, each citation was marked as: (1) eligible for review as full-text article or (2) ineligible for full-text review. Teams consisted of one senior member (the team leader) and two junior members. All team members initially examined at least one training set (n=100) of representative titles and abstracts for each Key Question to assure uniform application of screening criteria. They assessed a subsequent set, establishing concordance among the team. All team members performed title and abstract screening. A reference was excluded only when the senior and either junior team member made a concordant decision to exclude it. In case of disagreement between junior members, the team leader adjudicated in consensus discussion with all team members. A record of the reason for exclusion of each reference retrieved was kept in the DistillerSR database. A reference could be excluded for multiple reasons but only one reason was recorded.

A data abstraction guide was created that detailed the process and defined key data elements to ensure accuracy and consistency in the data abstraction procedure across the team. Junior and senior team membersevaluated a test set of three references relevant to the three Key Questions to ensure that selection criteria were applied correctly. Subsequently, two junior team members and the team leader reviewed full-text articles independently to determine their inclusion in the systematic review. Team meetings were held regularly to discuss progress and to ensure that the team leader was aware of difficulties or problems in this process.

The main data elements for the CER were abstracted directly into Microsoft Word® tables. Other elements and the study risk-of-bias assessments were abstracted in DistillerSR. The evidence tables were divided by Key Question and assigned for abstraction to all team members. One reviewer performed primary data abstraction of all data elements into the evidence tables, and a second reviewed the articles and evidence tables for accuracy. Disagreements were resolved by discussion, and if necessary, by consultation with a third reviewer.

In adherence with the Methods Guide,[29] the risk of bias of individual comparative studies was assessed by the U.S. Preventive Services Task Force (USPSTF) criteria.[31] The quality of the abstracted studies was assessed by one reviewer and examined by the senior team member.

The quality of comparative studies was assessed on the basis of the following criteria:

- Initial assembly of comparable groups: adequate randomization, including concealment and equal distribution among groups of potential confounders (e.g., other concomitant care)
- Maintenance of comparable groups (including attrition, crossovers, adherence, and contamination)
- Important differential loss to followup or overall high loss to followup
- Equal, reliable, and valid measurements (including masking of outcome assessment)
- Clear definition of interventions
- Consideration of all important outcomes
- Analysis:
  - For RCTs: intention-to-treat, covariate adjustment
  - For cohort studies: adjustment for potential confounders

Comparative studies were rated according to one of three quality categories:

Good. Studies are graded "good" if they meet all criteria; comparable groups are assembled initially and maintained throughout the study (followup at least 80%); reliable and valid measurement instruments are used and applied equally to the groups; interventions are spelled out clearly; all important outcomes are considered; and appropriate attention is given to confounders in analysis. In addition, intention-to-treat analysis was used for RCTs.

Fair. Studies are graded "fair" if any or all of the following problems occur, without the fatal flaws noted in the "poor" category below: In general, comparable groups are assembled initially, but some questions remain about whether some (although not major) differences occurred with followup; measurement instruments are acceptable (although not the best) and are generally applied equally; some but not all important outcomes are considered; and some but not all potential confounders are accounted for. Intention-to-treat analysis was used for RCTs.

Poor. Studies are graded "poor" if any of the following fatal flaws exists: Groups assembled initially are not close to being comparable or are not maintained throughout the study; unreliable or invalid measurement instruments are used or measures are not applied at all equally among groups; key confounders are given little or no attention; there is a lack of masked outcome assessment; and, for RCTs, intention-to-treat analysis is lacking.

The quality of the single-arm intervention studies was assessed by Carey and Boden criteria.[32] These include eight criteria, as follows:

- Clearly defined study questions
- Well-described study population
- Well-described intervention
- Use of validated outcome measures
- Appropriate statistical analyses
- Well-described results
- Discussion and conclusion supported by data
- Acknowledgement of the funding source

We created thresholds for converting the Carey and Boden risk-assessment tool into the AHRQ format of standard quality ratings (good, fair, and poor). This allowed us to differentiate the quality of single-arm studies as good, fair, or poor. For a study to be ranked good quality, all eight Carey and Boden criteria mentioned above had to be met. For a fair quality assessment, seven of eight criteria had to be met. A study that met fewer than seven of eight criteria was rated as poor quality. The quality rankings for these studies can be found in Appendix C of the full report.

Data Synthesis and Analysis

Given the lack of appropriate comparative studies for all Key Questions, this evidence review did not incorporate formal data synthesis involving meta-analysis. The quality of individual studies was assessed as outlined in the preceding section, and the strength of evidence (SOE) for each Key Question was evaluated as follows.

Assessment of the Strength of Evidence

We graded the strength of the overall body of evidence for overall survival, symptom relief, quality of life, and harms. The system used for rating the strength of the overall body of evidence is outlined in the AHRQ Methods Guide[29] and based on a system developed by the Grading of Recommendations Assessment, Development and Evaluation (GRADE) Working Group.[33] We also used the GRADE guideline on assessing the risk of bias.[34] This system explicitly addresses four required domains: risk of bias, consistency, directness, and precision. Two independent reviewers rated all studies on domain scores and resolved disagreements by consensus discussion; the same reviewers also used the domain scores to assign an overall SOE grade.

The process of grading the body of evidence[33] was as follows. A body of evidence represented by RCT(s) would have a starting strength of high. A body of evidence represented by nonrandomized comparative studies would generally have a starting strength of low. For all study designs, the strength of evidence would be reduced by one level if there was high risk of bias, inconsistency or unknown consistency, indirectness, and imprecision. Further, based on GRADE guidelines on assessing the risk of bias,[34] when the evidence was generated from studies that had very serious risk of bias, the strength of evidence was rated down by two levels. Case series or single-arm studies were deemed indirect, imprecise, and "unknown" for the domains of directness, precision, and consistency.

The grade of evidence strength was classified into the following four categories:
- **High.** High confidence that the evidence reflects the true effect. Further research is very unlikely to change our confidence in the estimate of effect.
- **Moderate.** Moderate confidence that the evidence reflects the true effect. Further research may change our confidence in the estimate of effect and may change the estimate.
- **Low.** Low confidence that the evidence reflects the true effect. Further research is likely to change our confidence in the estimate of effect and is likely to change the estimate.
- **Insufficient.** Evidence was either unavailable or did not permit estimation of an effect.

Additional domains, including strength of association, publication bias, coherence, dose-response relationship, and residual confounding, were not addressed in this review.

Results

Overview

Of the 4,648 unique titles identified, we screened 1,178 in full text. Of these, 55 met the CER inclusion criteria; 35 were relevant to Key Question 1, 6 were relevant to Key Question 2, and 17 were relevant to Key Question 3. Three studies addressed both Key Questions 1 and 2. Details are given in the Preferred Reporting Items for Systematic Reviews and Meta-Analyses (PRISMA)[35] diagram (Figure C). All studies relevant to Key Questions 1 and 2 were single-arm design, prospective (n=15), retrospective (n=21), or not specified (n=2). Among 17 papers included for Key Question 3, 5 were RCTs, 1 was a nonrandomized comparative study, and 11 were single-arm studies.

Figure C. PRISMA diagram for disposition of literature search results

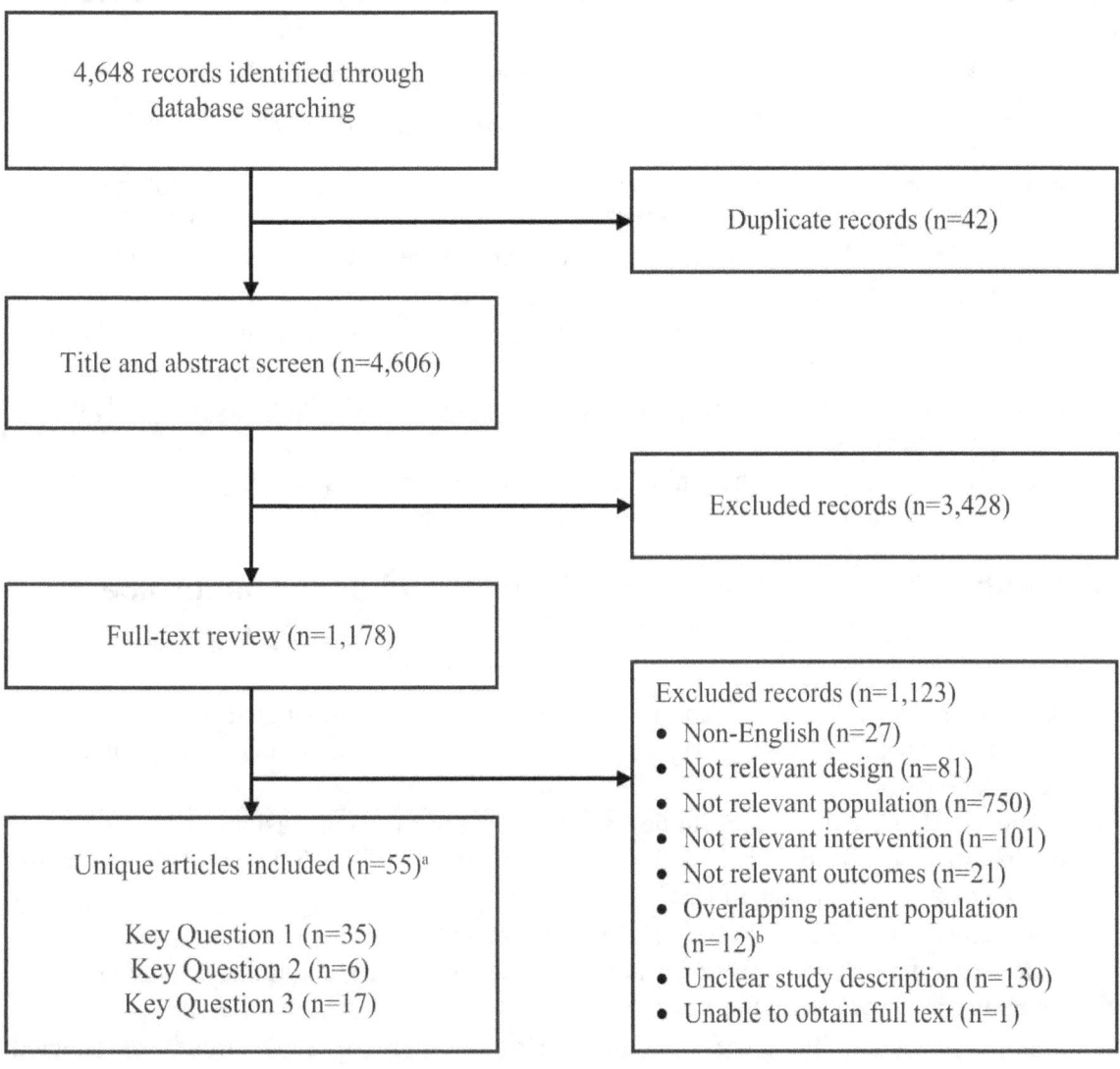

PRISMA = Preferred Reporting Items for Systematic Reviews and Meta-Analyses
[a]Three studies addressed both Key Questions 1 and 2.
[b]Overlapping patient population refers to the studies in which the same patients were included in more than 1 study. In all such cases, only 1 study was included to avoid oversampling. The decision to include a study was based on the nature of the study design (preference of randomized controlled trials over observational study designs) and the clarity in reporting relevant patients and/or outcomes.

Key Points

Key Question 1: Comparative Effectiveness of Local Nonsurgical Definitive Interventions for Stage I NSCLC in Medically Inoperable Patients

- All evidence included in this report for Key Question 1 is from single-arm studies. No evidence is available from any type of direct comparative study of one intervention versus another.
- Evidence from 35 single-arm studies is insufficient to form conclusions about the comparative benefits or harms of SBRT (24 reports), 3DRT (7 reports), PBRT (3 reports), or RFA (1 report) in medically inoperable patients with stage I NSCLC.
- The results of interest for this report comprise direct outcomes (overall survival and cancer-specific survival), an indirect outcome (local control), and radiation-associated toxicities, as shown in Figure A.
- Post-treatment toxicities were reported across studies, but no relative trend was detected among interventions.
- We are uncertain whether the limited evidence on AEs reflects that they were absent or that the investigators did not systematically collect data or report them.

Key Question 2: Comparative Effectiveness of Local Nonsurgical Definitive Interventions for Stage I NSCLC in Medically Operable Patients

- All evidence included in this report for Key Question 2 is from single-arm studies. No evidence is available from any type of direct comparative study of one intervention versus another.
- Evidence from six single-arm studies is insufficient to form conclusions about the comparative benefits or harms of SBRT (five reports) or PBRT (one report) in medically operable patients with stage I NSCLC.
- The results of interest for this report comprise direct outcomes (overall survival and cancer-specific survival), an indirect outcome (local control), and radiation-associated toxicities, as shown in Figure A.
- Post-treatment toxicities were not common across studies. No relative trend was detected among interventions.
- We are uncertain whether the limited evidence on AEs reflects that they were absent or that the investigators did not systematically collect data or report them.

Key Question 3: Comparative Effectiveness of Local Nonsurgical Therapies for Symptoms Secondary to an Inoperable Obstructive Endoluminal NSCLC

- All six RCTs included in this report were of poor quality according to the USPSTF rating criteria. Further analysis is provided in the Discussion section that follows.
- Evidence from six comparative studies is insufficient to draw conclusions about relative benefits and harms of six unique treatment comparisons (brachytherapy plus EBRT vs. brachytherapy alone, brachytherapy plus EBRT vs. EBRT alone, brachytherapy vs.

EBRT, laser plus brachytherapy vs. laser alone, laser vs. electrocautery, and laser vs. PDT) for local nonsurgical therapies in symptomatic inoperable patients with obstructive endoluminal NSCLC. Evidence from three single-arm studies of debridement and stenting is insufficient to draw conclusions about the effectiveness of those interventions.

- The results of interest for this report comprise direct outcomes (overall survival), symptom relief (cough, dyspnea, hemoptysis), and AEs (radiation toxicities, other intervention-associated AEs), as shown in Figure B.

- Overall, treatment-related toxicities varied according to the type of intervention. Hemoptysis was the most common toxicity reported across studies. There may be underreporting of treatment-related toxicities, as three comparative studies did not describe the frequency, process of data collection, or assessment of severity of treatment-related toxicities.

Discussion

Strength of Evidence

To evaluate the SOE, we used an approach that was specifically developed by the EPC program and referenced in the Methods Guide.[29] This approach is based on a system developed by the GRADE Working Group.[33] It explicitly addresses four required domains: risk of bias, consistency, directness, and precision, as outlined in the Methods section.

Key Question 1

As shown in Table B, the overall SOE is insufficient to form conclusions about the comparative beneficial effects or toxicities of 3DRT, PBRT, RFA, or SBRT in the treatment of stage I NSCLC in medically inoperable patients. Direct outcomes of interest were overall survival, cancer-specific survival, and toxicities.

Thirty-five single-arm studies were available. The risk of bias was high. The consistency of effect size direction is unknown in the absence of comparative studies. No direct comparative evidence is available among interventions, but the outcomes reported are direct. Precision cannot be determined in the absence of direct comparative evidence among interventions; therefore, the evidence was deemed imprecise.

Table B. Strength of evidence for local nonsurgical interventions in medically inoperable stage I NSCLC patients

Treatment and Evidence Base	Risk of Bias	Consistency	Directness	Precision	Overall Strength of Evidence
SBRT (24 single-arm studies, total n=1,665 patients)	High	Unknown	Indirect	Imprecise	Insufficient
3DRT (7 single-arm studies, total n=240 patients)	High	Unknown	Indirect	Imprecise	Insufficient
PBRT (3 single-arm studies, total n=144 patients)	High	Unknown	Indirect	Imprecise	Insufficient
RFA (1 single-arm study, n=19 patients)	High	Unknown	Indirect	Imprecise	Insufficient

3DRT = three-dimensional radiotherapy; NSCLC = non–small-cell lung cancer; PBRT = proton beam radiotherapy; RFA = radiofrequency ablation; SBRT = stereotactic body radiotherapy

Key Question 2

As shown in Table C, the overall SOE is insufficient to form conclusions about the comparative beneficial effects or toxicities of PBRT or SBRT in the treatment of stage I NSCLC in medically operable patients. Direct outcomes of interest were overall survival, cancer-specific survival, and toxicities.

Six single-arm studies were available. The risk of bias was high. The consistency of effect size direction is unknown in the absence of comparative studies. No direct comparative evidence is available among interventions, but the outcomes reported are direct. Precision cannot be determined in the absence of direct comparative evidence among interventions; therefore, the evidence was deemed imprecise.

Table C. Strength of evidence for local nonsurgical interventions in medically operable stage I NSCLC patients

Treatment and Evidence Base	Risk of Bias	Consistency	Directness	Precision	Overall Strength of Evidence
SBRT (5 single-arm studies, total n=378)	High	Unknown	Indirect	Imprecise	Insufficient
PBRT (1 single-arm study, n=28)	High	Unknown	Indirect	Imprecise	Insufficient

NSCLC = non–small-cell lung cancer; PBRT = proton beam radiotherapy; SBRT = stereotactic body radiotherapy

Key Question 3

Overall, the evidence from RCTs is insufficient to form conclusions about the benefits (symptom relief, survival) and harms (treatment-related toxicities) of local nonsurgical therapies (brachytherapy plus EBRT vs. brachytherapy alone, brachytherapy plus EBRT vs. EBRT alone, brachytherapy vs. EBRT, laser plus brachytherapy vs. laser alone, laser vs. electrocautery, laser vs. PDT) in symptomatic inoperable patients with obstructive endoluminal NSCLC. The strength of evidence for the six included RCTs is summarized in Table D.

Evidence from three single-arm studies of debridement and stenting is insufficient to draw conclusions about the effectiveness of those interventions. The SOE for the noncomparative studies included in the report is summarized in Table E.

Brachytherapy Plus EBRT Versus Brachytherapy Alone

The evidence for this comparison comprised one small RCT[36] (n=45, 15 patients per treatment arm). This trial was considered to have a high risk of bias because it failed to provide details of randomization and allocation concealment. The consistency of the evidence was unknown, as it was a single RCT without confirmation from any other study. The outcomes measured in the study—symptom relief, QOL and treatment-related toxicities—were all direct. The evidence for symptom relief, QOL, and treatment-related toxicities was imprecise.

Because the evidence base that addressed these outcomes consisted of an RCT, the starting level of SOE was high. SOE was reduced by one level each based on the high risk of bias, unknown consistency, and imprecision. Therefore, the SOE is insufficient that, compared with brachytherapy alone, brachytherapy plus EBRT improves symptom relief and QOL and reduces treatment-related toxicities.

Brachytherapy Plus EBRT Versus EBRT Alone

The evidence for this comparison comprised one small RCT[37] (n=95). This trial was considered to have a high risk of bias, primarily because the trial was discontinued prematurely due to lack of patient accrual and was underpowered to detect a difference in the rate of the primary endpoint (rate of dyspnea). The consistency of the evidence was unknown, as it was a single RCT without confirmation from any other study. The outcomes measured in the study—symptom relief, survival, and treatment-related toxicities—were all direct. The evidence for symptom relief, survival, and treatment-related toxicities was imprecise.

Because the evidence base that addressed these outcomes consisted of an RCT, the starting level of SOE was high. SOE was reduced by one level each based on the high risk of bias, unknown consistency, and imprecision. Therefore, the SOE is insufficient that, compared with EBRT alone, brachytherapy plus EBRT improves symptom relief and survival and reduces treatment-related toxicities.

Brachytherapy Versus EBRT

The evidence for this comparison comprised one small RCT[38] (n=99). This trial was considered to have a very serious risk of bias because the study failed to adjust for potential confounding resulting from crossover of a large proportion of patients between treatment arms during the trial period. The consistency of the evidence was unknown, as it was a single RCT without confirmation from any other study. The outcomes measured in the study—symptom relief, survival, and treatment-related toxicities—were all direct. The evidence for symptom relief and treatment-related toxicities was imprecise, while the evidence for survival was precise.

Because the evidence base that addressed these outcomes consisted of an RCT, the starting level of SOE was high. SOE was reduced by two levels based on very serious risk of bias, by one level for unknown consistency, and by one level for imprecision (only for symptom relief and treatment toxicity). Therefore, the SOE is insufficient that, compared with EBRT, brachytherapy improves symptom relief and survival and reduces treatment-related toxicities.

Laser Plus Brachytherapy Versus Laser Alone

The evidence for this comparison comprised one small RCT[39] (n=29). This trial was considered to have a high risk of bias, primarily due to failure to provide details of randomization, allocation concealment, and NSCLC staging of patients at the baseline. The consistency of the evidence was unknown, as it was a single RCT without confirmation from any other study. The outcomes measured in the study—symptom relief, survival, and treatment-related toxicities—were all direct. The evidence for symptom relief, survival, and treatment-related toxicities was imprecise.

Because the evidence base that addressed these outcomes consisted of an RCT, the starting level of SOE was high. SOE was reduced by one level each based on the high risk of bias, unknown consistency, and imprecision. Therefore, the SOE is insufficient that, compared with laser alone, laser plus brachytherapy improves symptom relief and survival and reduces treatment-related toxicities.

Laser Versus PDT

The evidence for this comparison comprised one small RCT[40] (n=31). This trial was considered to have a serious risk of bias, primarily because the treatment arms had imbalances at the baseline. The proportion of patients with stage III–IV cancer was much smaller in the PDT group (57%, 8 of 14) than the laser group (88%, 15 of 17) at the baseline. The consistency of the evidence was unknown, as it was a single RCT without confirmation from any other study. The outcomes measured in the study—survival and treatment-related toxicities—were all direct. The evidence for treatment-related toxicities was imprecise, while it was precise for survival.

Because the evidence base that addressed these outcomes consisted of an RCT, the starting level of SOE was high. SOE was reduced by two levels based on very serious risk of bias, by one level for unknown consistency, and by one level for imprecision (only for treatment-related toxicity). Therefore, the SOE is insufficient that, compared with photodynamic therapy, laser therapy improves survival and reduces treatment-related toxicities.

Laser Versus Electrocautery

The evidence for this comparison comprised one small nonrandomized comparative study[41] (n=29). This study was considered to have serious risk of bias, primarily because of lack of adjustment for any potential confounders. A disproportionate number of patients had received previous treatment in the laser-treated group (93%) compared with the electrocautery group (53%). Further, the mean time from diagnosis to study treatment was different in the two groups (4.7 months in the laser group vs. 7.5 months in the electrocautery group). The consistency of the evidence was unknown, as it was a single nonrandomized comparative study without confirmation from any other study. The outcomes measured in the study—survival and symptom relief—were direct. The evidence for symptom relief and survival was imprecise.

Because the evidence base that addressed these outcomes consisted of a nonrandomized comparative study, the starting level of SOE was low. SOE was reduced by two levels based on very serious risk of bias and by one level each for unknown consistency and imprecision. Therefore, the SOE is insufficient that, compared with electrocautery, laser therapy improves survival and symptom relief.

Table D. Strength of comparative evidence for local nonsurgical therapies for symptoms secondary to an inoperable obstructive endoluminal NSCLC

Treatment and Evidence Base	Outcome	Unit of Measure	Risk of Bias	Consistency	Directness	Precision	Overall Strength of Evidence
Brachytherapy plus EBRT vs. brachytherapy alone (1 RCT, n=45)	Symptom relief	Incidence and response rate	High	Unknown	Direct	Imprecise	Insufficient
	QOL	EORTC QLQ-C30 & LC 13 V3.0 instruments					
	Treatment toxicity	Incidence of Grade ≥II RTOG morbidity scoring criteria					
Brachytherapy plus EBRT vs. EBRT alone (1 RCT, n=95)	Symptom relief	Response rate	High	Unknown	Direct	Imprecise	Insufficient
	Survival	Overall survival					
	Treatment toxicity	Incidence					
Brachytherapy vs. EBRT (1 RCT, n=99)	Symptom relief	% improvement	High	Unknown	Direct	Imprecise	Insufficient
	Survival	Overall survival	High	Unknown	Direct	Precise	Insufficient
	Treatment toxicity	Incidence	High	Unknown	Direct	Imprecise	Insufficient

Table D. Strength of comparative evidence for local nonsurgical therapies for symptoms secondary to an inoperable obstructive endoluminal NSCLC (continued)

Treatment and Evidence Base	Outcome	Unit of Measure	Risk of Bias	Consistency	Directness	Precision	Overall Strength of Evidence
Nd-YAG plus brachytherapy vs. Nd-YAG alone (1 RCT, n=29)	Symptom relief	Speiser's index	High	Unknown	Direct	Imprecise	Insufficient
	Survival	Overall survival					
	Treatment toxicity	Incidence					
Photodynamic therapy vs. laser (1 RCT, n=31)	Survival	Overall survival	High	Unknown	Direct	Precise	Insufficient
	Treatment toxicity	Incidence	High	Unknown	Direct	Imprecise	Insufficient
Nd-YAG vs. electrocautery (1 NRC, n=29)	Survival	Mean survival	High	Unknown	Direct	Imprecise	Insufficient
	Symptom relief	% response					

EBRT = external-beam radiotherapy; EORTC QLQ = European Organization for Research and Treatment of Cancer Quality of Life Questionnaire; Nd-YAG = neodymium-doped yttrium aluminum garnet; NRC = nonrandomized comparative study; NSCLC = non–small-cell lung cancer; QOL = quality of life; RCT = randomized controlled trial; RTOG = Radiation Therapy Oncology Group

Table E. Strength of noncomparative evidence for local nonsurgical therapies for symptoms secondary to an inoperable obstructive endoluminal NSCLC

Treatment and Evidence Base	Risk of Bias	Consistency	Directness	Precision	Overall Strength of Evidence
RFA (1 study, n=33)	High	Unknown	Indirect	Imprecise	Insufficient
BT + STNT (1 study, n=10)	High	Unknown	Indirect	Imprecise	Insufficient
LASR + STNT (1 study, n=52)	High	Unknown	Indirect	Imprecise	Insufficient

BT = brachytherapy; LASR = laser; NSCLC = non–small-cell lung cancer; RFA = radiofrequency ablation; STNT = stenting

Applicability of the Findings

Our results show no direct comparative evidence to support a decision among 3DRT, PBRT, RFA, or SBRT in stage I NSCLC patients. Comparative evidence is sparse among any of the interventions considered in Key Question 3. In the absence of direct comparative effectiveness data, additional factors may be considered in making a treatment decision. Those could include relative convenience and cost, issues outside the scope of this CER.

Key Questions 1 and 2

In general, applicability assessment would depend on a body of evidence sufficient to permit conclusions about the comparative outcomes of local nonsurgical therapies for stage I NSCLC. The evidence for Key Questions 1 and 2 does not reach that level, so we have primarily limited comments to the relevance of the PICOTS elements. The PICOTS format is a practical and useful structure to review applicability in a systematic manner. With the exception of cost, factors potentially affecting the applicability of the findings of this CER are summarized in Table F for Key Questions 1 and 2.

The degree to which the data presented in this report are applicable to clinical practice is a function of the similarity between populations in the included studies and the patient population that receives clinical care in diverse settings. It also is related to the relative availability of the interventions. The literature base is observational, lacking comparative evidence. Case series are descriptive studies that are limited in their ability to control for biases. Selection bias is of particular concern, as patients receive treatment based on clinician preferences, center resources, and patient characteristics and preference rather than random allocation. This evidence base is therefore insufficient to support any attempt to draw comparative conclusions.

Table F. Summary of applicability of evidence for Key Question 1 and Key Question 2

Domain	Applicability of Evidence
Populations	• Overall, the patients included in the single-arm studies were not suitable for surgery or were suitable for surgery but declined it. • Patients with stage I NSCLC in the studies included in this report appear to be representative of cases that would be considered for a local nonsurgical intervention. • Patients typically were in their late 60s to mid-70s, congruent with the incidence of stage I NSCLC, which tends to rise with age. • The medically inoperable patients of KQ1 had compromised cardiopulmonary reserves or other comorbidities that preclude surgical resection. • The medically operable patients of KQ2 were often not substantially different from the inoperable population of KQ1, but neither group is considered as healthy as the population that undergoes surgery.
Interventions	• 3DRT, IMRT, and SBRT represent different technological approaches to the delivery of conformal photon radiotherapy. The major advantage of these interventions compared with traditional wide-field 2DRT is the ability to deliver tightly focused cytotoxic radiation by delineating the shape and size of the tumor using a CT-based or other imaging planning system. • 3DRT represents a minimum technical standard for delivery of conformal radiotherapy. It involves static fields with a fixed shape, modified by compensators (wedges and segments). 3DRT is widely available. • IMRT offers beam strength attenuation through a multileaf collimator (tungsten), with dynamic field shapes for each beam angle. IMRT is not as widely available as 3DRT and requires a higher level of inverse planning effort and quality assurance. • SBRT is a hypofractionated technique administered in 5 or fewer fractions; 3DRT and IMRT typically deliver radiation in many more fractions than SBRT. • SBRT is not as widely available as 3DRT or IMRT, but its use is growing. It may soon supplant other technologies in the KQ1 and KQ2 settings. The institutional programmatic requirements for SBRT are similar to those for IMRT. • This CER did not allow for a rigorous and systematic comparison of the relative performance of local nonsurgical therapies stratified by technological factors. The impact of these factors on health outcomes remains unclear. • Applicability of the evidence for PBRT and RFA is unknown due to limited evidence.
Comparators	• See above for Interventions.
Outcomes	• The major beneficial health outcomes in this CER are OS, CSS, and LCT, typically reported over a period of 1 to 5 years. • OS is the primary direct outcome for any cancer intervention study. • CSS reflects the absolute effect of a cancer intervention on the disease. CSS is a highly relevant direct outcome in the KQ1 practice setting, in that such patients are generally fragile and susceptible to succumbing to underlying comorbidities. Its relevance in KQ2 patients may be slightly less than in KQ1, as the former may be relatively healthier than the latter, but they still are not as healthy as good surgical candidates. • LCT is of interest to patients because it measures the effectiveness of an intervention in disease control. Upon local failure, patients enter into a new category centered on systemic chemotherapy. This is a potentially perilous position for the medically frail patients considered in KQ1, and perhaps many of those in KQ2.
Timing	• The relevant periods occur from the time of treatment through followup over months (palliation) or years (overall survival).

Table F. Summary of applicability of evidence for Key Question 1 and Key Question 2 (continued)

Domain	Applicability of Evidence
Setting	• The evidence for KQ1 and KQ2 is international, primarily obtained in tertiary institutional settings. More sophisticated interventions such as IMRT and SBRT require an institutional commitment to quality assurance and ongoing training that may be difficult to achieve in smaller community-based centers. • We did not collect or analyze information to examine these issues.

2DRT = two-dimensional radiotherapy; 3DRT = three-dimensional radiotherapy; CER = Comparative Effectiveness Review; CSS = cancer-specific survival; CT = computer tomography; IMRT = intensity-modulated radiotherapy; KQ = Key Question; LCT = local control; NSCLC = non–small-cell lung cancer; OS = overall survival; PBRT = proton beam radiotherapy; RFA = radiofrequency ablation; SBRT = stereotactic body radiotherapy

Key Question 3

Multiple shortcomings of the current evidence base for Key Question 3 preclude interpretation about general applicability. First, the comparative benefits and harms of various endobronchial treatments are still unknown because of the lack of good-quality RCTs. The available studies were all poor quality, and often were small and not powered to detect a prespecified clinically meaningful difference in a standardized outcome of interest. Second, patient characteristics were poorly defined. The majority of studies did not report performance status, and therefore it is difficult to assess the relative health and activity level of these patients and to whom this limited evidence applies. Third, there was a wide variation in the outcome measures to report symptom relief in the current studies. Fourth, many studies did not report the frequency, process, or method of assessing severity of treatment-related toxicities, and therefore the true harms associated with these interventions are likely to be underrepresented in the current data. Some factors that affect applicability of the findings of this CER are summarized in Table G for Key Question 3.

Table G. Summary of applicability of evidence for Key Question 3

Domain	Applicability of Evidence
Populations	• The patients in the studies included in this report appear to be representative of cases that would be considered for a bronchoscopic intervention. All patients included in the 6 studies had histologically confirmed NSCLC with airway obstruction that required a bronchoscopic intervention. The mean age of patients included in these studies ranged from 61 to 68 years, and this is congruent with the incidence of NSCLC, which tends to rise with age.
Interventions	• The single-modality nonsurgical interventions (brachytherapy, EBRT, electrocautery, laser, photodynamic, debridement, and stenting) and 2 dual-modality interventions (laser plus brachytherapy and brachytherapy plus EBRT) represent a general landscape of current treatment options for patients with endoluminal obstructive NSCLC and therefore are applicable.
Comparators	• See above for Interventions.
Outcomes	• The major outcomes of interest were symptom relief, OS, disease-specific survival, QOL, and treatment-related toxicity. • Although OS is the primary direct outcome for any cancer intervention study, it may not be the best measure of the efficacy of a palliative intervention in symptomatic patients. • Immediate relief of obstructive symptoms and improvement in QOL provide reasonable and pertinent justification for use of endobronchial intervention in such patients. • According to the structured review by the Patient Reported Outcome Measurement Group-Oxford on the use of PROMs (Patient Reported Outcome Measures), both generic and disease-specific instruments exist that can be used in patients with lung cancer to assess the impact of interventions on QOL. These measures include generic measures such as SF-36 and EQ-5D and lung cancer–specific measures such as the EORTC QLQ-C30 and EORTC QLQ-LC13 instruments, and FACT-L. However, QOL data were reported only by 1 small study out of the 6 comparative studies. Therefore, the applicability of the current evidence base on QOL cannot be determined.

Table G. Summary of applicability of evidence for Key Question 3 (continued)

Domain	Applicability of Evidence
Timing	• The relevant periods occur from the time of treatment through followup over months (palliation) or years (overall survival).
Setting	• The outcomes of local bronchoscopic therapies largely depend on the expertise of the provider and the center providing these services. We could not assess the impact of such operating characteristics on the treatment outcomes because these data were not available in the published papers.

EBRT = external beam radiotherapy; EORTC QLQ = European Organization for Research and Treatment of Cancer Quality of Life Questionnaire; EQ-5D = EuroQOL 5 dimension; FACT-L = Functional Assessment of Cancer Therapy- Lung; NSCLC = non–small-cell lung cancer; OS = overall survival; QOL = quality of life; SF-36 = Short Form 36 Health Survey

Findings in Relationship to What Is Already Known

We sought credible sources of evidence-based information on the use of the local interventions assessed in this CER to treat NSCLC. Our systematic literature search and review revealed no relevant evidence-based guidelines we could compare with our findings for Key Questions 1 and 2, and two publications relevant to Key Question 3.[27,42] Our report offers the first comprehensive systematic review on this topic.

Limitations of Current Review and Evidence Base

Key Questions 1 and 2

The primary limitation for Key Questions 1 and 2 is lack of comparative trials of any design. Percutaneous image-guided RFA has been investigated as an option for the treatment of stage I NSCLC. In our review, we found that RFA studies in lung primarily comprise heterogeneous case series that are complicated by several factors. First, many reports included metastatic and primary lesions from nonlung and lung sites, but did not stratify outcomes such as overall survival according to tumor stage or type. Second, the technical details of RFA, such as the type of equipment used, the power settings or wattage delivered, and details of followup assessment and subsequent therapy, were not consistent or consistently reported across studies. These factors conspired to severely limit RFA study selection in the report.

Although the body of evidence we included for the conformal radiotherapy techniques addressed in Key Questions 1 and 2, particularly SBRT, was more substantial in quantity than the evidence for RFA, we have similar concerns about interstudy heterogeneity, with variability in radiotherapy dose, schedule of treatment, patient selection criteria, tumor size and location, and so forth. In a systematic review in general, heterogeneous noncomparative evidence makes it very difficult to assess the benefits and harms of any intervention. In this CER, the type of evidence we identified for Key Questions 1 and 2 precludes comparative assessment among the interventions we investigated. We therefore believe further careful study of the interventions we considered in this CER is needed in the settings of Key Question 1 or 2 to establish optimal technical protocols and patient selection criteria, perhaps standardizing and comparing them across institutions. These data and methods could, in theory, be applied to the design and conduct of comparative studies of the local nonsurgical interventions for stage I NSCLC, as outlined in the Research Gaps section below.

Key Question 3

The body of evidence available for Key Question 3 comprised five RCTs, one nonrandomized comparative study, and three relevant single arms from three otherwise comparative studies. We included the latter three study arms because we did not have higher level evidence for the interventions in question, debridement and stenting. Significant limitations in the quality and quantity of the evidence base led us to conclude that the evidence was insufficient to make conclusions about the comparative effectiveness of local nonsurgical interventions to treat endobronchial obstructions in NSCLC patients. There was only one comparative study available to draw inferences about comparative effectiveness for six unique treatment comparisons. Therefore, the consistency domain for SOE was unknown. All six studies received a low rating in terms of USPSTF study quality; often the studies were small and not powered to detect a prespecified clinically meaningful difference in a standardized outcome of interest, thereby limiting their utility beyond hypothesis generation. Most studies lacked details about randomization and allocation concealment. The one nonrandomized comparative study available for Key Question 3 did not use statistical adjustment to reduce confounding; such adjustment for confounding should be consistently used in nonrandomized studies.

Research Gaps

Key Questions 1 and 2

The primary research gap we identified in preparing this CER is the lack of evidence from comparative studies to draw conclusions as to the relative clinical benefits and harms of the local nonsurgical interventions used in the stage I NSCLC setting of medically inoperable or operable patients. We also identified some feasibility issues associated with the interventions that are potential impediments to the type of rigorous comparative studies we suggest are necessary to determine their comparative effectiveness. In this section, we first describe characteristics of ideal comparative studies we believe are needed to compare these technologies. Some potential impediments to such studies are discussed subsequently in this section.

Lack of Clinical Trial Evidence on Local Nonsurgical Interventions for Stage I NSCLC

As part of this review, we searched for ongoing clinical trials of these technologies in stage I NSCLC. In the process, we identified two international randomized phase 3 clinical trials of surgical resection versus SBRT that are recruiting patients (NCT 01336894 and NCT 00840749). However, neither of these trials will reveal relative outcomes among local nonsurgical interventions in stage I NSCLC. Thus, we suggest that prospective studies are needed to properly evaluate the relative clinical benefits and harms of the technologies evaluated in this CER, taking into account the potential impediments to study we discuss below. Ideally, comparative studies in medically inoperable or operable stage I NSCLC patients would incorporate the following:

- To assure comparability of patients and minimize bias, standardized patient selection criteria would be used that involve consultation, including a thoracic surgeon, medical oncologist, and radiation oncology specialist. Key factors to consider include comorbidity status (particularly cardiopulmonary function and capacity), age, performance status, tumor size, and tumor location.
- Standardized intervention protocols with training and quality assurance programs within and across participating institutions are necessary for the best study. For radiotherapy, key factors would include the imaging and planning method, immobilization method, dose and fractionation schedule, and the biologically effective dose (BED) for comparisons of different modalities (e.g., SBRT, 3DRT, IMRT, and PBRT). For RFA,

issues would include treatment power and duration in the context of tumor size and location.

- Prespecified followup criteria and methods—in particular, notation of subsequent systemic therapy administered at recurrence—are key considerations. Subsequent systemic therapy is a key concern because it is impossible to discern the effect of an intervention followed by systemic therapy at progression from that achieved with the intervention alone. Is the effectiveness a function of the systemic therapy, the intervention, or the combination?

- Rigorous and standardized reporting is needed to account for all patients and treatments received. Data for operable and inoperable patients would be reported separately. We urge that rigorous methods be used for the conduct of RCTs, particularly intent-to-treat analysis and adjustment of survival data to account for patients who develop recurrent disease and subsequently receive systemic chemotherapy as part of their treatment plan.

- Primary outcomes would include overall survival, cancer-specific survival, and local control. Prespecified systematic collection of AEs using validated criteria (e.g., Common Terminology Criteria for Adverse Events [CTCAE]) is necessary to permit accurate assessment of relative benefits and risks of the interventions.

Potential Impediments to Comparative Studies of Local Nonsurgical Interventions for Stage I NSCLC

The general dissemination of conformal radiotherapy technologies into community clinical practice, most lately and specifically SBRT,[43,44] is a potential impediment to comparative study of those technologies. Published survey results show that nearly 40 percent of solo practitioners already treat patients with SBRT, which suggests that this technology is accessible and its efficacy accepted in the broader radiation oncology community.[43,44] The shorter hypofractionated SBRT course is more "patient friendly" than those associated with conventionally fractionated conformal radiotherapy methods. This patient-specific advantage may represent an additional reason that SBRT has rapidly disseminated into clinical practice in the absence of direct comparative clinical trial evidence to support its reputation of clinical superiority over conventionally fractionated conformal techniques. We also recognize a number of other significant, perhaps insurmountable, technical impediments to conducting adequate comparative studies among the most widely available conformal radiotherapy-based modalities and other interventions such as RFA. These are outlined below.

Several practical limitations would complicate comparative study of RFA and conformal radiotherapy modalities in the stage I NSCLC setting. Although we did not evaluate these issues in this CER, it is generally thought that a tumor size greater than 4 cm or a tumor location less than 1 cm from the hilum or large vessels precludes the use of RFA.[22,45] Current clinical wisdom suggests that RFA is best suited for patients with peripherally located, smaller lesions due to the "heat sink" effect of large blood vessels that dissipates heat from the tumor and reduces efficacy.[45-47] By contrast, although we also did not investigate any relationship in our systematic review, conformal radiotherapy-based modalities, particularly SBRT, have been used in patients with either peripheral or central tumors, as well as tumors > 4 and up to 7 cm in diameter, the latter corresponding to stage IB (T2N0M0).[4] Furthermore, radiotherapy-based modalities are not subject to a heat sink effect that limits their efficacy. Given those caveats, recruitment and accrual of sufficient numbers of well-matched stage I NSCLC patients to make meaningful, clinically relevant comparisons between RFA and conformal radiotherapy-based treatments could be difficult.

A key technical issue in comparing the radiotherapy interventions likely is the significant difference in the BED of radiation that can be safely delivered by SBRT compared with IMRT or 3DRT delivered with conventional fractionation protocols. In brief, radiation therapy for NSCLC typically is delivered to a total dose of 60-70 Gy; SBRT delivers that dose in three to five fractions of 20 Gy each (estimated BED = 180 Gy_{10} using standard principles), whereas conventionally fractionated IMRT or 3DRT delivers 60-70 Gy in 30 fractions of 2 Gy each in 4 to 5 weeks, yielding an estimated BED of 72 Gy_{10}. The difference in attainable BED is considered to have potential efficacy implications.[48] The higher BED causes tumor ablation, rather than tumor cell kill, allowing for little to no tumor cell repopulation between doses of radiation.

In this CER, we did not systematically investigate whether a higher BED delivered by any conformal radiotherapy modality can be associated with better clinical outcomes, such as overall survival, compared with a lower BED. This has been reported in published single-arm studies reviewed in this CER—for example, the large multicenter retrospective series on SBRT in Japan by Onishi and colleagues.[49] However, we are not aware of any direct comparative evidence on this topic for any of the conformal radiotherapy technologies, so it is not possible to make even indirect comparisons between the delivered BED and clinical outcomes in any case. Furthermore, we are aware of no published clinical trial evidence to ascertain whether a higher BED delivered by SBRT is associated with differences in patient outcomes compared with a lower BED delivered either by SBRT or by a conventionally fractionated conformal radiotherapy modality. We acknowledge that the difference in delivered BED has biologically plausible clinical implications, and perhaps ethical implications, that would need to be addressed in designing any type of study to compare conformal radiotherapy-based technologies. However, it is not clear to us that the BED issue under discussion here is settled.

In summary, we acknowledge the views of some members of the radiation oncology and interventional radiology communities that clinical trials of local nonsurgical modalities, including RFA, SBRT, and other conformal radiotherapy modalities (e.g., 3DRT, IMRT, PBRT), in stage I NSCLC patients may be very difficult to recruit and conduct, based on technical and potential ethical issues related to perceptions of unequal clinical benefit among the interventions. However, we maintain that current evidence is insufficient to support a view that clinical outcomes achieved with one technology are superior or inferior to those achieved with other modalities. Clinical evidence from comparative studies is needed to establish the standard of care for local nonsurgical treatment of stage I NSCLC patients.

Key Question 3

Lack of Clinical Trial Evidence on Local Nonsurgical Interventions for Endoluminal Obstructive NSCLC

- Key Question 3 compared outcomes of available local endobronchial interventions used with curative or palliative intent to treat airway obstruction as a result of NSCLC. Evidence on the patient outcomes is limited and, as such, is insufficient to make conclusions. We identified a number of research gaps during the course of review:

- Lack of comparative evidence generated from adequately powered RCTs regarding the benefits and harms of various bronchoscopic interventions used for treating endoluminal obstructions in patients with NSCLC
- Lack of comparative evidence generated from good-quality RCTs regarding the QOL data from patients who receive various bronchoscopic interventions used for treating endoluminal obstructions in patients with NSCLC
- Need for systematic collection of treatment-related toxicity data from various bronchoscopic interventions used for treating endoluminal obstructions from actual clinical practice settings

During our review, we identified two RCTs that aimed to compare local endobronchial interventions in patients with endobronchial NSCLC. However, neither of these trials were completed due to lack of patient accrual. Of these two RCTs, the trial by Moghissi and colleagues[50] is notable. The objective of this trial was to compare two treatment policies in terms of symptom relief, respiratory function, performance status, QOL, and survival. This study planned to recruit 400 patients in 3 years at 24 clinical centers in the United Kingdom. Even though the study organizers had successfully conducted many RCTs in the past, they failed to recruit patients in this clinical setting. Moreover, 20 percent of those randomized did not receive the assigned treatment. A study by Langendijk and colleagues,[37] which randomized patients to a brachytherapy plus EBRT or EBRT-alone arm, was discontinued due to lack of patient accrual before completing the planned enrollment of 160 patients.

Potential Impediments to Comparative Studies of Local Nonsurgical Interventions for Endoluminal Obstructive NSCLC

NSCLC patients with endoluminal obstructions are particularly difficult to randomize in trials because of many reasons, particularly ethical issues. Most of these bronchoscopic interventions are considered complementary and are used sequentially in a clinical setting,[51] and therefore randomizing critically ill patients to either therapy alone has ethical implications. Further, many of these patients present with an impending obstruction, and immediate symptom relief is foremost. Obtaining informed consent in such a situation is a barrier in patient recruitment. These reasons are likely to obviate successful conduct of a future RCT.

A prospective cohort study may be able to answer some questions about relative harms and benefits of local endobronchial interventions. Although concerns about selection bias and unknown confounders always exist in such a study design, addressing and collecting data about most relevant confounders a priori can provide much-needed information about comparative benefits and harms of these therapies in the population of interest. We recommend that the research team for conducting such a study be multidisciplinary, including oncologists experienced in treating NSCLC patients with endobronchial obstruction, a methodologist with expertise in QOL measurement, clinical researchers with expertise in the planning and conduct of large cohort multicentric studies, and ethicists. Relevant outcomes that would be measured in such a study include symptom control, QOL, survival, and treatment-related AEs. Data related to symptom control would be captured using a standardized validated tool applied uniformly across all interventions. Generic instruments such as the Short Form 36 Health Survey (SF-36) and EuroQOL 5 dimension (EQ-5D) would be used in conjunction with lung cancer–specific measures such as European Organization for Research and Treatment of Cancer Quality of Life Questionnaire (EORTC QLQ) modules C30 and LC13 and Functional Assessment of Cancer Therapy-Lung (FACT-L) to measure QOL data.

Treatment-related AEs would be assessed from the date of the procedure extending to a reasonable time, preferably until death, using standardized and well-defined criteria with an independent causality analysis. The process to capture AEs that occur when patients are not under direct medical supervision (such as at home or in a long-term care facility) would also be prespecified in the study protocol. Data on all potential prognostic covariates would include, but not be limited to, patient characteristics (age, sex, race, performance status, comorbidities); disease characteristics (tumor stage, histopathology, location, size, blockage); and technical attributes of the procedure (technical success, technical variables related to use of procedures, type of instrument used) as well as data on the operator (expertise, years of experience, size of the facility).

Conclusions

Evidence is insufficient to permit conclusions on the comparative effectiveness of local nonsurgical therapies for inoperable or operable patients with stage I NSCLC or inoperable NSCLC patients with endoluminal tumor causing pulmonary symptoms. Important outcomes of therapy include overall survival, AEs, and QOL.

References

1. Goldstraw P, Ball D, Jett JR, et al. Non-small-cell lung cancer. Lancet. 2011 Nov 12;378(9804):1727-40. PMID: 21565398.

2. Jemal A, Siegel R, Xu J, et al. Cancer statistics, 2010. CA Cancer J Clin. 2010 Sep-Oct;60(5):277-300. PMID: 20610543.

3. Pfister DG, Johnson DH, Azzoli CG, et al. American Society of Clinical Oncology treatment of unresectable non-small-cell lung cancer guideline: update 2003. J Clin Oncol. 2004 Jan 15;22(2):330-53. PMID: 14691125.

4. Detterbeck FC, Boffa DJ, Tanoue LT. The new lung cancer staging system. Chest. 2009 Jul;136(1):260-71. PMID: 19584208.

5. Rankin SC. Staging of non-small cell lung cancer (NSCLC). Cancer Imaging. 2006;6:1-3. PMID: 16478697.

6. Christie NA, Pennathur A, Burton SA, et al. Stereotactic radiosurgery for early stage non-small cell lung cancer: rationale, patient selection, results, and complications. Semin Thorac Cardiovasc Surg. 2008 Winter;20(4):290-7. PMID: 19251167.

7. Crino L, Weder W, van Meerbeeck J, et al. Early stage and locally advanced (non-metastatic) non-small-cell lung cancer: ESMO Clinical Practice Guidelines for diagnosis, treatment and follow-up. Ann Oncol. 2010 May;21 Suppl 5:v103-15. PMID: 20555058.

8. Decker RH, Tanoue LT, Colasanto JM, et al. Evaluation and definitive management of medically inoperable early-stage non-small-cell lung cancer. Part 1: Assessment and conventional radiotherapy. Oncology (Williston Park). 2006 Jun;20(7):727-36. PMID: 16841796.

9. Robinson CG, Bradley JD. The treatment of early-stage disease. Semin Radiat Oncol. 2010 Jul;20(3):178-85. PMID: 20685580.

10. McGarry RC, Song G, des Rosiers P, et al. Observation-only management of early stage, medically inoperable lung cancer: poor outcome. Chest. 2002 Apr;121(4):1155-8. PMID: 11948046.

11. Raz DJ, Zell JA, Ou SH, et al. Natural history of stage I non-small cell lung cancer: implications for early detection. Chest. 2007 Jul;132(1):193-9. PMID: 17505036.

12. Mohiuddin MM, Choi NC. The role of radiation therapy in non-small cell lung cancer. Semin Respir Crit Care Med. 2005 Jun;26(3):278-88. PMID: 16052429.

13. Patel RR, Mehta M. Three-dimensional conformal radiotherapy for lung cancer: promises and pitfalls. Curr Oncol Rep. 2002 Jul;4(4):347-53. PMID: 12044245.

14. Powell JW, Dexter E, Scalzetti EM, et al. Treatment advances for medically inoperable non-small-cell lung cancer: emphasis on prospective trials. Lancet Oncol. 2009 Sep;10(9):885-94. PMID: 19717090.

15. Widesott L, Amichetti M, Schwarz M. Proton therapy in lung cancer: clinical outcomes and technical issues. A systematic review. Radiother Oncol. 2008 Feb;86(2):154-64. PMID: 18241945.

16. Martel MK. Advanced radiation treatment planning and delivery approaches for treatment of lung cancer. Hematol Oncol Clin North Am. 2004 Feb;18(1):231-43. PMID: 15005291.

17. Low DA, Moran JM, Dempsey JF, et al. Dosimetry tools and techniques for IMRT. Med Phys. 2011 Mar;38(3):1313-38. PMID: 21520843.

18. Heinzerling JH, Kavanagh B, Timmerman RD. Stereotactic ablative radiation therapy for primary lung tumors. Cancer J. 2011 Jan-Feb;17(1):28-32. PMID: 21263264.

19. Santos RS, Raftopoulos Y, Keenan RJ, et al. Bronchoscopic palliation of primary lung cancer: single or multimodality therapy? Surg Endosc. 2004 Jun;18(6):931-6. PMID: 15108108.

20. Zhu JC, Yan TD, Morris DL. A systematic review of radiofrequency ablation for lung tumors. Ann Surg Oncol. 2008 Jun;15(6):1765-74. PMID: 18368456.

21. Haasbeek CJ, Senan S, Smit EF, et al. Critical review of nonsurgical treatment options for stage I non-small cell lung cancer. Oncologist. 2008 Mar;13(3):309-19. PMID: 18378542.

22. Das M, Abdelmaksoud MH, Loo BW Jr., et al. Alternatives to surgery for early stage non-small cell lung cancer-ready for prime time? Curr Treat Options Oncol. 2010 Jun;11(1-2):24-35. PMID: 20577833.

23. Dagnault A, Ebacher A, Vigneault E, et al. Retrospective study of 81 patients treated with brachytherapy for endobronchial primary tumor or metastasis. Brachytherapy. 2010 Jul-Sep;9(3):243-7. PMID: 20122873.

24. Ernst A, Feller-Kopman D, Becker HD, et al. Central airway obstruction. Am J Respir Crit Care Med. 2004 Jun 15;169(12):1278-97. PMID: 15187010.

25. Amjadi K, Voduc N, Cruysberghs Y, et al. Impact of interventional bronchoscopy on quality of life in malignant airway obstruction. Respiration. 2008;76(4):421-8. PMID: 18758153.

26. Morris CD, Budde JM, Godette KD, et al. Palliative management of malignant airway obstruction. Ann Thorac Surg. 2002 Dec;74(6):1928-32; discussion 32-3. PMID: 12643375.

27. Cardona AF, Reveiz L, Ospina EG, et al. Palliative endobronchial brachytherapy for non-small cell lung cancer. Cochrane Database Syst Rev. 2008;(2):CD004284. PMID: 18425900.

28. Yerushalmi R, Fenig E, Shitrit D, et al. Endobronchial stent for malignant airway obstructions. Isr Med Assoc J. 2006 Sep;8(9):615-7. PMID: 17058411.

29. Methods Guide for Effectiveness and Comparative Effectiveness Reviews. AHRQ Publication No. 10(11)-EHC063-EF. Rockville, MD: Agency for Healthcare Research and Quality; March 2011. Chapters available at www.effectivehealthcare.ahrq.gov.

30. Pham B, Klassen TP, Lawson ML, et al. Language of publication restrictions in systematic reviews gave different results depending on whether the intervention was conventional or complementary. J Clin Epidemiol. 2005 Aug;58(8):769-76. PMID: 16086467.

31. Harris RP, Helfand M, Woolf SH, et al. Current methods of the US Preventive Services Task Force: a review of the process. Am J Prev Med. 2001 Apr;20(3 Suppl):21-35. PMID: 11306229.

32. Carey TS, Boden SD. A critical guide to case series reports. Spine (Phila Pa 1976). 2003 Aug 1;28(15):1631-4. PMID: 12897483.

33. Owens DK, Lohr KN, Atkins D, et al. AHRQ series paper 5: grading the strength of a body of evidence when comparing medical interventions--Agency for Healthcare Research and Quality and the effective health-care program. J Clin Epidemiol. 2010 May;63(5):513-23. PMID: 19595577.

34. Guyatt GH, Oxman AD, Vist G, et al. GRADE guidelines: 4. Rating the quality of evidence—study limitations (risk of bias). J Clin Epidemiol. 2011;64(4):407-15.

35. Moher D, Liberati A, Tetzlaff J, et al. Preferred reporting items for systematic reviews and meta-analyses: the PRISMA statement. PLoS Med. 2009 Jul 21;6(7):e1000097. PMID: 19621072.

36. Mallick I, Sharma SC, Behera D, et al. Optimization of dose and fractionation of endobronchial brachytherapy with or without external radiation in the palliative management of non-small cell lung cancer: a prospective randomized study. J Cancer Res Ther. 2006 Jul-Sep;2(3):119-25. PMID: 17998689.

37. Langendijk H, de Jong J, Tjwa M, et al. External irradiation versus external irradiation plus endobronchial brachytherapy in inoperable non-small cell lung cancer: a prospective randomized study. Radiother Oncol. 2001 Mar;58(3):257-68. PMID: 11230886.

38. Stout R, Barber P, Burt P, et al. Clinical and quality of life outcomes in the first United Kingdom randomized trial of endobronchial brachytherapy (intraluminal radiotherapy) vs. external beam radiotherapy in the palliative treatment of inoperable non-small cell lung cancer. Radiother Oncol. 2000 Sep;56(3):323-7. PMID: 10974381.

39. Chella A, Ambrogi MC, Ribechini A, et al. Combined Nd-YAG laser/HDR brachytherapy versus Nd-YAG laser only in malignant central airway involvement: a prospective randomized study. Lung Cancer. 2000 Mar;27(3):169-75. PMID: 10699690.

40. Diaz-Jimenez JP, Martinez-Ballarin JE, Llunell A, et al. Efficacy and safety of photodynamic therapy versus Nd-YAG laser resection in NSCLC with airway obstruction. Eur Respir J. 1999 Oct;14(4):800-5. PMID: 10573224.

41. Boxem T, Muller M, Venmans B, et al. Nd-YAG laser vs bronchoscopic electrocautery for palliation of symptomatic airway obstruction: a cost-effectiveness study. Chest. 1999 Oct;116(4):1108-12. PMID: 10531180.

42. Kvale PA, Selecky PA, Prakash UB. Palliative care in lung cancer: ACCP evidence-based clinical practice guidelines (2nd edition). Chest. 2007 Sep;132(3 Suppl):368S-403S. PMID: 17873181.

43. Pan H, Rose BS, Simpson DR, et al. Clinical practice patterns of lung stereotactic body radiation therapy in the United States: a secondary analysis. Am J Clin Oncol. 2012 Apr 6; Epub ahead of print. PMID: 22495454.

44. Pan H, Simpson DR, Mell LK, et al. A survey of stereotactic body radiotherapy use in the United States. Cancer. 2011 Oct 1;117(19):4566-72. PMID: 21412761.

45. Dupuy DE. Image-guided thermal ablation of lung malignancies. Radiology. 2011 Sep;260(3):633-55. PMID: 21846760.

46. Goldberg SN, Hahn PF, Tanabe KK, et al. Percutaneous radiofrequency tissue ablation: does perfusion-mediated tissue cooling limit coagulation necrosis? J Vasc Interv Radiol. 1998 Jan-Feb;9(1 Pt 1):101-11. PMID: 9468403.

47. Gomez FM, Palussiere J, Santos E, et al. Radiofrequency thermocoagulation of lung tumours. Where we are, where we are headed. Clin Transl Oncol. 2009 Jan;11(1):28-34. PMID: 19155201.

48. Nguyen NP, Garland L, Welsh J, et al. Can stereotactic fractionated radiation therapy become the standard of care for early stage non-small cell lung carcinoma. Cancer Treat Rev. 2008 Dec;34(8):719-27. PMID: 18657910.

49. Onishi H, Shirato H, Nagata Y, et al. Hypofractionated stereotactic radiotherapy (HypoFXSRT) for stage I non-small cell lung cancer: updated results of 257 patients in a Japanese multi-institutional study. J Thorac Oncol. 2007 Jul;2(7 Suppl 3):S94-100. PMID: 17603311.

50. Moghissi K, Bond MG, Sambrook RJ, et al. Treatment of endotracheal or endobronchial obstruction by non-small cell lung cancer: lack of patients in an MRC randomized trial leaves key questions unanswered. Medical Research Council Lung Cancer Working Party. Clin Oncol (R Coll Radiol). 1999;11(3):179-83. [Erratum in Clin Oncol (R Coll Radiol); 1999(11(5):365.] PMID: 10465472.

51. Lee P, Kupeli E, Mehta AC. Therapeutic bronchoscopy in lung cancer. Laser therapy, electrocautery, brachytherapy, stents, and photodynamic therapy. Clin Chest Med. 2002 Mar;23(1):241-56. PMID: 11901914.

Introduction

Background

Non–Small-Cell Lung Cancer (NSCLC)

NSCLC refers to any type of epithelial lung cancer other than small-cell lung cancer.[1] The disease arises from epithelial cells of the lung, from the central bronchi to terminal alveoli. The histological type correlates with site of origin, reflecting the variation in respiratory tract epithelium by location. The most common types of NSCLC are adenocarcinoma, squamous cell carcinoma, and large cell carcinoma, but several other types occur less frequently; all types can occur in unusual histological variants. Squamous cell carcinoma typically originates near a central bronchus. Adenocarcinoma and adenocarcinoma in situ (formerly bronchioloalveolar carcinoma) usually arise in peripheral lung tissue. Adenocarcinomas are frequently associated with cigarette smoke, but may occur in patients who have never smoked.

Over 1 million deaths are attributed per year to NSCLC, making it the leading cause of cancer-related mortality worldwide.[2] In the United States, lung cancer is the leading cause of cancer death, and in 2010, an estimated 222,520 cases were expected to be diagnosed, with 157,300 deaths due to the disease.[2]

NSCLC may be symptomatic at presentation or it may be incidentally discovered at a routine chest imaging examination. The most common symptoms at presentation are progressive cough or chest pain. Other presenting symptoms include hemoptysis, malaise, weight loss, dyspnea, and hoarseness. Symptoms may result from local invasion or compression of adjacent thoracic structures such as compression involving the esophagus causing dysphagia, compression of laryngeal nerves causing hoarseness, or compression of the superior vena cava causing facial edema and distension of the superficial veins of the head and neck. Symptoms from distant metastases may also be present and include neurological defect or personality change from brain metastases or pain from bone metastases. Physical examination may identify enlarged supraclavicular lymphadenopathy, pleural effusion or lobar collapse, unresolved pneumonia, or signs of associated disease such as chronic obstructive pulmonary disease or pulmonary fibrosis.

NSCLC Staging

The prognosis of an NSCLC patient, and the subsequent treatment plan, are a function of disease stage.[3] NSCLC stage is defined by the TNM system, which was initially developed by the Union Internationale Contre le Cancer (UICC) and the American Joint Committee for Cancer Staging (AJCC). The TNM system takes into account the size of the primary tumor (T); the extent of regional lymph node involvement (N); and, the presence or absence of distant metastases (M).[4] The current Revised International System for Staging Lung Cancer, based on information from a clinical database of nearly 70,000 patients, was subsequently adopted by the AJCC and UICC.[4] Current TNM staging groups are summarized in Table 1.

Table 1. TNM staging groups

Overall Stage	T	N	M
Stage 0	Tis (in situ)	N0	M0
Stage IA	T1a, b	N0	M0
Stage IB	T2a	N0	M0
Stage IIA	T1a, b	N1	M0
	T2a	N1	M0
	T2b	N0	M0
Stage IIB	T2b	N1	M0
	T3	N0	M0
Stage IIIA	T1, T2	N2	M0
	T3	N1, N2	M0
	T4	N0, N1	M0
Stage IIIB	T4	N2	M0
	Any T	N3	M0
Stage IV	Any T	Any N	M 1a, b

M = presence of absence of distant metastases; N = extent of regional lymph node involvement; T = size of the primary tumor

Imaging methods used to stage NSCLC patients may include 18F-fluorodeoxyglucose positron emission tomography (FDG PET), computed tomography (CT) or magnetic resonance imaging (MRI).[5] The presence of symptoms, physical signs, laboratory findings, or perceived risk of distant metastasis ultimately drives evaluation for nodal and distant metastatic disease. Bone scans, FDG PET, CT, or MRI may be performed if initial assessments suggest nodal or more distant metastases or if a patient with more advanced disease is under consideration for aggressive local nonsurgical and combined modality treatments. Surgical staging of the mediastinum is considered the standard to evaluate local nodal status.

Treatment Options for NSCLC

Patients who are diagnosed with NSCLC can be divided into three general groups that reflect the extent of disease, which in turn dictates the initial treatment approach, not considering systemic therapies, which are not typically used in this setting until or unless a patient develops recurrence or distal disease:

- Surgically resectable disease (generally stage I, stage II, and selected stage III tumors).
- Potentially operable or inoperable locally (T3–T4) or regionally (N2–N3) advanced disease.
- Inoperable distant metastatic disease (includes distant metastases [M1] that are found at the time of diagnosis).

Surgical Resection for Stage I NSCLC

Based on the International Association for the Study of Lung Cancer (IASLC) database of more than 100,000 patients treated between 1990 and 2002, about 20–-25 percent of NSCLC patients present with stage I (T1N0M0, T2N0M0) disease.[6] Resection is considered the standard of care for surgically eligible patients in this setting. This would preferably be a lobectomy for most patients, alternatively a pneumonectomy for tumors in which sleeve resection or bronchoplasty would not allow achievement of adequate margins.[7] Data from the IASLC database of patients shows 5-year overall survival rates may range from 71 to 77 percent for stage IA NSCLC and 35 to 58 percent for stage IB disease.[8] Improvements in the use of staging methods including FDG PET and CT have led to improved surgical outcomes, exemplified by a report including 405 stage IA and Stage IB patients who had a 5-year overall survival of 80 percent and 72 percent, respectively.[9]

2

A comprehensive preoperative assessment must be performed to assess the risk for morbidity and mortality in NSCLC stage I patients being considered for curative-intent surgery.[10] Surgical morbidity and mortality are typically low in most modern series in the stage I setting, with major complications reported in about 6 percent of lobectomy cases and 18 percent in pneumonectomy cases.[11] The estimated risk of surgical mortality should be less than 4 percent for lobectomy and less than 9 percent for pneumonectomy in order to proceed to surgery.[7,10]

Local Nonsurgical Treatment Options for Stage I NSCLC

Surgery is the standard of care for patients with resectable stage I NSCLC. However, alternative treatments are needed for two subsets of stage I NSCLC patients. First is a subset that comprises about 20-30 percent of stage I patients, who have resectable tumors but are deemed medically inoperable due to comorbidities such as diminished cardiac reserve, poor pulmonary function, and poor performance status.[7,12-14] A second, much less common subset comprises patients who are deemed operable but decline surgery. Medically inoperable patients are more likely to die from intercurrent illness than from lung cancer; however, evidence exists to question this assumption.[7] For example, among a group of 128 patients with stage I or II NSCLC treated between 1994 and 1999, 49 received no treatment because they were deemed medically inoperable; 53 percent of the latter succumbed to lung cancer.[15] Among 1,432 untreated medically inoperable stage I NSCLC patients reported to a registry in California, the lung cancer-specific survival rate at 5 years was 16 percent, suggesting the need for alternative interventions in such patients.[16]

A recent systematic review reported postsurgical 30-day mortality ranged from 7 percent to 25 percent among patients with poor ventilatory function, with a weighted mean of 10 percent.[17] These patients would not be considered for surgery, but would be offered nonsurgical options that are outlined in the following section of this report.

Radiotherapy

External-beam radiotherapy (EBRT) has a role in the definitive treatment of patients with stage I NSCLC who are deemed medically inoperable, or in those who decline surgery.[7,13] Ideally, EBRT balances delivery of a cytotoxic dose of ionizing radiation to the tumor volume, attempting to minimize adverse effects (AEs) of radiation on adjacent normal lung tissue and thoracic structures. A "standard" total dose is typically 60 to 70 Gray (Gy), delivered in increments (fractions) over variable periods, depending on the technology that is used and the therapeutic intent. All available radiotherapy platforms use a medical linear accelerator to deliver photon radiation, typically in the energy range of 6-10 MeV. Several modalities have been used to treat patients with stage I NSCLC, as follows.

Conventional Two-Dimensional External-Beam Radiotherapy (2DRT)

Conventional wide-field 2DRT has been used extensively to treat medically inoperable patients with stage I NSCLC. Delivery of radiation to a total dose that ranged from 31 to 103 Gy, in daily fractions of 1.8-2 Gy, has been reported to produce overall survival rates of 17 percent to 42 percent among patients with early stage disease.[14] However, this technique is no longer in routine use in modern radiation oncology practice in this setting. Thus, it was not considered for the stage I setting in this comparative effectiveness review (CER).

External-Beam Conformal Radiotherapy Options

A quest to improve upon survival rates achieved with conventional 2DRT has led to development of conformal radiotherapy methods for definitive (curative) treatment of inoperable patients with stage I NSCLC. Conformal radiotherapy refers to modalities in which cytotoxic radiation beams are "shaped" to cover the tumor volume plus a surrounding tissue margin to treat microscopic disease that may reside there. Photon-based modalities include three-dimensional conformal radiation therapy (3DRT); intensity-modulated radiation therapy (IMRT); and stereotactic body radiation therapy (SBRT), which is also known as stereotactic ablative radiotherapy.[18-20] For purposes of this report, we will use the term "SBRT." Charged particle-based therapy such as proton beam radiotherapy (PBRT) is also available.[21]

Three-dimensional Conformal Radiation Therapy (3DRT)

3DRT employs CT simulation, allowing for more accurate dose calculations by taking into account axial anatomy and complex tissue contours. Three-dimensional anatomic information from diagnostic CT scans are used to deliver multiple highly focused beams of radiation that converge at the tumor site.12 This allows accurate and precise conformity of the radiation to the tumor volume, with very rapid dose fall-off in surrounding normal lung parenchyma. A 3DRT treatment protocol typically comprises 25-40 fractions (usually 1.8-2 Gy) delivered over a period of 5-10 weeks.

Intensity-Modulated Radiation Therapy (IMRT)

IMRT allows for the modulation of both the number of fields and the intensity of radiation within each field, allowing for greater control of the dose distribution to the target.[17,20,21] A potential theoretical benefit of IMRT is the ability to deliver higher doses to the tumor than with other methods, with greater tumoricidal effectiveness. A typical total dose of 60 to 70 Gy is usually delivered in 25-40 fractions over a period of 5-10 weeks. Dose-volume histogram studies suggest IMRT allows better conformality of the high-dose volume to the tumor. However, questions continue about the relative benefits and harms of this technique because a larger volume of lung receives a low radiation dose with IMRT, which may actually increase the rate of injury.[19]

Stereotactic Body Radiation Therapy (SBRT)

SBRT delivers very high, conformal ablative doses of radiation in fewer treatment sessions than other conformal modalities, with the potential to cause less damage to surrounding normal tissue.[22] SBRT regimens generally deliver a total dose of 60 Gy at greater than 10 Gy per fraction. Four-dimensional monitoring of tumor motion during the breathing cycle is accomplished by using a number of imaging techniques (CT, X-ray, ultrasound) that depend on the platform, tracking on bony structures or implanted fiducials. SBRT can deliver very high biologically effective doses (BED) above 100 Gray equivalent (GyE) that are needed to ablate the tumor and sterilize the tumor margins, minimizing damage to adjacent normal tissue. Conventionally fractionated schemes, delivering a similar total dose in 25-40 fractions, typically do not reach a similar BED range.

Proton Beam Radiotherapy (PBRT)

PBRT delivers high doses of radiation to the tumor. Proton beams enter the body with a low radiation dose, stop at the tumor, match its shape and volume or depth, and deposit the bulk of their cytotoxic energy within the tumor; thus this type of treatment may cause less damage to surrounding healthy tissue.[21] Analysis of the application of PBRT to NSCLC presents challenges secondary to the small number of institutions that have experience with this technique and small reported patient numbers.[21]

Summary: Radiotherapy

The optimal definitive external radiotherapy modality is not defined for patients with medical contraindications (medically inoperable patients) or for those with stage I NSCLC who elect nonsurgical treatment.[20] 3DRT and IMRT are distinguished from SBRT therapeutically primarily as a function of the fractionation schemes employed and the higher BED delivered to the tumor with SBRT compared to either 3DRT or IMRT. Technological distinctions include the methods or equipment used in patient positioning, patient immobilization, tumor tracking methods, control systems, beam collimation, and treatment-planning software. Conformal radiotherapy procedures are generally time-intensive, require significant training, and necessitate substantial advance planning.[19,23] Institutional quality control processes are required to assure their safe and effective use, in particular IMRT.[24]

Interventional Treatment Options

Interventional treatment options for stage I NSCLC include radiofrequency ablation (RFA).[22,25] Percutaneous RFA is a minimally invasive technique that uses high-frequency electric currents to heat and destroy tumor and is typically performed in a single session.[26] The most frequent complication of RFA is pneumothorax.[27]

Analysis of the application of RFA to NSCLC presents challenges secondary to the small number of institutions that have experience with this technique and limited patient data.[21,26,28]

Earlier brachytherapy was used as a definitive treatment of stage I nonsurgical patients, but is now considered appropriate only as an adjunct to surgery.[29] It was not considered in the stage I setting in this CER.

Local Nonsurgical Treatment Options for Symptomatic Malignant Endobronchial NSCLC

About 20 percent to 30 percent of NSCLC patients experience airway obstruction from non-resectable primary or recurrent lesions, with symptoms that may include disabling dyspnea, cough, and hemoptysis.[30,31] Up to 40 percent of lung cancer deaths may be attributed to such locoregional disease. Management of these patients is a significant challenge. The ability to promptly alleviate airway distress may be lifesaving, as some patients may succumb to suffocation within hours of presentation.[31-33] Patients in this situation often require emergency treatment to relieve airway obstruction or to stop bleeding. Intervention typically is palliative, but may be performed with curative intent in some cases.

Radiotherapy

Patients with good performance status may benefit from EBRT (conventional 2DRT or conformal methods outlined above) to quickly ameliorate symptoms (e.g., hemoptysis, cough, chest pain, dyspnea, obstructive pneumonia, dysphagia, etc.) associated with an airway obstructive tumor.[33] However, if they have already been heavily pretreated or the tumor is located close to radiosensitive organs or other anatomic structures, interventional options may become necessary.

Interventional Options

Brachytherapy

Brachytherapy is another option for treating airway obstruction and can be used alone, or in combination with EBRT to boost the total dose of irradiation used.[33,34] It has been used in combination with high-dose EBRT as a potential curative primary treatment in selected cases. Serious complications have been described with brachytherapy, including massive hemoptysis, tracheoesophageal fistulas, bronchial stenosis and radiation bronchitis.[34]

The role of brachytherapy for the palliative treatment of symptomatic patients with airway obstruction is unclear. It has been used as a palliative treatment in case of endobronchial tumor recurrence after EBRT. Brachytherapy also may be an option for patients in whom EBRT fails to relieve symptoms, or those with endobronchial disease who require lung re-expansion before or in conjunction with radiotherapy.[33]

Bronchoscopy and Stents, Cryoablation and Photodynamic Therapy (PDT)

Several interventional methods are used to palliate symptoms in patients with an obstructive endobronchial NSCLC.[25,32,33,35] Interventional bronchoscopy with mechanical tumor debridement and stent placement can rapidly reestablish airway patency and relieve dyspnea and respiratory distress in patients with airway obstruction due to a malignant endoluminal tumor.[32,35] In a large cryosurgery series, 86 percent of 521 patients experienced improvement in one or more symptoms including cough, dyspnea, hemoptysis, and chest pain.[36] Laser resection involving the neodymium-doped yttrium aluminum garnet (Nd-YAG) laser and PDT using porfimer sodium have been investigated in this setting with suggestion of symptomatic improvement in some cases.[25] RFA also has been used in this setting.

Scope of the Review

This Agency for Healthcare Research and Quality (AHRQ) -sponsored CER of local nonsurgical therapies for stage I (T1N0M0, T2N0M0) NSCLC and airway obstruction due to NSCLC is intended as a comprehensive systematic review of the relative benefits and harms of lung-directed nonsurgical therapies in two disease settings encompassing four distinct patient populations (see PICOTS, below). Several local nonsurgical therapies are available for definitive treatment of inoperable stage I NSCLC, or those with operable lesions who decline surgery. These include conformal radiation modalities (3DRT, IMRT, SBRT, PBRT), and interventional methods such as RFA. Likewise, numerous methods are used to treat patients with symptomatic malignant airway obstruction, including EBRT methods, brachytherapy, surgical debridement and stent placement, and others (e.g., Nd-YAG laser, RFA, cryoablation).

Rationale

Surgery is currently regarded as the standard of care for eligible patients with stage I NSCLC. However, alternative treatments are needed for a subset of stage I NSCLC patients for whom surgery is contraindicated because of underlying comorbidities. Alternatives also are needed for another smaller proportion of stage I patients who are medically operable but decline surgery. Comparison of outcomes with alternative procedures to those achieved with surgery is outside the scope of the CER. Instead, the CER is focused on local nonsurgical modalities for inoperable patients in Key Question 1, and in operable patients who decline surgery in Key Question 2.

Key Question 3 addresses the comparative benefits and harms of local nonsurgical therapies in patients with inoperable NSCLC who have symptoms secondary to the presence of an endoluminal lesion. The optimal approach in these patients is not established. These patients often require urgent care; typically have a short expected life span and interventions are often palliative.

All of the alternative modalities under consideration are clinically relevant and merit comparative evaluation due to uncertainty surrounding their optimal use in these settings. They are important to health care providers, patients, and policy makers given the substantial disease burden of NSCLC, especially in the elderly population.

Key Questions

The Key Questions and CER analytical frameworks (Figure 1 and Figure 2) are structured consistent with the PICOTS (Populations, Interventions, Comparators, Outcomes, Timeframes, Settings) framework, as laid out in the AHRQ Evidence-based Practice Center (EPC) "Methods Guide for Effectiveness and Comparative Effectiveness Reviews"[37] (hereafter Methods Guide).

Key Question 1. What are the comparative benefits and harms of local nonsurgical definitive therapies for documented (clinical or biopsy) stage I (T1N0M0, T2N0M0) NSCLC in adult patients (age 18 years or older) who are not surgical candidates because of the presence of contraindications to major surgery, for example, cardiac insufficiency, poor pulmonary function, presence of severe intercurrent illness, or poor performance status?

Key Question 2. What are the comparative benefits and harms of local nonsurgical definitive therapies for documented (clinical or biopsy) stage I (T1N0M0, T2N0M0) NSCLC in adult patients (age 18 years or older) who are deemed operable but decline surgery?

Key Question 3. What are the comparative short- and long-term benefits and harms of local nonsurgical therapies given with palliative or curative intent to patients with endoluminal NSCLC causing obstruction of the trachea, main stem, or lobar bronchi and recurrent or persistent thoracic symptoms such as hemoptysis, cough, dyspnea, and post obstructive pneumonitis?

Figure 1. Analytical framework for comparative effectiveness of local nonsurgical definitive therapies for adult patients (age 18 years or older) with documented (clinical or biopsy) stage I (T1N0M0 or T2N0M0) medically inoperable NSCLC or those with documented stage I NSCLC who are deemed operable but decline surgery

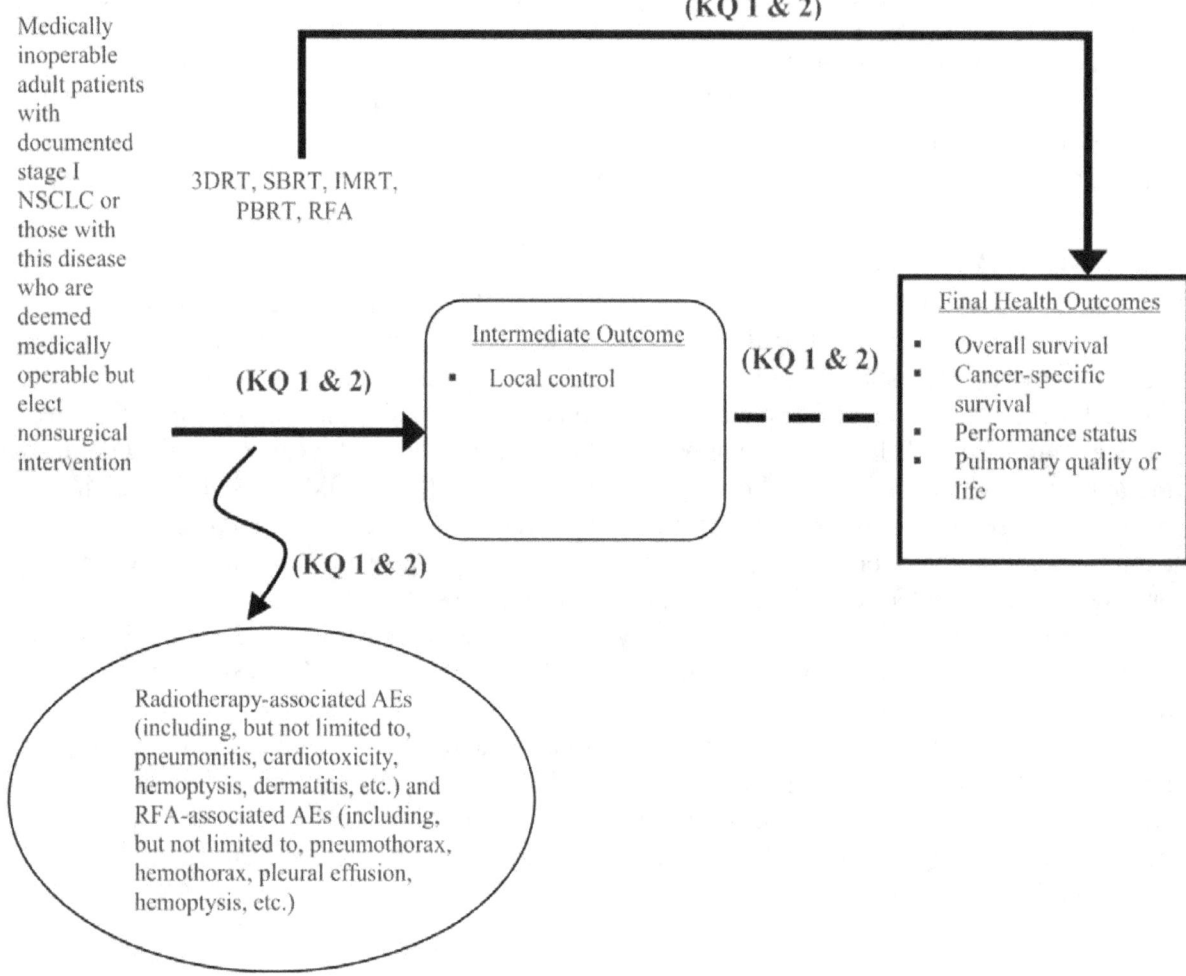

3DRT = three-dimensional radiotherapy; AE = adverse event; IMRT = intensity-modulated radiotherapy; KQ = Key Question; NSCLC = non–small-cell lung cancer; PBRT = proton beam radiotherapy; RFA = radiofrequency ablation; SBRT = stereotactic body radiotherapy

Figure 2. Analytical framework for comparative effectiveness of local nonsurgical curative or palliative therapies for adult patients (age 18 years or older) with symptomatic inoperable endobronchial obstruction due to NSCLC

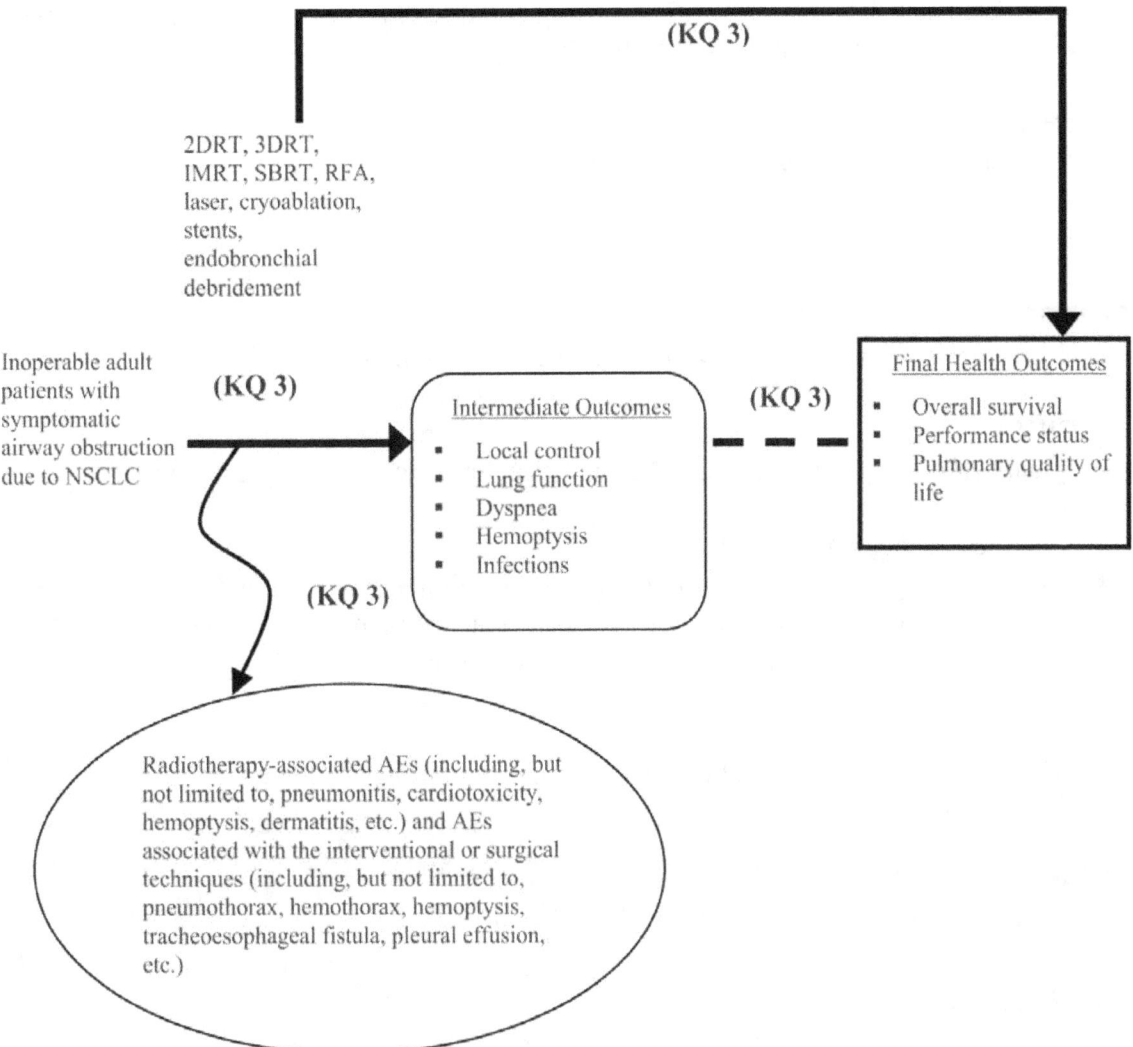

2DRT = two-dimensional, wide-field radiotherapy; 3DRT = three-dimensional radiotherapy; AE = adverse event; FEV = forced expiratory volume; IMRT = intensity-modulated radiotherapy; KQ = Key Question; NSCLC = non–small-cell lung cancer; PBRT = proton beam radiotherapy; RFA = radiofrequency ablation; SBRT = stereotactic body radiotherapy; YAG = yttrium aluminum garnet

PICOTS Framework

Key Questions 1 and 2

Population(s)

Key Question 1: Adult patients (age 18 years or older) with documented (clinical or biopsy) stage I (T1N0M0 and T2N0M0) NSCLC who were not deemed surgical candidates because of the documented presence of contraindications to major surgery, for example, cardiac

9

insufficiency, poor pulmonary function, presence of severe intercurrent illness, or poor performance status.

Key Question 2: Adult patients (age 18 years or older) with documented (clinical or biopsy) stage I (T1N0M0 and T2N0M0) NSCLC who would otherwise be deemed surgical candidates according to current clinical criteria but decline surgery.

Interventions
- Conformal radiotherapy methods (including SBRT, 3DRT, IMRT)
- PBRT
- RFA

Comparators
- Interventions were compared with each other as noted above.

Outcomes
- <u>Final health outcomes</u>: Overall survival, cancer-specific survival, performance status, pulmonary quality of life
- <u>Intermediate outcomes</u>: Local control
- <u>Adverse outcomes</u>: Includes, but not limited to, radiotherapy-associated AEs (e.g., pneumonitis, cardiotoxicity, hemoptysis, dermatitis, etc.), non-radiotherapy-associated AEs (e.g., pneumothorax, hemothorax, pleural effusion)

Timing
- The relevant periods occur at the time of treatment through followup over months (palliation) or years (overall survival).

Settings
- Inpatient and outpatient

Key Question 3

Population
Adult patients (age 18 years or older) with NSCLC with endoluminal obstruction of the trachea, main stem, or lobar bronchi and recurrent or persistent thoracic symptoms such as hemoptysis, cough, dyspnea and post obstructive pneumonitis, who were treated with curative or palliative intent.

Interventions
- Conventional 2DRT
- Conformal radiotherapy methods (including SBRT, 3DRT, IMRT)
- Brachytherapy
- RFA
- Cryoablation
- Laser therapy
- Endobronchial debridement and stents

- Electrocautery
- Combinations were considered, for example endobronchial debridement plus a stent, compared with debridement alone; or, combination of 2DRT with brachytherapy compared with radiotherapy alone.

Comparators
- Interventions were compared with each other as noted above.

Outcomes
- <u>Final health outcomes</u>: Overall survival, performance status, pulmonary quality of life
- <u>Intermediate outcomes</u>: Local control, lung function (e.g., forced expiratory volume [FEV1]), symptom relief (e.g., dyspnea, hemoptysis), respiratory tract infection
- <u>Adverse outcomes</u>: Includes, but not limited to, radiotherapy-associated AEs (e.g., pneumonitis, cardiotoxicity, hemoptysis, dermatitis, etc.), non-radiotherapy-associated AEs (e.g., pneumothorax, pleural effusion, transesophageal fistula, pericardial effusion)

Timing
- The relevant periods occur at the time of treatment through followup over months (palliation) or years (overall survival).

Settings
- Inpatient and outpatient

Organization of This Report

This report is organized into three chapters: Methods, Results and Discussion. The Methods chapter describes the search strategy used to identify the published and unpublished evidence relevant to Key Questions, the processes used to systematically review and assess individual clinical studies for inclusion or exclusion, data elements that were abstracted from these articles to compile evidence tables and method use to assess quality ratings for individual studies as well as strength of evidence (SOE) ratings. The Results chapter is structured to sequentially address Key Questions 1, 2 and 3. Results of each Key Question include evidence summary tables, an analysis of the quality and risk of bias of individual clinical studies, key points of evidence for the patient-important clinical outcomes, and a detailed synthesis of compiled evidence for each outcome according to Key Question. The Discussion chapter addresses key findings and the strength of evidence for all Key Questions using standard systematic review procedures outlined by AHRQ, a discussion of how the findings relate to or compare to existing standards, and the applicability of the body of evidence for each Key Question in terms of the PICOTS framework. The Discussion chapter also addresses implications for policy decisions, in the context of limitations of the systematic review processes used and the evidence itself. This chapter concludes with a section devoted to outlining the gaps in the available evidence base for each Key Question, and a Conclusions section that interprets the findings in the context of all considered factors.

Detailed electronic search strategy for this report is located in Appendix A. A list of excluded studies with reasons for exclusion is provided in Appendix B. Data abstraction tables for each Key Question can be found in Appendix C.

Methods

This chapter describes the methods used to produce this comparative effectiveness review (CER). Methodological practices followed in this review were derived from the Methods Guide[37] and its subsequent updates. The main sections in this chapter reflect the elements of the protocol established for the CER; certain methods map to the Preferred Reporting Items for Systematic Reviews and Meta-Analyses (PRISMA) checklist.[38]

Topic Refinement and Review Protocol

The topic for this report and preliminary Key Questions arose through a public process involving the public and various stakeholder groups. Initially a panel of Key Informants gave input on draft Key Questions. Key Informants are the end users of research, including patients and caregivers, practicing clinicians, relevant professional and consumer organizations, purchasers of health care, and others with experience in making health care decisions. Within the Evidence-based Practice Center (EPC) program, the role of Key Informant is to provide input in identifying relevant Key Questions for research that inform healthcare decisions. The EPC solicits input from the Key Informants when developing questions for systematic review or when identifying high priority research gaps and to identify topics for future research. Key Informants were not involved in analyzing the evidence or writing the report and have not reviewed the report except through the peer or public review mechanism. Key Informants had to disclose any financial conflicts of interest greater than $10,000 and any other relevant business or professional conflicts of interest. The Agency for Healthcare Research and Quality (AHRQ) Task Order Officer (TOO) and the EPC worked to balance, manage, or mitigate any potential conflicts of interest identified.

The draft Key Questions were posted on AHRQ's website for public comment on October 5, 2011 for 4 weeks. During this period, the EPC drafted a protocol for the CER and recruited a Technical Expert Panel (TEP) that comprised individuals with clinical expertise in radiation oncology, thoracic surgery and surgical oncology, pulmonology, and general oncology. The TEP provided input throughout the development of the review but was not involved in subsequent evidence analysis or drafting the report.

We received comments on the draft Key Questions, scope, and content of the proposed CER from several individuals and specialty societies. We addressed all the comments in discussions with the TOO and during conference calls with the TEP. Specifically, we eliminated a Key Question aimed at "technically inoperable" patients, and expanded the list of adverse events (AEs) we would attempt to capture for each intervention. The final protocol was posted on AHRQ's website on February 22, 2012.

Literature Search Strategy

Search Strategy

The databases listed below were searched electronically by a medical librarian for citations from January 1995 through July 25, 2012:

- MEDLINE®
- Embase®
- Cochrane Controlled Trials Register

The search was limited to English language studies based on the following rationale. First, evidence suggests that language restrictions do not change results of systematic review for conventional medical interventions.[39] Second, input from the TEP suggested that most if not all of the pivotal studies in this area would be captured in the English language evidence base and that restriction to English language would not introduce bias.

Our search strategy used the National Library of Medicine's Medical Subject Headings (MeSH®) keyword nomenclature developed for MEDLINE® and adapted for use in other databases. The searches were limited to studies of human subjects and those published in English. The full search strings and strategies can be found in Appendix A.

Grey Literature

Grey literature was sought by searching for clinical trials (Clinicaltrials.gov), the Food and Drug Administration website, and relevant conference abstracts (American Society of Clinical Oncology, and American Society for Radiation Oncology). We limited the grey literature search until 2010. We reviewed Scientific Information Packets provided by the Scientific Resource Center. Study authors were not contacted for unpublished results. Our goal was to include only phase 3 randomized controlled trials (RCTs) that we had not identified in our main electronic or hand searches.

Study Selection

Inclusion Criteria

Studies of any design were included if they fulfilled all of the following inclusion criteria.

Key Questions 1 and 2
1. Inclusion of medically inoperable NSCLC stage I patients (T1N0M0 and T2 N0M0) or medically operable NSCLC stage I patients (T1N0M0 and T2N0M0) who refuse surgery.
2. Such patients received only 1 of the following interventions:
   - Conformal radiotherapy methods (including stereotactic body radiotherapy (SBRT), three-dimensional conformal radiotherapy (3DRT), intensity-modulated radiotherapy (IMRT))
   - Proton beam radiotherapy (PBRT)
   - Radiofrequency ablation (RFA)
3. Reported data on one or more of the following outcome data for such patients:
   - Survival outcome (overall survival or cancer-specific survival)
   - Local control (an outcome defined as the arrest of cancer growth at the site of origin)
   - Pulmonary quality of life (QOL)
   - AEs

Key Question 3
1. Inclusion of NSCLC patients of any stage with a symptomatic endoluminal obstruction.
2. Such patients received 1 or more of the following interventions:
   - Conformal radiotherapy methods (including SBRT, 3DRT, IMRT)
   - Conventional 2D external beam radiotherapy (2DRT)
   - PBRT

- RFA
- Brachytherapy
- Cryoablation
- Laser Therapy
- Electrocautery
- Endobronchial debridement and stents

3. Reported data on one or more of the following outcome data for such patients:
   - Survival outcome (overall survival or disease specific survival)
   - Local control (an outcome defined as the arrest of cancer growth at the site of origin)
   - Symptom relief
   - Pulmonary QOL
   - AEs

Exclusion Criteria

- Editorials, commentaries, abstracts, animal studies, case report, non-English language and diagnostic accuracy study.
- On advice of our TEP, primary studies published prior to January 1, 1995 were excluded, to assure we considered current techniques and methods.
- Other reasons used to exclude studies were based on an assessment of the presence of duplicate patients in more than one paper; in that event, we included the article that included the same patients at longest follow up, cross-indexing that in the abstraction tables.
- No definitive surgical intervention was considered for any Key Question.
- For Key Questions 1 and 2, we compared single interventions, for example two different conformal radiotherapy methods, or RFA compared with a conformal radiotherapy method. We excluded studies that used any post-intervention systemic (e.g., chemotherapy) or local nonsurgical therapy but did not define the therapy or disaggregate the clinical outcomes of such patients.

A list of excluded primary studies and reasons for exclusion is provided in Appendix B.

Study Selection Process

Electronic search results were transferred to EndNote® and subsequently into Distiller SR® for study screening and selection. Using the study selection criteria (outlined above in this section) for screening titles and abstracts, each citation was marked as: 1) eligible for review as full-text articles; or 2) ineligible for full-text review. At least one training set (n=100) of representative titles and abstracts for each Key Question was examined initially by all team members to assure uniform application of screening criteria. A subsequent set was assessed to establish concordance among the team. Title and abstract screening was performed by two junior and one senior level team members. A reference was excluded only when both team members made independent decision to exclude it. In case of disagreement, the team leader adjudicated in consensus with all team members.

A test set of three references relevant to the three Key Questions was evaluated in full-text by junior and senior team members, including the team leader, to ensure selection criteria were applied correctly. Subsequently, two junior team members and the team leader reviewed full-text articles independently to determine their inclusion in the systematic review. The reason for exclusion of each full-text article reviewed was recorded in the Distiller SR® database. A paper could have been excluded for multiple reasons but only one reason was recorded. Team meetings were held regularly to discuss progress and to ensure the team leader was aware of difficulties or problems in this process. The process is shown schematically in Figure 3.

Figure 3. Schematic for data management

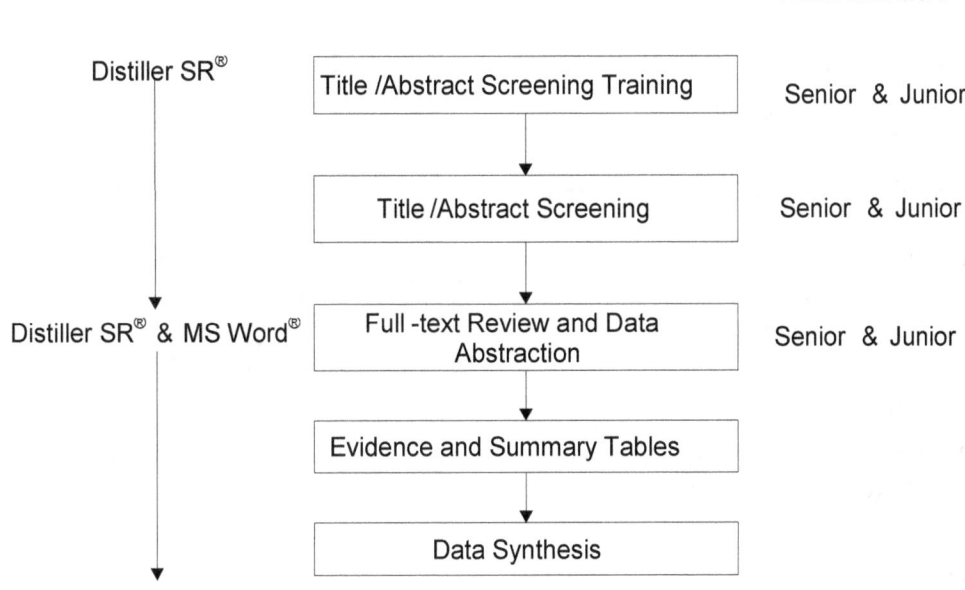

Data Extraction and Management

The main data elements for the CER were abstracted directly into Microsoft Word® tables. Other elements and the study risk of bias assessments were abstracted in Distiller SR.® A data abstraction guide was created that detailed the process of abstraction of data and definition of key data elements to ensure accuracy and consistency in data abstraction procedure across the team. The evidence tables were divided by Key Question and assigned for abstraction to all team members. One reviewer performed primary data abstraction of all data elements into the evidence tables, and a second reviewer reviewed the articles and evidence tables for accuracy. Disagreements were resolved by discussion, and if necessary, by consultation with a third reviewer.

Data Elements

- Study Attributes
  - Design
  - Author
  - Country
  - Year
  - Study start date
  - Study end date
  - Study setting
  - Treatment setting
  - Institution setting(s):

- o Criteria for staging:
- o Conflict of interest
- o Study funding
- Patient Characteristics
  - o Patients Enrollment numbers
  - o Lost to followup/Excluded
  - o Inclusion/Exclusion Criteria
  - o Stage Distribution
  - o Tumor Location
  - o Tumor Histopathology
  - o Age
  - o Women
  - o Race
  - o Comorbidities
  - o Performance status
  - o Histopathology confirmation
- Study Objective
- Primary Outcome
- Secondary Outcome(s)
- List of Outcome(s)
- Cause of Death
- Length of Followup
- Treatment Details
  - o Intervention name
  - o Vendor name
  - o Dose/frequency/details
  - o Technical details
  - o Treatment Intention
- Followup and Evaluation Criteria
- Study Outcomes
  - o Survival
    - Overall survival
    - Disease-specific survival
    - Local control
  - o Lung Outcomes
    - Lung function
    - Obstructive symptoms
    - QOL
    - Performance status
    - Others
  - o AEs

Quality (Risk of Bias) Assessment of Individual Studies

In adherence with the Methods Guide,[37] the risk of bias of individual comparative studies was assessed by the U.S. Preventive Services Task Force (USPSTF) criteria.[40] The quality of the abstracted studies was assessed by one reviewer, and examined by the senior team member. Assessment of the quality of included nonrandomized comparative intervention studies by this approach was informed by a selection of items proposed by Deeks et al.[41]

- The quality of comparative studies was assessed on the basis of the following criteria:
  - Initial assembly of comparable groups: adequate randomization, including concealment and whether potential confounders (e.g., other concomitant care) were distributed equally among groups.
  - Maintenance of comparable groups (includes attrition, crossovers, adherence, and contamination).
  - Important differential loss to followup or overall high loss to followup.
  - Measurements: equal, reliable, and valid (includes masking of outcome assessment).
  - Clear definition of interventions.
  - All important outcomes considered.
  - Analysis:
    - For RCTs: intention-to-treat, covariate adjustment
    - For cohort studies: adjustment for potential confounders for cohort studies

Comparative studies were rated according to one of three quality categories:

Good. Meets all criteria; comparable groups are assembled initially and maintained throughout the study (followup at least 80 percent); reliable and valid measurement instruments are used and applied equally to the groups; interventions are spelled out clearly; all important outcomes are considered; and appropriate attention is given to confounders in analysis. In addition, intention-to-treat analysis was used for RCTs.

Fair. Studies are graded "fair" if any or all of the following problems occur, without the fatal flaws noted in the "poor" category below: In general, comparable groups are assembled initially, but some questions remain about whether some (although not major) differences occurred with followup; measurement instruments are acceptable (although not the best) and are generally applied equally; some but not all important outcomes are considered; and some but not all potential confounders are accounted for. Intention-to-treat analysis has been done for RCTs.

Poor. Studies are graded "poor" if any of the following fatal flaws exists: Groups assembled initially are not close to being comparable or maintained throughout the study; unreliable or invalid measurement instruments are used or not applied at all equally among groups; and key confounders are given little or no attention; lack of masked outcome assessment; and for RCTs, intention-to-treat analysis is lacking.

The quality of the single-arm intervention studies was assessed by Carey and Boden criteria.[42] These include eight criteria, which are as follows:

1. Clearly defined study questions
2. Well-described study population
3. Well-described intervention
4. Use of validated outcome measures
5. Appropriate statistical analyses
6. Well-described results
7. Discussion and conclusion supported by data
8. Acknowledgement of the funding source

We created thresholds for converting the Carey and Boden risk assessment tool into the AHRQ format of standard quality ratings (good, fair, and poor). This allowed us to differentiate the quality of single-arm studies as good, fair, or poor. For a study to be ranked good quality, all eight Carey and Boden criteria mentioned above had to be met. For a fair quality assessment, 7 of 8 criteria had to be met. A study that met fewer than 7 of 8 criteria was rated as poor quality. These quality rankings for these studies can be found in Appendix C.

Data Synthesis

Given the lack of appropriate comparative studies for all Key Questions, this evidence review did not incorporate formal data synthesis involving meta-analysis. The quality of individual studies was assessed as outlined above, and the strength of the body of evidence for each Key Question was evaluated as follows.

Strength of the Body of Evidence

We graded the strength of the overall body of evidence for overall survival, symptom relief, quality of life and harms. The system used for rating the strength of the overall body of evidence is outlined in the AHRQ Methods Guide[37] and based on a system developed by the Grading of Recommendations Assessment, Development and Evaluation (GRADE) Working Group.[43] Further, we also used the GRADE guideline on assessing the risk of bias.[44] This system explicitly addressed four required domains: risk of bias, consistency, directness, and precision. Two independent reviewers rated all studies on domain scores and resolved disagreements by consensus discussion; the same reviewers also used the domain scores to assign an overall strength of evidence (SOE) grade.

The process of grading the body of evidence[43] was as follows. A body of evidence represented by RCT(s) would have a starting strength of high. A body of evidence represented by nonrandomized comparative studies would generally have a starting strength of low. For all study designs, the strength of evidence would be reduced by one level if there was high risk of bias, inconsistency or unknown consistency, indirectness and imprecision. Further, based on GRADE guidelines on assessing the risk of bias,[44] when the evidence was generated from studies that had very serious risk of bias, the strength of evidence was rated down by two levels. Case series or single-arm studies were deemed "indirect," "imprecise" and "unknown" for the domains of "directness," "precision" and "consistency."

The grade of evidence strength was classified into the following four categories:

- **High.** High confidence that the evidence reflected the true effect. Further research was very unlikely to change our confidence in the estimate of effect.
- **Moderate.** Moderate confidence that the evidence reflected the true effect. Further research may have changed our confidence in the estimate of effect and may have changed the estimate.
- **Low.** Low confidence that the evidence reflected the true effect. Further research was likely to change our confidence in the estimate of effect and was likely to change the estimate.
- **Insufficient.** Evidence was either unavailable or did not permit estimation of an effect.

Additional domains including strength of association, publication bias, coherence, dose-response relationship, and residual confounding were not addressed in this review.

Applicability

Applicability of findings in this review was assessed according to the AHRQ Comparative Effectiveness Methods Guide using the PICOTS (Population, Intervention, Comparator, Outcome, Timing, Setting) framework.[37,45,46] Included studies were assessed for relevance against target populations, interventions and comparators of interest, and outcomes of interest.

Peer Review and Public Commentary

Peer Reviewers were invited to provide written comments on the draft report based on their clinical, content, or methodological expertise. Peer review comments on the preliminary draft of the report were considered by the EPC in preparation of the final draft of the report. Peer Reviewers did not participate in writing or editing of the final report or other products. The synthesis of the scientific literature presented in the final report does not necessarily represent the views of individual reviewers. The dispositions of the peer review comments were documented and published after the publication of the evidence report.

Potential reviewers disclosed any financial conflicts of interest greater than $10,000 and any other relevant business or professional conflicts of interest. Invited Peer Reviewers did not have any financial conflict of interest greater than $10,000. Peer Reviewers who disclose potential business or professional conflicts of interest could submit comments on draft report through the public comment mechanism.

Results

Introduction

Overview

This chapter presents the results of this comparative effectiveness review (CER) on local nonsurgical interventions for patients with non–small-cell lung cancer (NSCLC) in three distinct settings. Key Question 1 addresses interventions in patients with stage I disease who are deemed medically inoperable due to comorbidities that preclude definitive resection. Key Question 2 addresses local nonsurgical intervention in patients with stage I disease who are deemed medically operable but refuse surgery. Key Question 3 addresses evidence for the use of local nonsurgical interventions in patients with symptoms secondary to an inoperable obstructive endoluminal NSCLC.

The results from the electronic literature search enumerate studies that were included and excluded from the review based on full-text examination. The excluded studies are shown in Appendix B. We did not perform a quantitative data synthesis for any Key Question.

Results of Literature Searches

Electronic Search

Of the 4,648 unique titles identified, we screened 1,178 in full-text. Of these, 55 met the CER inclusion criteria: 35 were relevant to Key Question 1, six were relevant to Key Question 2 and 17 were relevant to Key Question 3. Three studies[47-49] addressed both Key Questions 1 and 2. Details are given in the Preferred Reporting Items for Systematic Reviews and Meta-Analyses (PRISMA)[38] diagram (Figure 4). All studies relevant to Key Questions 1 and 2 were single-arm design, prospective (n=15), retrospective (n=21) or not specified (n=2). Among 17 papers included for Key Question 3, five were randomized controlled trials (RCTs), one was a nonrandomized comparative study and 11 were single-arm studies.

Grey Literature (Publication Bias)

Following review of 759 potentially relevant abstracts in the American Society of Clinical Oncology, and the American Society and American Society for Radiation Oncology proceedings over the past two years, and other sources including Clinicaltrials.gov, we identified one RCT that met the criteria for inclusion based on our protocol. This study (NCT00020709) is a phase 3 RCT of surgery versus stereotactic body radiotherapy (SBRT) in patients with Stage IA NSCLC who were fit to undergo primary resection. This study was terminated due to poor recruitment. After a MEDLINE search of the NCT number and title, we did not find any published results; it is unknown if any data have been reported. In examination of the U.S. Food and Drug Administration website and the Scientific Information Packets received from device manufacturers, we identified no additional RCTs that were relevant to this CER.

Figure 4. PRISMA diagram for identified trials

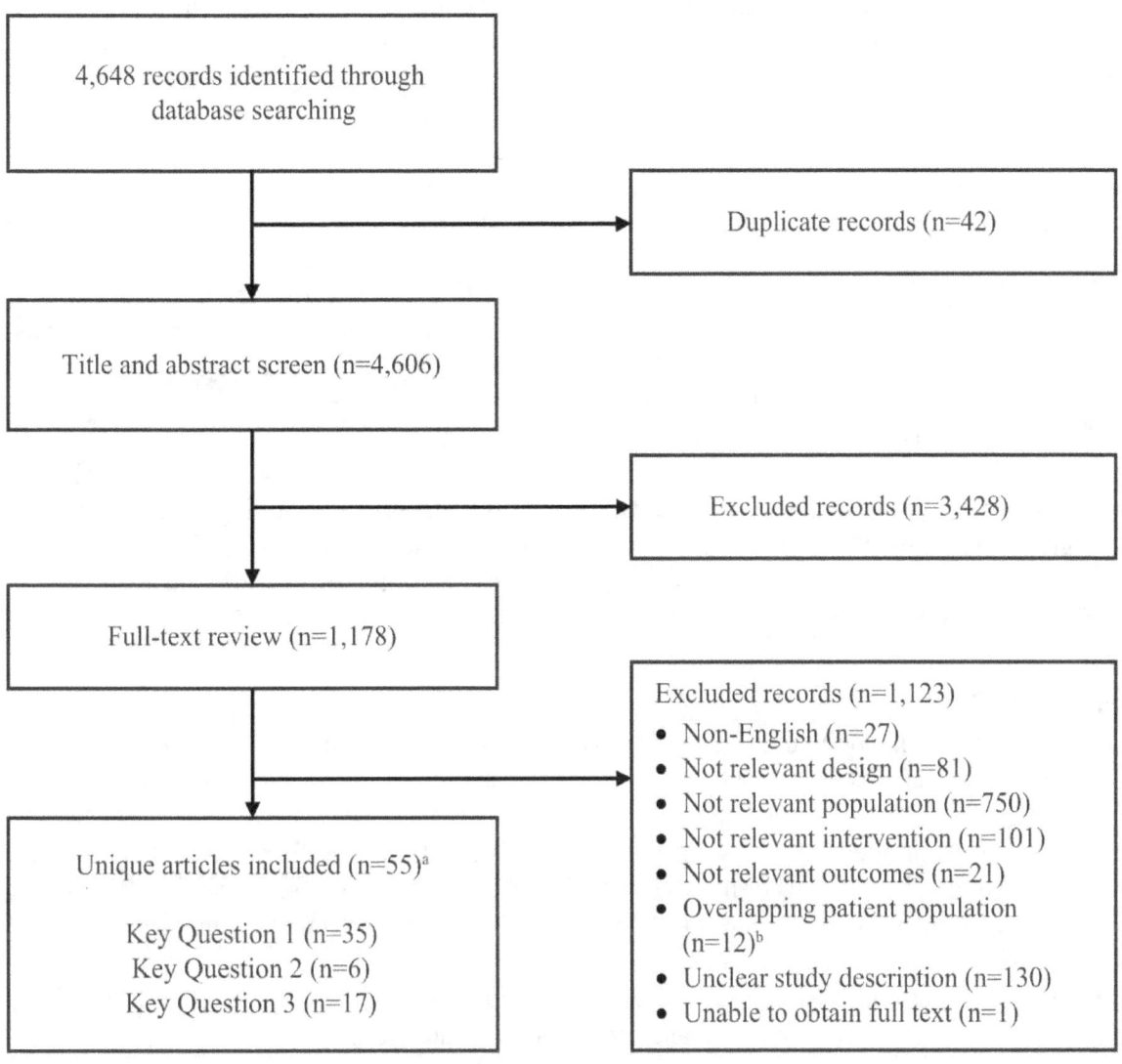

[a]Three studies addressed both Key Questions 1 and 2.
[b]Overlapping patient population refers to the studies in which the same patients were included in more than one study. In all such cases, only one study was included to avoid over sampling. Decision to include a study was based on the nature of the study design (preference of RCT over observational study designs) and the clarity in reporting relevant patients and/or outcomes.

Key Question 1. Comparative Effectiveness of Local Nonsurgical Interventions for Stage I NSCLC in Medically Inoperable Patients

Description of Included Studies

Table 2 provides a summary of characteristics of 35 single-arm studies that met our selection criteria for Key Question 1. Fourteen studies were prospective.[17,47,49-59] Interventions included SBRT (24 studies, total n=1665 patients),[17,48,49,53,56-75] three-dimensional radiotherapy (3DRT) (7 studies, total n=240 patients),[50,51,54,55,76-78] proton beam radiotherapy (PBRT) (three studies, total n=144 patients)[47,52,79] and radiofrequency ablation (RFA) (1 study, n=19 patients).[80] More detailed information on the interventions is provided in Appendix C. Patients included in these studies were typically in their 70s, with median ages ranging from 67-81 years, and an overall range from 31-93 years. Common reasons for medical inoperability included presence of pulmonary disease (chronic obstructive pulmonary disease), insufficient predicted post-therapy lung function, cardiovascular disease, and other comorbidities that in total preclude surgical resection. Sex distribution was uneven, with proportions of females ranging from 9-80 percent across studies. Karnofsky performance status (KPS) of enrollees ranged from 40-100 in 11 studies,[51,52,54,56,60,61,63-66,71,74] Eastern Cooperative Oncology Group (ECOG),[50,57,69,70,72,74,76,77] World Health Organization (WHO)[48,49,53,75], or European Organization for Research and Treatment of Cancer (EORTC)[79] KPS ranged from 0-3 across 11 studies. Perfomance status was not reported in 11 studies.[17,47,55,58,59,62,67,68,73,78,80] Sixteen studies (46 percent) reported histological confirmation of NSCLC cell types in 100 percent of patients.[47,49,50,52-54,56,60,61,66,67,71,76-78] The remaining nineteen (54 percent) studies[17,48,54,56-58,61-64,67-69,71-75,79,80] included patients without histological confimation of NSCLC. In 18 of such studies, a median 26 percent of patients did not have histologically confirmed NSCLC. Such studies used the rate of tumor growth in sucessive computed tomography (CT) scans and presence of 18F-fluorodeoxyglucose activity as a diagnostic marker of NSCLC rather than histological confirmation of NSCLC.

Key Points

- All evidence included in this report for Key Question 1 is from single-arm studies. No evidence is available from any type of direct comparative study of one intervention versus another.
- Evidence compiled from 35 single-arm studies is insufficient to form conclusions about the comparative benefits or harms of SBRT (24 studies), 3DRT (seven studies), PBRT (three studies) and RFA (one study) in medically inoperable patients with stage I NSCLC.
- The evidence comprises direct outcomes overall survival and cancer-specific survival; an indirect outcome, local control; and radiation-associated toxicities.
- Overall, post-treatment toxicities were reported across studies, but no relative trend was detected among interventions.
- We are uncertain whether the limited evidence on adverse events (AEs) reflects their absence, or that the investigators did not systematically collect those data or report them.

Table 2. Summary of characteristics for studies that address Key Question 1

Treatment	Author, Year, Country	Design (Quality)[42]	Number of Patients	Intervention Details	100% Histopathology Confirmation (% Not Confirmed)	Age, Years	% Female
3DRT	Bogart et al, 2010, USA[50]	Prospective (Poor)	39	70 Gy 17-29 frs	Yes	75 (48-87)	53%
	Bradley et al, 2003, USA[51]	Prospective (Fair)	56	70 Gy 5 frs	Yes	73 (52-90)	57%
	Campeau et al, 2009, Australia[76]	Retrospective (Fair)	34	60 Gy 30 frs	Yes	81 (54-88)	41%
	Graham et al, 2006, Australia[77]	Retrospective (Fair)	Total: 39 (100%) Medically inoperable: 36 (92%) Refused surgery or NR: 3 (8%)	65 Gy 35 frs Concurrent end-phase boost	Yes	72[B] (53-84)	38%
	Jimenez et al, 2010, Spain[78]	Retrospective (Poor)	47	79Gy 44 frs (calculated)	Yes	68±10	23%
	Mirri et al, 2009, Italy[54]	Prospective (Poor)	15	40 Gy BED: 72 Gy 5 frs	No (27%)	76[B]	NR
	Narayan et al, 2004, USA[55]	Prospective (Poor)	13	92 or 103 Gy 44-49 frs (calculated)	Yes	67±18	9%
PBRT	Bush et al, 2004, USA[52]	Prospective (Good)	Total: 68 (100%) Medically inoperable: 63 (93%) Refused surgery: 5 (7%)	51 CGE 10 frs 60 CGE 10 frs	Yes	72 (52-87)	56%
	Iwata et al, 2010, Japan[47]	Prospective (Good)	Total: 57 (100%) Medically inoperable: 29 (51%) Refused surgery: 28 (49%)	80 or 60 Gy BED: 96- 112 Gy 20 frs	Yes	76 (48-89)	29%
	Nakayama et al, 2010, Japan[79]	Retrospective (Poor)	Total: 55 (100%) Medically inoperable: 52 (94%) Refused surgery: 3 (6%)	66-73 GyE, 10-22 frs	No (12%)	74±9	26%
RFA	Pennathur et al, 2007, USA[80]	Retrospective (Good)	19	RF3000: power 5-10W increments until system impedance > 400 ohm RITA: power 35-50 W, target temperature 90 degrees C	Yes	78 (68-88)	58%

23

Table 2. Summary of characteristics for studies that address Key Question 1 (continued)

Treatment	Author, Year, Country	Design (Quality)[42]	Number of Patients	Intervention Details	100% Histopathology Confirmation (% Not Confirmed)	Age, Years	% Female
SBRT	Andratschke et al, 2011, Germany[60]	Retrospective (Poor)	92	24-45 Gy 3-5 frs	Yes	75 (53-93)	30%
	Baumann et al, 2006, Denmark[62]	Retrospective (Poor)	Total: 141 (100%) Medically inoperable: 136 (96%) Refused surgery: 5 (4%)	30-48 Gy 2-4 frs	No (24%)	74 (56-90)	51%
	Baumann et al, 2009, Denmark[61]	Retrospective (Good)	Total: 57 (100%) Medically inoperable: 56 (99%) Refused surgery: 1 (2%)	45 Gy BED: 112 Gy	No (33%)	75 (59-87)	54%
	Bollineni et al, 2012, Netherlands[75]	Retrospective (Poor)	132	60 Gy 3-8 frs	No (70%)	75 (46-90)	28%
	Burdick et al, 2010, USA[63]	Retrospective (Fair)	72	50-60 Gy 3-10 frs	No (32%)	73 (52-90)	NR
	Coon et al, 2008, USA[64]	Retrospective (Poor)	Total: 26 (100%) Medically inoperable: 24 (92%) Refused surgery: 2 (8%)	60 Gy 3 frs	No (38%)	76.5[a]	NR
	Dunlap et al, 2010, USA[65]	Retrospective (Fair)	Total: 40 (100%) Medically inoperable: 37 (92%) Refused surgery: 3 (8%)	30-60 Gy BED: 78-180 Gy 3-5 frs	Yes	73 (54-87)	NR
	Fritz et al, 2008, Germany[66]	Retrospective (Fair)	Total: 40 (100%) Medically inoperable: 37 (92%) Refused surgery: 3 (8%)	BED: 100 Gy	Yes	74 (59-82)	20%
	Kopek et al, 2009, Denmark[53]	Prospective (Good)	88	45 or 68 Gy 3 frs	Yes	73 (47-88)	49%
	Nyman et al, 2006, Sweden,[56]	Prospective (Fair)	45	45 Gy 3 frs	No (20%)	74[b] (58-84)	44%
	Olsen et al, 2011, USA[67]	Retrospective (Poor)	Total: 130 (100%) Medically inoperable: 117 (90%) Refused surgery: 13 (10%)	45-54 Gy 3-5 frs	No (15%)	75 (31-92)	50%

24

Table 2. Summary of characteristics for studies that address Key Question 1 (continued)

Treatment	Author, Year, Country	Design (Quality)[42]	Number of Patients	Intervention Details	100% Histopathology Confirmation (% Not Confirmed)	Age, Years	% Female
SBRT (continued)	Palma et al, 2011, Netherlands[17]	Prospective (Poor)	Total: 176 (100%) Medically inoperable: 169 (96%) Refused surgery or NR: 7 (4%)	54-64 Gy 3-8 frs	No (68%)	70 (47-86)	45%
	Pennathur et al, 2009, USA[68]	Retrospective (Fair)	21	20-60 Gy BED: 60-70 Gy 1-3 frs	No (5%)	71 (61-85)	57%
	Ricardi et al, 2010, Italy[57]	Prospective (Poor)	Total: 62 (100%) Medically inoperable: 56 (90%) Refused surgery: 6 (10%)	45 Gy BED: 124 Gy 3 frs	No (36%)	74[b] (53-83)	16%
	Scorsetti et al, 2007, Italy[69]	NR (Poor)	43	20-32 Gy BED: 40-117 Gy 2-4 frs	No (5%)	75 (52-90)	21%
	Shibamoto et al, 2012, Japan[49]	Prospective (Good)	Total: 180 (100%) Medically inoperable: 120 (67%) Refused surgery: 60 (33%)	44-52 Gy 4 frs	Yes	77 (29-89)	32%
	Song et al, 2009, Korea[70]	Prospective (Good)	Total: 32 (100%) Medically inoperable: 31 (97%) Refused surgery: 1 (3%)	40-60 Gy 3-4 frs	Yes	72 (58-89)	19%
	Stephans et al, 2009, USA[71]	Retrospective (Good)	86	50-60 Gy 3-5 frs	No (29%)	73 (40-90)	56%
	Takeda et al, 2009, Japan[48]	Retrospective (Fair)	Total: 63 (100%) Medically inoperable: 49 (78%) Refused surgery: 14 (22%)	50 Gy 5 frs	No (17%)	78 (56-91)	36%
	Taremi et al, 2011, Canada[58]	Prospective (Fair)	108	48-60 Gy 3-10 frs	No (29%)	73 (48-90)	51
	Turzer et al, 2011, Norway[72]	Retrospective (Fair)	Total: 36 (100%) Medically inoperable: 35 (97%) Refused surgery: 1 (3%)	45 Gy 3 frs	No (26%)	74 (54-85)	64%

25

Table 2. Summary of characteristics for studies that address Key Question 1 (continued)

Treatment	Author, Year, Country	Design (Quality)[42]	Number of Patients	Intervention Details	100% Histopathology Confirmation (% Not Confirmed)	Age, Years	% Female
SBRT (continued)	Vahdat et al, 2010, USA[59]	Prospective (Poor)	20	42-60 Gy 3 frs	Yes	75 (64-86)	80%
	van der Voort van Zyp et al, 2009, Netherlands[73]	NR (Poor)	Total: 70 (100%) Medically inoperable: 65 (93%) Refused surgery: 5 (7%)	36-60 Gy 3 frs	No (49%)	76 (54-90)	NR
	Videtic et al, 2010, USA[74]	Retrospective (Fair)	26	50 Gy 5 frs	No (29%)	74 (49-88)	50%

3DRT = three dimensional radiotherapy; BED = biologically effective dose; CGE = cobalt gray equivalent; frs = fractions; Gy = gray; GyE = gray equivalent; NR = not reported; PBRT = proton beam radiotherapy; RFA = radiofrequency ablation; SBRT = stereotactic body radiotherapy
Values are median (range) or mean (±SD) unless specified.
[a]Median.
[b]Mean.

Detailed Synthesis

All survival outcomes abstracted for this CER are compiled in Appendix C. In Table 3, we have aggregated evidence from studies with the longest followup period.

Table 3. Survival and local control outcomes for local nonsurgical interventions in medically inoperable patients with stage I NSCLC

Intervention	Reported Overall Survival Rates, Number of Studies (Number of Patients)[a]	Reported Cancer-Specific Survival Rates, Number of Studies (Number of Patients)[a]	Reported Local Control Rates, Number of Studies (Number of Patients)[a]
3DRT	3-years: 33-61% 4 studies[51,54,55,78] (n=131) 5-years: 30% 1 study[77] (n=36)	3-years: 48%, 51% 2 studies[51,55] (n=69) 5-years: 53% 1 study[77] (n=36)	3-years: 63%, 72% 2 studies[51,54] (n=71) 5-years: NR
SBRT	3-years: 52-77% 7 studies[48,49,57,61,62,66,74] (n=480) 5-years: 17-44% 6 studies[17,49,53,56,60,62] (n=650)	3-years: 57-94% 6 studies[48,57,61,62,65,66] (n=371) 5-years[56,60,62]: 40-48% 3 studies[47,51,53] (n=273)	3-years: 81-94% 5 studies[17,57,61,66,74] (n=344) 5-years: 83% 1 study[60] (n=92)
PBRT	3-years: 44%, 65% 2 studies[47,52] (n=92)	3-years: 72% 1 study[52] (n=63)	3-years: 74% 1 study[52] (n=63)
RFA	2-years: 68% 1 study[80] (n=19)	83% at FU 1 study[80] (n=19)	58% at FU 1 study[80] (n=19)

3DRT = three dimensional radiotherapy; FU = followup; n = number; NSCLC = non–small-cell lung cancer; NR = not reported; PBRT = proton beam radiotherapy; RFA = radiofrequency ablation; SBRT = stereotactic body radiotherapy
[a]Number of patients represents only inoperable.

The evidence summarized in Table 3 reflects single-arm studies that report direct outcomes-overall survival and cancer-specific survival and an indirect outcome- local control. Rates for overall survival, cancer-specific survival, and local control for SBRT at 3-years followup suggest a possible trend toward exceeding those reported with 3DRT. However, the reported ranges overlap. Furthermore, as this evidence comprises single-arm studies with no direct comparisons, conclusions are precluded. The nature of the evidence – no RCTs- does not support making indirect comparisons among interventions.

Intervention-Associated Adverse Events

Intervention-related toxicities reported in at least 2 percent of the study population are shown in Appendix C. The reported toxicities are grade 2 or greater (moderate) on a standardized crietria such as Common Toxicity Criteria for Adverse Events (CTCAE), or the WHO scale. They are all similar with respect to their grades and definitions. For Key Questions 1 and 2, these included radiation-associated pneumonitis and pulmonary toxicity, dyspnea, esophagitis, thoracic wall pain, pericardial or pleural effusion, bronchial stricture, and rib fracture. Rib fractures were reported in nine (41 percent) SBRT studies[17,53,56,57,60-62,65,66] and one PBRT study.[79] One death was attributed to grade 5 pericardial effusion at 3 months post-treatment in a 3DRT study.[54] A second death was attributed to grade 5 hemoptysis in an SBRT study.[70] Complications associated with RFA included pneumothorax and prolonged air leak from the lung.

As shown in Table 4, no relative difference in the proportion of studies reporting toxicities is evident among or across interventions, with the possible exception of rib fractures mentioned above.

Table 4. Percentage of studies reporting intervention-associated toxicities in stage I medically inoperable NSCLC patients

Toxicity	SBRT n=24 Studies (%)	3DRT n=7 Studies (%)	PBRT n=3 Studies (%)	RFA n=1 Study (%)
None	4 (17)	2 (29)	1 (33)	0
Grade 2	9 (38)	3 (43)	1 (33)	NA
Grade > 2	13 (54)	2 (29)	1 (33)	NA
Rib Fracture	9 (38)	0	1 (33)	NA
Mortality	1 (4)	0	1 (33)	1 (100)

3DRT = three dimensional radiotherapy; NA = not applicable; NSCLC = non–small-cell lung cancer; PBRT = proton beam radiotherapy; RFA = radiofrequency ablation; SBRT = stereotactic body radiotherapy

Overall, post-treatment toxicities were not commonly reported across studies in the body of evidence. We are uncertain whether the limited evidence on AEs reflects absence, or that the investigators did not systematically collect data or report them.

Key Question 2. Comparative Effectiveness of Local Nonsurgical Interventions for Stage I NSCLC in Medically Operable Patients

Description of Included Studies

Table 5 provides a summary of characteristics of six single-arm studies that address Key Question 2. Three studies were prospective.[47,49,81] Three studies[81-83] used SBRT and enrolled only operable patients and two studies[48,49] used SBRT and enrolled inoperable and operable patients but reported outcomes separately. One study[47] used PBRT. Overall, patients were typically in their mid-70s, with median ages ranging from 74[83] to 78[48] years, and overall range from 43-91 years. Sex distribution was uneven, with proportions of females ranging from 40 percent[81] to 72 percent[83] across studies. ECOG and WHO performance status ranged from 0-3 across studies. Four studies reported 100 percent histological confirmation of NSCLC cell type.[47,49,81,83] Details on the included studies are provided in Appendix C.

Key Points

- All evidence included in this report for Key Question 2 is from single-arm studies. No evidence is available from any type of direct comparative study of one intervention versus another.
- Evidence compiled from six single-arm studies is insufficient to form conclusions about the comparative benefits or harms of SBRT (five studies) or PBRT (one study) in medically operable patients with stage I NSCLC.
- The results of interest for this report comprise direct outcomes overall survival and cancer-specific survival; an indirect outcome, local control; and radiation-associated toxicities as shown in Figure A.
- Post-treatment toxicities were not common across studies. No relative trend was detected among interventions.

- We are uncertain whether the limited evidence on AEs reflects absence, or that the investigators did not systematically collect data or report them

Table 5. Summary of characteristics for studies that address Key Question 2

Treatment	Author, Year, Country	Design (Quality)[42]	Number of Patients	Intervention Details	100% Histopathology Confirmation (% Not Confirmed)	Age, Years (Range)[a]	% Female
PBRT	Iwata et al, 2010, Japan[47]	Prospective (Good)	Total: 57 (100%) Medically inoperable: 29 (51%) Refused surgery: 28 (49%)	80 or 60 Gy BED: 96-112 Gy 20 frs	Yes	76 (48-89)	29%
SBRT	Chen et al, 2012, USA[81]	Prospective (Poor)	40	50 Gy 3 frs	Yes	76 (63-87)	60%
SBRT	Lagerwaard et al, 2011, Netherlands[82]	Retrospective (Poor)	177	60 Gy BED > 100 Gy for all frs 3, 5, or 8 frs	No (66%)	76 (50-91)	43%
SBRT	Onishi et al, 2011, Japan[83] (longer FU to Onishi et. al, 2007)[84]	Retrospective (Good)	87	45-72 Gy BED:116 Gy (100-141) 3-10 frs	Yes	74 (43-87)	28%
SBRT	Shibamoto et al, 2012, Japan[49]	Prospective (Good)	Total: 180 (100%) Medically inoperable: 120 (67%) Refused surgery: 60 (33%)	44-52 Gy 4 frs	Yes	77 (29-89)	32%
SBRT	Takeda et al, 2009, Japan[48]	Retrospective (Fair)	Total: 63 (100%) Medically inoperable: 49(78%) Refused surgery: 14 (22%)	50 Gy 5 frs	No (18%)	78 (56-91)	36%

BED = biologically effective dose; frs = fractions; FU = followup; Gy = gray; NR = not reported; PBRT = proton beam radiotherapy; SBRT = stereotactic body radiotherapy
[a]Values are median (range).

Detailed Synthesis

Appendix C shows survival and local control outcomes with PBRT or SBRT in four studies relevant to Key Question 2. Survival outcomes were not reported in these the studies. Table 6 shows survival and local control outcomes for each intervention.

Table 6. Survival and local control outcomes for local nonsurgical interventions in medically operable patients with stage I NSCLC

Intervention	Reported Overall Survival Rates, Number of Studies (Number of Patients)[a]	Reported Cancer-Specific Survival Rates, Number of Studies (Number of Patients)[a]	Reported Local Control Rates, Number of Studies (Number of Patients)[a]
PBRT	3-years: 80% 1 study[47] (n=28)	NR	NR
SBRT	3-years: 74%- 91% 4 studies[48,49,81,82] (n=291) 5-years: 70%, 70% 2 studies [49,83] (n= 87)	3-years: 91% 1 study[48] (n=14) 5-years: 76% 1 study[83] (n=87)	3-years: 93% 1study[82] (n=177) 5-years: 87% 1 study[83] (n= 87)

NR = not reported; NSCLC = non–small-cell lung cancer; PBRT = proton beam radiotherapy; SBRT = stereotactic body radiotherapy
[a]Number of patients who were operable but refused surgery.

The evidence summarized in Table 6 above comprises single-arm studies that report direct outcomes overall survival and cancer-specific survival and an indirect outcome, local control. No direct comparative evidence is available to suggest any relative difference between the technologies in overall survival, cancer-specific survival or local control rates.

Intervention-Associated Adverse Events

Appendix C shows intervention-related grade 2 or greater toxicities reported in at least 2 percent of the study population. Toxicities enumerated included radiation-associated pneumonitis and pulmonary toxicity, dermatitis, and rib fracture. Rib fractures were reported in two (67 percent) SBRT studies[82,83] and in the PBRT study.[47] The toxicity reporting criteria for each study (when provided by the authors) are shown in Appendix C. Definitions used to grade toxicities vary, which further complicates any possible assessment. Table 7 shows the distribution of reporting post-treatment toxicities across studies.

Table 7. Percentage of studies reporting intervention-associated toxicities in stage I medically operable NSCLC patients

Toxicity	SBRT n=5 Studies (%)	PBRT n=1 Study (%)
None	2 (40)	0
Grade 2	2 (40)	1 (100)
Grade > 2	3 (60)	1 (100)
Rib Fracture	2 (40)	1 (100)
Other	NR	NR

NR = not reported; PBRT = proton beam radiotherapy; SBRT = stereotactic body radiotherapy

No relative trend in reporting toxicities was discerned among interventions. We are uncertain whether the limited evidence on AEs reflects absence, or that the investigators did not systematically collect data or report them.

Risk of Bias for Individual Studies Addressing Key Question 1 and Key Question 2

We used the convention described by Carey and Boden[42] to assess the risk of bias of individual single-arm studies included to address Key Question 1 and Key Question 2 (see

Methods chapter). Our ratings of good, fair and poor are shown in Table 8. Studies that met 8 of 8 criteria were classified as good, studies that met 7 of 8 criteria were classified as fair and studies that met fewer than 7 criteria were classified as poor.

Among 38 unique single-arm studies, all reported the use of validated outcomes. Study quality was most often downgraded because authors did not acknowledge the funding source in 23 studies (60 percent).[48,51,54,56,57,59,62-69,72-74,76-79,81,82] In eleven studies (29 percent)[17,54,55,57,59,60,67,75,78,79,81] it was unclear whether or not the conclusions and discussion were supported by the data. Eight studies (23 percent)[17,50,54,55,58,59,67,73] did not adequately describe the study population. Six (16 percent)[54,55,59,78,79,81] did not describe results well. Four (10 percent)[50,75,79,82] did not adequately describe the intervention. Three (9 percent)[54,60,64] did not report the use of appropriate statistical analysis. The only consistent reason for which a study was downgraded was "failure to report the funding source."

Table 8. Carey and Boden study quality rating summaries for Key Questions 1 and 2

Key Question (Number of Unique Studies)	Good (8 of 8 "Yes")	Fair (7 of 8 "Yes")	Poor (< 7 of 8 "Yes")
Key Question 1 (n=35)	8[47,49,52,53,61,70,71,80]	12[48,51,56,58,63,65,66,68,72,74,76, 77]	15[17,50,54,55,57,59,60,62,64,67,69,73,75,78,79]
Key Question 2 (n=3)	1[83]	0	2[81,82]
Total	9 (24%)	12 (32%)	17 (44%)

Key Question 3. Comparative Effectiveness of Local Nonsurgical Therapies for Symptoms Secondary to an Inoperable Obstructive Endoluminal NSCLC

Overview

This section describes the literature that evaluates the efficacy and safety of local nonsurgical therapies for palliation or treatment of endobronchial NSCLC. After an overview of the literature, the results are described for outcomes in three categories: outcomes related to obstructive symptom resolution, survival outcomes, and safety outcomes. Improvement in obstructive symptoms was the primary outcome of interest because palliative interventions are most proximately expected to have an impact on obstructive symptoms. We specifically looked for resolution or improvement in dyspnea, cough, hemoptysis, and pneumonitis and abstracted all other symptoms in the "other" category. In addition, we also abstracted survival outcomes that included overall survival (reported as both median overall survival and time specific survival), disease specific survival and local control. Among the outcomes related to treatment-related toxicities, we focused on hemoptysis, pneumothorax and radiation bronchitis. We only abstracted toxicities that were grade 2 or greater or necessitated an active intervention or considered serious by the authors.

Overall, 17 studies were abstracted for this review. The evidence base consisted of six comparative studies[85-90] and 11 noncomparative studies.[91-101] Overall data for these studies is presented in Appendix C. Table 9 and Table 22 summarize the comparative and noncomparative studies reviewed for Key Question 3, respectively.

Study Characteristics of Comparative Studies

Among the six comparative studies that address Key Question 3, five were RCTs and one was a retrospective nonrandomized comparative study. Three hundred and forty-two patients were randomized in these six studies[85-90] that compared six distinct treatment combinations. Additionally, we did not report data for one RCT[102] as it reported outcome data for three different endobronchial treatments cumulatively. The detailed outcomes related to symptom improvement, survival and AEs for all six comparative studies are presented in Appendix C. All six studies included patients with a histologically confirmed NSCLC. Four studies[85,86,89,90] reported staging of lung cancer patients but only one study[86] reported the criteria used for staging NSCLC. The duration of the study enrollment period was reported by four studies[85,87,88,90] and ranged from 2 to 4 years. Three studies[85,87,88] were conducted in an outpatient setting; one[90] was conducted in the inpatient setting and for two studies[86,89] study setting was not reported. Four[85,88-90] were single-center studies, the remaining two[86,87] were multicenter studies. Four studies[87-90] did not state whether there existed a conflict of interest or not, the remaining two studies[85,86] stated no conflict of interest. Three studies[87,88,90] did not state the source of funding, one each was manufacturer sponsored,[89] professional scientific society sponsored[86] and investigator initiated.[85]

All six[85-90] comparative studies were rated as poor quality, five studies[85-88,90] reported data on symptom relief, five studies[85-88,90] reported survival data, two studies reported quality of life (QOL) data[85,87] and six studies[85-90] reported data related to treatment-related toxicity. Detailed characteristics of patients included in the six studies are summarized in Table 10.

Table 9. Overview of comparative studies that address Key Question 3

Treatment	Author, Year, Country	Design	N	GQ	FQ	PQ	OS	DSS	LCT	SC	QOL	TOX
BT + EBRT vs. BT alone	Mallick-2006, India[85]	RCT	45			•				•	•	•
BT + EBRT vs. EBRT alone	Langendjik-2001, Netherlands[86]	RCT	98			•	•			•		•
BT vs. EBRT	Stout-2000, UK[87]	RCT	108			•	•			•	•	•
Laser + BT vs. laser alone	Chella-2000, Italy[88]	RCT	29			•	•			•		•
Laser vs. photodynamic therapy	Jimenez-1999, Spain[89]	RCT	31			•	•					•
Laser vs. Electrocautery	van Boxem-1999, Netherlands[90]	NRC	31			•	•			•		•
	Overall	6	342	0	0	6	5	0	0	5	2	6

BT = brachytherapy; DSS = disease specific survival; EBRT = external beam radiotherapy; FQ = fair quality; GQ = good quality; KQ = Key Question; LCT = local control; N = total sample size of the study; NRC = nonrandomized comparative study; OS = overall survival; PQ = poor quality; QOL = quality of life; RCT = randomized controlled trial; SC = symptom control; TOX = toxicity

Key Points

- All RCTs included in this report were of poor quality according to the U.S. Preventive Services Task Force (USPSTF) rating criteria.
- Evidence from six comparative studies is insufficient to draw conclusions about relative benefits and harms of six unique treatment comparisons (brachytherapy plus external-beam radiotherapy (EBRT) versus brachytherapy alone; brachytherapy plus EBRT versus EBRT alone; brachytherapy versus EBRT; laser plus brachytherapy versus laser alone;

laser versus electrocautery or photodynamic therapy (PDT) for local nonsurgical therapies in symptomatic inoperable patients with obstructive endoluminal NSCLC.

- None of the six comparative studies included interventions related to debridement and stenting and RFA. These interventions are addressed in three single-arm studies.
- The evidence comprises direct outcomes (overall survival), symptom relief and treatment-related toxicities.
- Overall, treatment-related toxicities varied according to type of intervention. Hemoptysis was the most common toxicity reported across studies. There may be underreporting of treatment-related toxicities, as three comparative studies did not describe the frequency, process of data collection, or assessment of severity of treatment-related toxicities.

Table 10. Study characteristics of comparative studies that address Key Question 3

Treatment	Author, Year, Country	N	Stage Distribution	Histopathology Confirmation	Age, Years[a]	Females	PS
BT + EBRT vs. BT alone	Mallick-2006, India[85] (RCT)	N: 45 (100%) EBRT+BT-16Gy: 15 (33.3%) EBRT+BT-10Gy: 15 (33.3%) BT-15Gy: 15 (33.4%)	III: 45 (100%)	Yes	64.5 (35-75)	Total: 2 (4%)	NR
BT + EBRT vs. EBRT alone	Langendijk-2001, Netherlands[86] (RCT)	N: 95 (100%) EBRT+BT: 47 (49%) EBRT: 48 (51%)	EBRT +BT vs. EBRT I: 4 (9%) vs. 5 (10%) III: 43 (91%) vs. 43 (90%)	Yes	EBRT+BT: 67 (±9) EBRT: 68 (±9)	EBRT+BT: 9 (19%) EBRT: 8 (17%)	NR
BT vs. EBRT	Stout-2000, UK[87] (RCT)	N: 108 (100%) BT: 49 (49%) EBRT: 50 (51%)	NR	Yes	68[b] (40-84)	20 (20%)	NR
Laser + BT vs. laser alone	Chella-2000, Italy[88] (RCT)	N: 29 (100%) YAGL+BT: 14 (48%) YAGL: 15 (52%)	NR	Yes	61[b] (47-76)	6 (21%)	WHO 0: 3 (10%) I: 11 (40%) II: 15 (52%)
Laser vs. PDT	Jimenez-1999, Spain[89] (RCT)	N: 31 (100%) PDT: 14 (45%) YAGL: 17 (55%)	PDT vs. YAGL I: 3 (21%) vs. 1 (6%) II: 1 (7%) vs. 0 III: 5 (36%) vs. 11 (65%) IV: 4 (24%) vs. 3 (21%) R: 2 (14%) vs. 1 (6%)	Yes	64 (±7)	0	NR
Laser vs. ECAU	van Boxem-1999, Netherlands[90] (NRC)	N: 31 (100%) YAGL: 14 (45%) ECAU: 17 (55%)	YAGL vs. ECAU IV: 6 (43%) vs. 6 (35%) IIIB: 6(43%) vs. 10 (59%) IIIA: 2 (14%) vs. 1 (6%)	Yes	YAGL: 61 (37-88) ECAU: 62 (47-79)	N: 10 (32%) YAGL: 3 (21%) ECAU: 7(41%)	NR

BT = brachytherapy; EBRT = external beam radiotherapy; ECAU = electrocautery; Gy = gray; N = total sample size of the study; NR = not reported; NRC = nonrandomized comparative study; PDT = photodynamic therapy; PS = performance status; R = recurrent; RCT = randomized controlled trial; WHO = World Health Organization; YAGL = yttrium aluminum garnet laser

[a]Values are mean (±SD) or median (range) unless specified.

[b]Mean (range).

34

Description of Comparative Studies According to Intervention(s)

Brachytherapy Plus EBRT Versus Brachytherapy Alone

One RCT[85] compared brachytherapy plus EBRT versus brachytherapy alone and included a total of 45 patients (Table 11 and 12). These 45 patients were randomized equally across three treatment groups; EBRT plus brachytherapy (16 Grays [Gy]), EBRT plus brachytherapy (10Gy) and brachytherapy (15Gy) alone. All patients in the first two treatment arms received the same dose of EBRT (30 Gy in 10 fractions over 2 weeks). The authors assessed treatment harms at a predefined periods (at weekly intervals for acute toxicities) using a standardized Radiation Therapy Oncology Group (RTOG) morbidity-scoring criterion. This was the strength of this trial. Weaknesses of the trial included lack of sample size calculation, small number of patients per treatment group, and lack of defined statistical adjustments for multiple comparisons. These weaknesses affected the USPSTF domain of "appropriate analysis of results" (Table 13). Further, no details were provided on randomization or allocation concealment, which adversely affected the USPSTF domain of "assembled comparable groups." Therefore, we judged this trial to have a poor USPSTF quality rating.

There was no statistical difference in the response rate of dyspnea, cough, hemoptysis and obstructive pneumonia among the 3 treatment groups. The authors did not provide clear definitions of what constituted a partial or complete response for obstructive symptoms. Though the authors reported significant improvement in obstruction scores as well as multiple QOL scores (including sub-domains) within treatment groups, they did not report the results of between treatment groups. Survival data was not reported. Using the RTOG morbidity scoring criteria, the authors did not observe any grade II-grade IV acute toxicities. One patient died due to hemoptysis in the treatment group that received brachytherapy alone.

Table 11. Comparative effect of brachytherapy plus EBRT versus brachytherapy alone on obstructive symptoms in the Mallick trial[85]

Treatment Groups	Time	Dyspnea n(%)	Cough n(%)	Hemoptysis n(%)	Obstructive Pneumonia n(%)
EBRT+BT-16Gy (n=15)	Baseline	15 (100)	15 (100)	9 (60)	9 (60)
	Post Rx*	14 (93)	12 (80)	9 (100)	9 (100)
EBRT+BT-10Gy (n=15)	Baseline	13 (87)	15 (100)	13 (87)	10 (67)
	Post Rx*	12 (92)	13 (87)	13 (100)	7 (70)
BT-15Gy (n=15)	Baseline	15 (100)	15 (100)	12 (80)	10 (67)
	Post Rx*	13 (87)	13 (87)	10 (82)	8 (80)

BT = brachytherapy; EBRT = external beam radiotherapy; Gy = gray; n = number; Rx = treatment
*Represents number of patient who had complete or partial response.
Note: There were no statistically significant differences between any treatment arms.

Table 12. Comparative effect of brachytherapy plus EBRT versus brachytherapy alone on quality of life outcomes in the Mallick trial[85]

Treatment Groups	Time	QLQ-C3 (Global Health Status)	QLQ-C3 (Physical Functioning)
EBRT+BT-16Gy (n=15)	Baseline	37	71
	Post Rx	75 (↑103%)	90 (↑27%)
EBRT+BT-10Gy (n=15)	Baseline	35	74
	Post Rx	63 (↑80%)	85 (↑15%)
BT-15Gy (n=15)	Baseline	34	56
	Post Rx	62 (↑82%)	78 (↑39%)

BT = brachytherapy; EBRT = external beam radiotherapy; Gy = gray; n = number; QLQ-C3 = quality of life questionnaire; QOL = quality of life; Rx = treatment

Table 13. USPSTF study quality ratings of the Mallick trial[85]

Assembled CG	Maintained CG	Minimal LTFU	Measurements Equal, Valid, and Reliable	Interventions Clearly Defined	Important Outcomes Considered	Appropriate Analysis of Results	Overall USPSTF Rating
No	Yes	Yes	No	Yes	Yes	No	Poor

CG = comparable groups; LTFU = loss to followup; USPSTF = U.S. Preventive Services Task Force

Brachytherapy Plus EBRT Versus EBRT Alone

One RCT[86] compared brachytherapy plus EBRT versus EBRT alone. The trial was planned to recruit a total of 160 patients with an 80 percent power to detect a 25 percent decrease in the rate of palliation of dyspnea with 0.05 type-I error (Table 14). However, the trial was discontinued prematurely due to lack of patient accrual. The authors reported results of 95 evaluable patients who were randomized to brachytherapy plus EBRT (n=47) or EBRT alone (n=48) using a central randomization process. The USPSTF trial quality rating was poor (Table 15). The analysis with 95 patients was underpowered to detect a prespecified difference in the rate of dyspnea (a primary outcome) and therefore adversely affected the USPSTF domain of "appropriate analysis of results." The authors did not report the frequency, the process or the method of assessing severity of treatment-related toxicity. This negatively affected the USPSTF domain of "valid measurement."

The results did not show any difference in the response rate of dyspnea in patients treated with EBRT plus brachytherapy versus EBRT alone (46 percent and 37 percent respectively). The median overall survival was similar across both groups; 7.0 (95% confidence interval (CI): 5.3 to 8.9) and 8.5 (95% CI: 5.4 to 11.6) months respectively. The authors assessed QOL scores (Dutch version of the EORTC Quality of Life Questionnaire (EORTC QLQ-C30) and lung cancer module QLQ-LC13) both before and after therapy with a 90 percent compliance rate, but the results were not reported in the paper. We were unable to find a citation in subsequent years. The proportion of patients with death due to hemoptysis was similar across the two treatment groups (15 percent and 13 percent in the EBRT plus brachytherapy versus EBRT alone group respectively).

Table 14. Comparative effect of brachytherapy plus EBRT versus EBRT alone on obstructive symptoms in the Langendijk trial[86]

Treatment Groups	Dyspnea	Cough	Hemoptysis	Others
EBRT + BT (% response)	18/39 (46%)	24%	86%	Chest pain: 80% Pain in arm/ shoulder: 74%
EBRT (% response)	16/43 (37%) (p=0.29)	38% (NS)	82%	Chest pain: 67% (NS) Pain in arm/ shoulder: 69%

BT = brachytherapy; EBRT = external beam radiotherapy; NS = nonsignificant

Table 15. USPSTF study quality ratings of the Langendijk trial[86]

Assembled CG	Maintained CG	Minimal LTFU	Measurements Equal, Valid, and Reliable	Interventions Clearly Defined	Important Outcomes Considered	Appropriate Analysis of Results	Overall USPSTF Rating
Yes	Yes	Yes	No	Yes	Yes	No	Poor

CG = comparable groups; LTFU = loss to followup; USPSTF = U.S. Preventive Services Task Force

Brachytherapy Versus EBRT

One controlled trial[87] randomly allocated 108 inoperable NSCLC patients with endobronchial tumors to two treatment arms: brachytherapy (n=49) or EBRT (n=50) (Table 16). Nine patients were excluded from the analysis. The primary aim of the trial was to evaluate symptom relief, treatment-related toxicities and impact on QOL. The strength of the trial was that it assessed treatment harms adequately at predefined periods using patient questionnaires but did not use standardized scoring criteria to rate severity of treatment-related toxicities. The trial was judged to have a poor quality on USPSTF rating for failing to appropriately take into account potential confounding—here fundamentally important for estimating an unbiased effect estimated owing to its time-dependent nature. Fifty-one percent in the brachytherapy arm received EBRT if the symptoms persisted or deteriorated or if the symptoms recurred. Similarly, 28 percent in the EBRT arm received brachytherapy. In the absence of taking into account this time-dependent confounding (a per-protocol analysis with appropriate censoring), it is impossible to judge the magnitude or even direction of potential bias. This fatal flaw negatively affected all three domains of USPSTF quality rating: "maintained comparable groups," "measurements valid" and "appropriate analysis of results" (Table 17) Further, lack of details about randomization and allocation concealment adversely affected the domain of "assembled comparable groups."

The response to treatment measured as positive symptom (improvement or no change in symptom severity from baseline to 4 and 8 weeks after treatment) by the physician was similar across two treatment arms. Though survival was not a planned endpoint, the EBRT treatment arm had a statistically significant higher survival than the brachytherapy arm (287 versus 250 days at 1 year, p=0.04). The authors did not report the treatment-related toxicities in detail except that they were similar across two treatment groups. Four (8 percent) and three (6 percent) patients died due to hemoptysis in the brachytherapy and EBRT group, respectively.

Table 16. Comparative effect of brachytherapy versus EBRT on obstructive symptoms in the Stout trial[87]

Treatment Groups	Time	Dyspnea	Hemoptysis	Breathlessness
BT (% of positive symptom endpoints)	4 weeks	59% (n=41)	85% (n=41)	78% (n=41)
	8 weeks	50% (n=46)	78% (n=46)	59% (n=46)
EBRT (% of positive symptom endpoints)	4 weeks	59% (n=29)	90% (n=29)	66% (n=29)
	8 weeks	67% (n=46)	89% (n=46)	78% (n=46)

BT = brachytherapy; EBRT = external beam radiotherapy; n = number
Note: There was not statistically significant difference between any treatment arms.

Table 17. USPSTF study quality ratings of the Stout trial[87]

Assembled CG	Maintained CG	Minimal LTFU	Measurements Equal, Valid, and Reliable	Interventions Clearly Defined	Important Outcomes Considered	Appropriate Analysis of Results	Overall USPSTF Rating
No	No	Yes	No	Yes	Yes	No	Poor

CG = comparable groups; LTFU = loss to followup; USPSTF = U.S. Preventive Services Task Force

EBRT Versus Endobronchial Treatments (Brachytherapy, Laser or Cryotherapy)

One RCT[102] randomly allocated patients to EBRT or endobronchial treatment (clinician choice of any one endobronchial treatment: brachytherapy, laser therapy or cryotherapy). This trial was designed to have a 90 percent power to detect a difference of 15 percent in the relief of breathlessness at 0.05 significance level with 400 patients randomized across four treatment arms. The trial[102] was discontinued before completion due to lack of patient accrual. The authors presented data for only 75 patients, of whom 16 patients did not receive the allocated treatment. As a result, the interpretation of available data for 59 patients distributed across four treatment arms poses significant limitations, namely small number per group and uncertainty about the preservation of randomization sequence. Further, the data for three different endobronchial treatment groups is reported cumulatively which does not allow comparison of treatment effects. Therefore, we did not report the data for this trial in this report. Details of this trial are provided in the abstraction tables in Appendix C.

Laser Plus Brachytherapy Versus Laser Alone

One RCT[88] compares combination treatment of laser plus brachytherapy versus laser therapy only (Table 18). This trial by Chella el al.,[88] randomized 29 patients across two treatment arms: laser plus brachytherapy (n=14) versus laser (n=15) alone. This small trial lacked details on randomization and allocation concealment. It did not report the NSCLC staging of patients, which is an important prognostic factor. These factors adversely affected the USPSTF domain of "assembled comparable groups." The authors did not report the frequency, the process or the method of assessing severity of treatment-related toxicity. This negatively affected the USPSTF domain of "measurements valid" (Table 19) We therefore rated this trial to have a poor USPSTF quality rating.

The reported median overall survival in the two treatment groups was not statistically significant different between the two treatment arms (10.3 months and 7.4 months respectively). Speiser's index (a semi-quantitative score in which a higher score indicates severe obstruction) was reduced by 4.2 and 3.4 points in the combined versus single treatment arms respectively. This reduction in score was not statistically different between the two arms. The authors also reported the pretreatment and post-treatment values of lung function tests but showed no statistically significant differences between the treatment arms. One patient died due to hemoptysis 12 months after treatment in the laser plus brachytherapy arm.

Table 18. Comparative effect of laser plus brachytherapy versus laser alone on obstructive symptoms in the Chella trial[88]

Treatment Groups	Speiser's Index
Laser + brachytherapy	Pre: 6.9 (±0.7) Post: 2.7 (±0.9)
Laser alone	Pre: 6.4 (±0.7) Post: 3.0 (±0.8)

N = total sample size of the trial

Table 19. USPSTF study quality ratings of the Chella trial[88]

Assembled CG	Maintained CG	Minimal LTFU	Measurements Equal, Valid, and Reliable	Interventions Clearly Defined	Important Outcomes Considered	Appropriate Analysis of Results	Overall USPSTF Rating
No	Yes	Yes	No	Yes	Yes	Yes	Poor

CG = comparable groups; LTFU = loss to followup; USPSTF = U.S. Preventive Services Task Force

Laser Versus Photodynamic Therapy

One controlled trial[89] randomized 31 NSCLC patients with airway obstruction to either PDT (n=14) versus laser therapy (n=17). The trial assessed treatment harms at predefined and regular periods and assessed causality but the authors did not report using standardized criteria to assess the severity of treatment-related toxicities. This small trial lacked details on randomization and allocation concealment. At the baseline, the proportion of patients with stage III–IV cancer in the PDT group and laser group was 57% (8 of 14) and 88% (15 of 17) respectively. The authors did not explain the imbalance in tumor stage distribution even though it was a randomized trial.

Further, the authors did not report whether they adjusted for the baseline differences in the outcomes. This negatively affected the USPSTF domain of "assembled comparable groups" and was considered a fatal flaw in the USPSTF quality rating (Table 20). We therefore judged this trial to have a poor USPSTF quality rating.

Median survival was reported to be longer in the PDT versus laser group (265 versus 95 days, p=0.007). Though quantitative symptom relief was not reported, the authors described amelioration of symptoms to be similar in both treatment groups. Two patients (one in each group) died from hemoptysis, and there was one probable death due to treatment in the PDT-treated group.

Table 20. USPSTF study quality ratings of the Jimenez trial[89]

Assembled CG	Maintained CG	Minimal LTFU	Measurements Equal, Valid, and Reliable	Interventions Clearly Defined	Important Outcomes Considered	Appropriate Analysis of Results	Overall USPSTF Rating
No	Yes	Yes	Yes	Yes	Yes	No	Poor

CG = comparable groups; LTFU = loss to followup; USPSTF = U.S. Preventive Services Task Force

Laser Versus Electrocautery

One nonrandomized retrospective study[90] conducted with 29 patients compared the effects of treatment with laser (n=14) versus electrocautery (n=17) on dyspnea relief in NSCLC patients with tracheobronchial obstruction due to an endobronchial tumor. The study was judged to have poor quality on USPSTF quality rating because of lack of adjustment for any potential confounders given that it was a nonrandomized retrospective study with imbalanced distribution of prognostic factors at the baseline. A disproportionate number of patients had received previous treatment in the laser treated group (93 percent) as compared with the electrocautery group (53 percent). Further, the mean time from diagnosis to study treatment was different in the two groups (4.7 versus 7.5 months in laser versus electrocautery group). These factors negatively affected the USPSTF domain of "assembled comparable groups" (Table 21).

The reported mean survival and percent improvement of symptoms was similar in both groups. The mean survival was 8.0±2.5 and 11.5±3.5 months in the laser and electrocautery treated groups respectively. The proportion of patients with symptom improvement (rated on a dichotomous scale by the treating clinician) was 10 (71 percent) and 13 (76 percent) in the laser and electrocautery treated groups respectively.

Table 21. USPSTF study quality ratings of the Boxem study[90]

Assembled CG	Maintained CG	Minimal LTFU	Measurements Equal, Valid, and Reliable	Interventions Clearly Defined	Important Outcomes Considered	Appropriate Analysis of Results	Overall USPSTF Rating
No	Unclear	Yes	No	Yes	Yes	No	Poor

CG = comparable groups; LTFU = loss to followup; USPSTF = U.S. Preventive Services Task Force

Study Characteristics of Noncomparative Studies

A total of 11 studies[91-101] included 858 patients given eight distinct treatment modalities (three single intervention: brachytherapy, PDT, RFA; five multiple interventions: brachytherapy plus EBRT, brachytherapy plus PDT plus chemotherapy, EBRT plus chemotherapy, stenting plus brachytherapy and stenting plus laser therapy). Data were abstracted from a single arm of three otherwise comparative studies.[91,93,96] In the latter, the comparator arms were not considered relevant and not abstracted, for reasons summarized in the section, "Description of Noncomparative Studies" below. Three studies (27 percent) originated in the United States, seven were from Europe (64 percent), and one (9 percent) was from former Yugoslavia. An overview of the noncomparative studies is given in Table 22.

Table 22. Overview of noncomparative studies of local nonsurgical endobronchial therapies

Treatment	Author, Year	Time	N	OS	DSS	LCT	SC	QOL	TOX
BT	Celebioglu-2002, Turkey[94]	R	95				•		•
BT	Guilcher-2011, France[95]	R	226	•	•	•			•
BT	Petera-2001, Czech Republic[96]	NR	41	•			•		
PDT	Jones-2001, USA[97]	R	10	•					
RFA	Lencioni-2008, Multiple Countries[91]	P	33	•	•			•	•
BT + EBRT	Muto-2000, Italy[98]	P	320	•			•		
BT + EBRT	Vucicevic-1999, Yugoslavia[99]	R	39	•			•		•
BT + STNT	Allison-2004, USA[92]	P	10	•		•		•	
LASR + STNT	Chhajed-2006, Switzerland[93]	R	52						•
EBRT + CHEM	Celikoglu-2006, Turkey[100]	P	23				•		
BT + CHEM + PDT	Weinberg-2010, USA[101]	NR	9	•					•

DSS = disease specific survival; LCT = local control; N = total sample size of the study; NSCLC = non–small-cell lung cancer; OS = overall survival; QOL = quality of life; RCT = randomized controlled trial; SAS = single-arm study; SC = symptom control; TOX = toxicity

Key Points

- Of the total 11 noncomparative studies that addressed Key Question 3, we focused on three studies that cover two unique interventions (RFA and debridement and stenting) for which comparative data was not available.
- These three noncomparative studies included 95 patients, two studies were prospective[91,92] and one was retrospective.[93]
- All three non-comparative studies were of poor quality according to Carey and Boden quality ratings.
- The evidence comprises of overall survival reported by all three studies, lung function tests and QOL by one study[91], performance status by one study[92] and treatment-related toxicities by two studies.[91,93]

Description of Noncomparative Studies

We do not present detailed study data (study characteristics and outcomes) of eight[94-100] noncomparative studies that utilize interventions for which comparative studies exists. These interventions include brachytherapy, EBRT, laser, electrocautery and PDT. Instead, we focused on three noncomparative studies[91-93] that cover two unique interventions (RFA and debridement and stenting) for which comparative data was not available. Table 23 provides a summary of patient characteristics of three single-arm studies that covers RFA and debridement and stenting. It includes two studies on combination treatment with stenting and one study on RFA.

Among these three noncomparative studies, two were prospective[91,92] and one was retrospective.[93] Ninety-five patients were included in these three studies. The Lencioni and Chhajed studies included patients which were not relevant to Key Question 3. The Lencioni study included 73 patients with non-NSCLC malignancy; the Chhajed study included 92 NSCLC patients that did not have endobronchial obstruction and received chemotherapy. The data presented in this report for these two studies exclude data of such non-relevant patient population. All but one study[93] included patients with a histologically non-confirmed NSCLC. One study[92] included only recurrent patients, one study[91] included recurrent and stage I patient, and the third study[93] did not report on tumor stage of patients. None of the three studies reported the criteria used for staging NSCLC. The duration of the study enrollment period was reported by only one study.[91] One study[92] was conducted in an outpatient setting; the remaining two studies[91,93] did not describe the study setting. Two[92,93] were single-center studies, the third[91] was a multicenter study. All three studies[91-93] stated no conflict of interest. Two studies[92,93] did not state the source of funding, the remaining study[91] was manufacturer sponsored. All three noncomparative studies were rated as poor quality. All three studies reported data on survival data. The Lencioni study[91] reported 1 and 2-year survival rates; Chhajed[93] reported 3, 9, and 12-month survival rates and median survival. However, of the 52 patients assessed in the Chhajed study, 13 each received laser and stenting alone respectively and remaining 26 patients received both laser and stenting. However, the authors did not present data of patients stratified by the treatment they received. This severely limited meaningful interpretation of the data. Mean survival for 10 patients included in the Allison study[92] was not reported in the published paper but calculated for this report. Among the miscellaneous outcomes related to symptom relief and quality of life, the Lencioni study[91] reported results of lung function tests and QOL and the Allison study [92] reported results on performance status. The detailed outcomes related to survival, symptom improvement and quality of life are presented in Table 24.

Table 23. Study characteristics of noncomparative studies that address Key Question 3

Treatment	Author, Year, Country	Design (Quality)[42]	N	Intervention Details	100% Histopathology Confirmation (% Not Confirmed)	Age, Years[a]	% Female
RFA	Lencioni-2008, Multiple Countries[91]	Prospective (Poor)	33	Ablation protocol to destroy visible tumor mass plus 0.5 cm safety of margin	Yes	67 (29-82)	24%
BT + STNT	Allison-2004, USA[92]	Prospective (Poor)	10	18Gy 3frs	Yes	66.5 (52-77)	20%
LASR + STNT	Chhajed-2006, Switzerland[93]	Retrospective (Poor)	52	Laser ablation through a rigid bronchoscope, stenting when significant airway obstruction (>50%)	No (17%)	61[b]	27%

BT = brachytherapy; frs = fractions; Gy = gray; N = total sample size of the study; RFA = radiofrequency ablation; STNT = stenting; LASR = laser
[a]Values are median (range) unless specified.
[b]Mean.

Table 24. Survival and local control outcomes for noncomparative studies that address Key Question 3

Intervention	Author, Year	Reported Overall Survival Rates (Number of Patients)	Reported Cancer-Specific Survival Rates (Number of Patients)	Miscellanous Outcomes
RFA	Lencioni-2008 (n=33)[91]	1 yr: 70% (95% CI: 51 to 83) 2 yr: 48% (95% CI: 30 to 65)	1 yr: 92% (95% CI: 78–98) 2 yr: 73% (95% CI: 54–86)	Lung function: (n=22) FEV, L 0 months: 1·9 (±0·9) 12 months: 1·5 (±0·7) FACT-G 0 months: 80·5 (±11·2) 12 months: 82·2 (±11·1)
BT + STNT	Allison-2004 (n=10)[92]	10.3 months (±4.1) (calculated)	NA	Baseline KPS: 45 (±7.1) Post Rx KPS: 77 (±9.5)
LASR + STNT	Chhajed-2006 (n=52)[93]	Median survival : 8.4 months (4.8-17.1) 3-months survival: 90% 6-months survival: 71% 12-months survival: 40%	NA	NR

BT = brachytherapy; CI = confidence interval; FACT-G = Functional Assessment of Cancer Therapy- General; FEV = forced expiratory volume; frs = fractions; Gy = gray; KPS = Karnofsky performance status; L = liter; LASR = laser; N = total sample size of the study; NR = not reported; RFA = radiofrequency ablation; Rx = treatment; STNT = stenting

Intervention-Associated Adverse Events

As per Agency for Healthcare Research and Quality (AHRQ) guidance on comparing harms about medical interventions,[103] data about harms from observational studies should always be assessed. This is because quantity and quality of harms reporting in clinical trials is frequently inadequate and hypotheses are usually designed to evaluate benefits than harms. Further, clinical trials usually are not large enough to capture rare adverse events nor are they long enough to capture late adverse events. Moreover, clinical trials tend to include homogenous and healthier subjects who are less likely to have AEs than the general population.[103] Therefore, we report the treatment-related toxicities data from all 11 noncomparative studies. These data are compiled in Table 25. In the largest prospective study[98] of 320 patients who were treated with a combination of brachytherapy and EBRT, radiation bronchitis was the most common treatment-related toxictiy observed. The incidence of grade 2, 3 and 4 radiation bronchitis was 7, 10 and 8 percent respectively. In the second largest single arm study by Guilcher,[95] 226 patients with endobronchial NSCLC treated with brachytherapy alone were analysed retrospectively. The incidence of radiation bronchitis was 12 percent. Six percent (n=13) of patients died due to complication (10 hemoptysis, 2 of necrosis and 1 of radiation stenosis). The authors of the study did not specify if these were treatment-related complications or not. There was only one study[91] that reported incidence of pneumothorax with use of RFA. Pneumothorax occurred in 13 percent of patients included in the study. The incidence of hemoptysis in more than 2 percent of study subjects was observed in four studies[93,95,98,99] and ranged from 2 to 7 percent. The toxicity reporting criteria for each study (when provided by the authors) are shown in Appendix C.

Table 25. Treatment-related toxicities in noncomparative studies that address Key Question 3

Treatment	Author, Year	Hemoptysis	Pneumothorax	Radiation Bronchitis	Death	Others
BT	Muto-2000 (N=320)[98]	10 (4%)	-	Grade 2: 20 (7%) Grade 3: 28 (10%) Grade 4: 23 (8%)	-	Bronchoesophageal fistulas: 3 (1%)
BT	Celebioglu-2002 (N=95)[94]		0	-		Fistula: 0 Cardiovascular problems: 0
BT	Guilcher-2011 (N=226)[95]	15 (7%)	3 (1%)	Grade II: 28 (12%)	Death due to complication: 13 (6%)	Bronchial stenosis: 21 (9%) Necrosis of bronchial wall: 7 (3%) Grade 2 mucitis: 9 (4%)
RFA	Lencioni-2008 (N=33)[91]	-	5 (13%)[a]	-	-	
BT + EBRT	Vucicevic-1999 (N=39)[99]	1/30 (3%)	-	-	-	Esophagitis: 3/39 (8%) Cardiac arrhythmia: 1/39 (3%) Pulmonary fibrosis: 4/39 (10%) Esophageal stricture: 1/39 (3%) Fistulae: 1/39 (3%)
STNT + LASR	Chhajed-2006 (N=52)[93]	1 (2%)	-	-	Death within 24 h of the procedure: 1 (2%)	Stent migration: 3 (6%) Mucous plugging of the airway stent: 2 (4%)
BT + CHEM + PDT	Weinberg-2010 (N=9)[101]	-	-	-	-	Bronchial contraction: 5/9 (56%) Occlusion from bronchial contraction: 2/9 (22%) Photosensitivity: 2/9 (22%)

BT = brachytherapy; CHEM = chemotherapy; EBRT = external beam radiotherapy; HDR = high-dose rate; N = total sample size of the study; NR = not reported; NRC = nonrandomized comparative study; PDT = photodynamic therapy; RFA = radiofrequency ablation; STNT = stenting

[a]This is procedure level and not patient data. Forty procedures were done in 33 patients and 5 procedures were associated with pneumothorax.

Risk of Bias for Noncomparative Studies Addressing Key Question 3

We used the convention described by Carey and Boden[42] to assess the risk of bias of individual noncomparative studies included to address Key Question 3 (see Methods chapter). We rated the quality of only three noncomparative studies that utilize interventions for which no comparative data was available. Our ratings of good, fair and poor are shown in Table 26. Studies that met 8 of 8 criteria were classified as good, studies that met 7 of 8 criteria were classified as fair and studies that met fewer than 7 criteria were classified as poor.

The reasons for not fullfilling Carey and Boden crietria were as follows: the Chhajed study[93] did not clearly define a research question, did not well describe the study population or the intervention used in the study nor did they describe the results well. One study[91] did not use valdiated outcome measure, two studies[91,92] did not use appropriate statistical analysis, discussion and conclusion was not supported by data for two studies[91,93] and two studies[92,93] did not describe their funding source.

Table 26. Carey and Boden quality rating summary

Key Question (Number of Studies)	Good (8 of 8 "Yes")	Fair (7 of 8 "Yes")	Poor (< 7 of 8 "Yes")
Key Question 3 (3)	0	0	3
Total	0	0	3 (100%)

Discussion

Overview

This chapter presents a discussion of the results of the comparative effectiveness review (CER) organized as follows:

- Key Findings
- Strength of Evidence (SOE)
- Relationship of the Findings to Existing Information
- Applicability of the Findings
- Implications for Clinical and Policy Decisionmaking
- Limitations of the CER Process
- Limitations of the Evidence Base
- Research Gaps and Conclusions
- In each of the above-mentioned sections, the results are organized by Key Questions 1, 2, and 3.

Key Findings

Key Question 1: Local Nonsurgical Interventions in Medically Inoperable Patients With Stage I Non–Small-Cell Lung Cancer (NSCLC)

- Thirty-five single-arm studies reported clinical benefits and harms associated with the use of three-dimensional radiotherapy (3DRT), proton beam radiotherapy (PBRT), radiofrequency ablation (RFA) and stereotactic body radiotherapy (SBRT) to treat patients with stage I NSCLC who were deemed to be medically inoperable. Clinical benefits included post-treatment overall survival, cancer-specific survival and local control rates. Harms were radiation-induced for 3DRT, PBRT and SBRT and procedural complications for RFA.
- No studies directly compared the relative benefits or harms of the interventions of interest in inoperable stage I NSCLC patients.
- The evidence is insufficient to answer Key Question 1.

Key Question 2: Local Nonsurgical Interventions in Medically Operable Patients With Stage I NSCLC

- Six single-arm studies reported clinical benefits and harms associated with the use of PBRT and SBRT to treat patients with stage I NSCLC who were deemed to be medically operable. Clinical benefits included post-treatment overal survival, cancer-specific survival and local control rates. Harms were radiation-induced for PBRT and SBRT.
- No studies directly compared the relative benefits or harms of the interventions of interest in medically operable stage I NSCLC patients.
- The evidence is insufficient to answer Key Question 2.

Key Question 3: Local Nonsurgical Interventions for Inoperable Patients With NSCLC and Symptoms Due to an Endoluminal Lesion

- Six comparative studies reported clinical benefits and harms associated with the use of local nonsurgical therapies (external-beam radiotherapy (EBRT), brachytherapy, laser therapy, photodynamic therapy (PDT) and electrocautery) for palliation in symptomatic inoperable patients with obstructive endoluminal NSCLC. Reported clinical benefits included post-treatment symptom relief and overall survival. Harms were hemoptysis, pneumothorax, radiation bronchitis, bronchoesophageal fistulas and photosensitivity.
- One comparative study was available per treatment comparison. All six comparative studies were of poor quality and therefore the evidence from these studies had a high risk of bias, consistency was unknown, evidence was direct and all were imprecise.
- Evidence from three single-arm studies of debridement and stenting is insufficient to draw conclusions about the effectiveness of those interventions.
- The evidence is insufficient to answer Key Question 3.

Strength of Evidence

To evaluate the SOE, we used an approach that was specfically developed for the Evidence-based Practice Center program and referenced in the Methods Guide.[37] This approach is based on a system developed by the Grading of Recommendations Assessment, Development and Evaluation (GRADE) Working Group.[43] This system explicitly addresses four required domains: risk of bias, consistency, directness, and precision, as outlined in the Methods section.

Key Question 1

As shown in Table 27 below, the overall SOE is insufficient to form conclusions about the comparative beneficial effects or toxicities of 3DRT, PBRT, RFA or SBRT in the treatment of stage I NSCLC in medically inoperable patients. Direct outcomes of interest were overall survival, cancer-specific survival, and toxicities.

Thirty-five single-arm studies were available. The risk of bias among the studies was inherently high. The consistency of effect size direction cannot be determined in the absence of comparative studies, so this domain was deemed unknown. No direct comparative evidence is available among interventions, so this domain was deemed indirect. Because precision cannot be determined in the absence of direct comparative evidence among interventions, we deemed the evidence to be imprecise.

Table 27. Strength of evidence for local nonsurgical interventions in medically inoperable stage I NSCLC patients

Treatment and Evidence Base	Risk of Bias	Consistency	Directness	Precision	Overall Strength of Evidence
SBRT (22 single-arm studies,[17,48,49,53,56-75] total n=1665 patients)	High	Unknown	Indirect	Imprecise	Insufficient
3DRT (7 single-arm studies,[50,51,54,55,75-77] total n=240 patients)	High	Unknown	Indirect	Imprecise	Insufficient
PBRT (3 single-arm studies,[47,52,79] total n=144 patients)	High	Unknown	Indirect	Imprecise	Insufficient
RFA (1 single-arm study,[80] n=19 patients)	High	Unknown	Indirect	Imprecise	Insufficient

3DRT = three dimensional radiotherapy; n = number; NSCLC = non–small-cell lung cancer; PBRT = proton beam radiotherapy; RFA = radiofrequency ablation; SBRT = stereotactic body radiotherapy

Key Question 2

As shown in Table 28, the overall SOE is insufficient to form conclusions about the comparative benefical effects or toxicities of PBRT or SBRT in the treatment of stage I NSCLC in medically operable patients. Direct outcomes of interest were overall survival, cancer-specific survival, and toxicities.

Six single-arm studies were available. The risk of bias among the studies was inherently high. The consistency of effect size direction cannot be determined in the absence of comparative studies, so this domain was deemed unknown. No direct comparative evidence is available among interventions, so this domain was deemed indirect. Because precision cannot be determined in the absence of direct comparative evidence among interventions, we deemed the evidence to be imprecise.

Table 28. Strength of evidence for local nonsurgical interventions in medically operable stage I NSCLC patients

Treatment and Evidence Base	Risk of Bias	Consistency	Directness	Precision	Overall Strength of Evidence
SBRT (5 single-arm studies,[48,49,81-83] total n=378)	High	Unknown	Indirect	Imprecise	Insufficient
PBRT (1 single-arm study,[47] total n=28)	High	Unknown	Indirect	Imprecise	Insufficient

n = number; NSCLC = non–small-cell lung cancer; PBRT = proton beam radiotherapy; SBRT = stereotactic body radiotherapy

Key Question 3

Overall, evidence from five randomized controlled trials (RCTs) and one nonrandomized comparative study is insufficient to form conclusions about the benefits (symptom relief, survival) and harms (treatment-related toxicities) of local nonsurgical therapies (brachytherapy plus EBRT versus brachytherapy alone; brachytherapy plus EBRT versus EBRT alone; brachytherapy versus EBRT; laser plus brachytherapy versus laser alone; laser versus electrocautery or PDT) in symptomatic inoperable patients with obstructive endoluminal NSCLC.

47

Evidence from three single-arm studies of debridement and stenting is insufficient to draw conclusions about the effectiveness of those interventions.

Strength of Evidence

Brachytherapy Plus EBRT Versus Brachytherapy Alone

The evidence for comparison of brachytherapy plus EBRT versus brachytherapy alone comprised of one small RCT[85] (n=45, 15 patients per treatment arm). This trial was considered to have a high risk of bias because it failed to provide details of randomization and allocation concealment. The consistency of the evidence was unknown as it was a single RCT without confirmation from any other study. The outcomes measured in the study – symptom relief, quality of life (QOL) and treatment-related toxicities were all direct. The evidence for symptom relief, QOL and treatment-related toxicities was imprecise.

Because the evidence base that addressed these outcomes consisted of one RCT, the starting level of SOE was high (Table 29). SOE was reduced by one level each based on the high risk of bias, unknown consistency and imprecision. Therefore, compared to brachytherapy alone, the SOE that brachytherapy plus EBRT improves symptom relief, QOL and reduces treatment-related toxicities is insufficient.

Brachytherapy Plus EBRT Versus EBRT Alone

The evidence for comparison of brachytherapy plus EBRT versus EBRT alone comprised of one small RCT[86] (n=95). This trial was considered to have a high risk of bias primarily because the trial was discontinued prematurely due to lack of patient accrual and was underpowered to detect a difference in the rate of primary endpoint (rate of dyspnea). The consistency of the evidence was unknown as it was a single RCT without confirmation from any other study. The outcomes measured in the study – symptom relief, survival and treatment-related toxicities were all direct. The evidence for symptom relief, survival and treatment-related toxicities was imprecise.

Because the evidence base that addressed these outcomes consisted of one RCT, the starting level of SOE was high. SOE was reduced by one level each based on the high risk of bias, unknown consistency and imprecision. Therefore, compared to EBRT alone, the SOE that brachytherapy plus EBRT improves symptom relief, survival and reduces treatment-related toxicities is insufficient.

Brachytherapy Versus EBRT

The evidence for comparison of brachytherapy versus EBRT comprised of one small RCT[87] (n=99). This trial was considered to have a very serious risk of bias because the study failed to adjust for potential confounding secondary to crossover of a large proportion of patients between treatment arms during the trial period. The consistency of the evidence was unknown as it was a single RCT without confirmation from any other study. The outcomes measured in the study – symptom relief, survival and treatment-related toxicities were all direct. The evidence for symptom relief and treatment-related toxicities was imprecise while the evidence for survival was precise.

Because the evidence base that addressed these outcomes consisted of one RCT, the starting level of SOE was high. SOE was reduced by two levels based on very serious risk of bias, by one level for unknown consistency and by one level for imprecision (only for symptom relief and treatment toxicity). Therefore, compared to EBRT, the SOE that brachytherapy improves symptom relief, survival and reduces treatment-related toxicities is insufficient.

Laser Plus Brachytherapy Versus Laser Alone

The evidence for comparison of laser plus brachytherapy versus laser alone comprised of one small RCT[88] (n=29). This trial was considered to have a high risk of bias primarily due to failure to provide details of randomization, allocation concealment and NSCLC staging of patients at the baseline. The consistency of the evidence was unknown as it was a single RCT without confirmation from any other study. The outcomes measured in the study—symptom relief, survival and treatment-related toxicities—were all direct. The evidence for symptom relief, survival and treatment-related toxicities was imprecise.

Because the evidence base that addressed these outcomes consisted of one RCT, the starting level of SOE was high. SOE was reduced by one level each based on the high risk of bias, unknown consistency and imprecision. Therefore, compared to laser alone, the SOE that laser plus brachytherapy improves symptom relief, survival and reduces treatment-related toxicities is insufficient.

Laser Versus Photodynamic Therapy

The evidence for comparison of laser versus PDT comprised of one small RCT[89] (n=31). This trial was considered to have a serious risk of bias primarily because the treatment arms had imbalances at the baseline. The proportion of patients with stage III–IV cancer was much smaller in the PDT group (57%, 8 of 14) than the laser group (88%, 15 of 17) at the baseline. The consistency of the evidence was unknown as it was a single RCT without confirmation from any other study. The outcomes measured in the study –survival and treatment-related toxicities were all direct. The evidence for treatment-related toxicities was imprecise while it was precise for survival.

Because the evidence base that addressed these outcomes consisted of one RCT, the starting level of SOE was high. SOE was reduced by two levels based on very serious risk of bias, by one level for unknown consistency and by one level for imprecision (only for treatment-related toxicity). Therefore, compared to PDT, the SOE that laser therapy improves survival and reduces treatment-related toxicities is insufficient.

Laser Versus Electrocautery

The evidence for comparison of laser versus electrocautery comprised of one small nonrandomized comparative study[90] (n=29). This study was considered to have serious risk of bias primarily because of lack of adjustment for any potential confounders. A disproportionate number of patients had received previous treatment in the laser treated group (93 percent) as compared with the electrocautery group (53 percent). Further, the mean time from diagnosis to study treatment was different in the two groups (4.7 versus 7.5 months in laser versus electrocautery group). The consistency of the evidence was unknown as it was a single nonrandomized comparative study without confirmation from any other study. The outcomes measured in the study –survival and symptom relief were direct. The evidence for symptom relief and survival was imprecise.

Because the evidence base that addressed these outcomes consisted of one nonrandomized comparative study, the starting level of SOE was low (Table 30). SOE was reduced by two levels based on very serious risk of bias and by one level each for unknown consistency and imprecision. Therefore, compared to electrocautery, the SOE that laser therapy improves survival and symptom relief is insufficient.

Table 29. Strength of comparative evidence for local nonsurgical therapies for symptoms secondary to an inoperable obstructive endoluminal NSCLC

Treatment and Evidence Base	Outcome	Unit of Measure	Risk of Bias	Consistency	Directness	Precision	SOE
Brachytherapy plus EBRT versus brachytherapy alone (1 RCT, n=45)[85]	Symptom relief	Incidence and response rate	High	Unknown	Yes	Imprecise	Insufficient
	QOL	EORTC QLQ-C30 & LC 13 V3.0					
	Treatment toxicity	Incidence of Grade ≥II RTOG morbidity scoring scriteria					
Brachytherapy plus EBRT versus EBRT alone (1 RCT, n=95)[86]	Symptom relief	Response rate	High	Unknown	Yes	Imprecise	Insufficient
	Survival	Overall survival					
	Treatment toxicity	Incidence					
Brachytherapy versus EBRT (1 RCT, n=99)[87]	Symptom relief	% improvement	High	Unknown	Yes	Imprecise	Insufficient
	Survival	Overall survival	High	Unknown	Yes	Precise	Insufficient
	Treatment toxicity	Incidence	High	Unknown	Yes	Imprecise	Insufficient
Nd-YAG plus Brachytherapy versus Nd-YAG alone (1 RCT, n=29)[88]	Symptom relief	Speiser's index	High	Unknown	Yes	Imprecise	Insufficient
	Survival	Overall survival					
	Treatment toxicity	Incidence					
Photodynamic Therapy versus Laser (1 RCT, n= 31)[89]	Survival	Overall survival	High	Unknown	Yes	Precise	Insufficient
	Treatment toxicity	Incidence	High	Unknown	Yes	Imprecise	Insufficient
Nd-YAG versus Electrocautery (1 NRC, n=29)[90]	Survival	Mean survival	High	Unknown	Yes	Imprecise	Insufficient
	Symptom relief	% response					

BT = brachytherapy; EBRT = external beam radiotherapy; EORTC QLQ = European Organization for Research and Treatment of Cancer Quality of Life Questionnaire; KQ = Key Question; n = number; N = total sample size of the study; Nd-YAG = neodymium-doped yttrium aluminum garnet; NSCLC = non–small-cell lung cancer; NRC = nonrandomized comparative study; QOL = quality of life; RCT = randomized controlled trial; RTOG = Radiation Therapy Oncology Group; SOE = strength of evidence

Table 30. Strength of noncomparative evidence for local nonsurgical therapies for symptoms secondary to an inoperable obstructive endoluminal NSCLC

Treatment and Evidence Base	Risk of Bias	Consistency	Directness	Precision	Overall Strength of Evidence
RFA (1 study, n=33)[91]	High	Unknown	Indirect	Imprecise	Insufficient
BT + STNT (1 study, n=10)[92]	High	Unknown	Indirect	Imprecise	Insufficient
LASR + STNT (1 study, n=52)[93]	High	Unknown	Indirect	Imprecise	Insufficient

BT = brachytherapy; LASR = laser; n = total sample size of the study; NSCLC = non–small-cell lung cancer; RFA = radiofrequency ablation; STNT = stenting

Relationship of the Findings to Existing Information

Key Questions 1 and 2

We sought credible sources of evidence-based information on the use of the local nonsurgical interventions assessed in this CER to treat stage I NSCLC. We identified a recent systematic review that examined the effectiveness of SBRT among patients with severe chronic obstructive pulmonary disease.[17] The authors of that review reported limited, noncomparative published data are available to assess outcomes in this setting. An Agency for Healthcare Research and Quality (AHRQ) Technical Brief reported on the state of the evidence for SBRT in a number of cancers, including NSCLC.[104] The authors of this Technical Brief did not identify any published RCTs or other comparative studies that compared SBRT to another modality. Our systematic literature search and review did not reveal any relevant evidence-based guidelines we could compare to our findings. Our report offers the first comprehensive systematic review on this topic.

Key Question 3

This systematic review sought RCTs that compared local nonsurgical bronchoscopic interventions in patients with an endobronchial NSCLC. We found five RCTs of poor quality and one nonrandomized comparative study that compared six unique combinations of bronchoscopic interventions in NSCLC patients. Evidence is insufficient to conclude relative benefits and harms of one therapy over another for the following six interventions:

- Brachytherapy plus EBRT versus brachytherapy alone
- Brachytherapy plus EBRT versus EBRT alone
- Brachytherapy versus EBRT
- Laser plus brachytherapy versus laser alone
- Laser versus electrocautery
- Laser versus PDT

Evidence from three single-arm studies of debridement and stenting is insufficient to draw conclusions about the effectiveness of those interventions.

We found one Cochrane systematic review[34] that compares endobronchial brachytherapy with palliative intent for NSCLC patients with other available treatments including EBRT, other bronchoscopic interventions, chemotherapy or best supportive care. The Cochrane review included only RCTs with only metastatic or advanced (stage IIIb and IV) NSCLC patients. The strength of this review is its broader scope as it included all NSCLC stages patients including recurrent patients. Further, we addressed all possible combination of local nonsurgical bronchoscopic therapies and all possible study designs except for case reports. However, unlike the Cochrane review, the present review excluded all studies published prior to 1995 and did not include data from studies that were published as abstracts only.

In concurrence with our findings, the Cochrane review also agreed that the evidence did not provide conclusive results that endobronchial brachytherapy plus EBRT improved symptom relief compared with EBRT alone or there was any conclusive evidence to recommend endobronchial brachytherapy in combination with EBRT, chemotherapy or laser therapy.

The second edition of American College of Chest Physicians (ACCP) Evidence Based Clinical Practice Guidelines[105] for palliative care of lung cancer patients relevant in part to the current context of local nonsurgical bronchoscopic interventions for endoluminal obstruction in NSCLC patients. These guidelines describe the general landscape of palliative bronchoscopic therapies including mechanical debridement, laser, argon plasma coagulation, brachytherapy, cryotherapy, balloon dilatation, PDT, electrocautery and stenting. The ACCP guidelines[105] state that all such interventions provide significant relief from dyspnea and hemoptysis in majority of patients but do not discuss comparative effectiveness (harms and benefits) of these therapies. The guideline recommends treatment with appropriate therapies (Grade 1C) for all lung cancer patients who complain of dyspnea with a potentially correctable cause. These guidelines also state that in all lung cancer patients with large volume hemoptysis, bronchoscopic evaluation of source of bleeding followed by endobronchial management options such as argon plasma coagulation, laser and electrocautery is recommended (Grade 1C).

Applicability of the Findings

Key Questions 1 and 2

In general, applicability assessment would depend on a body of evidence sufficient to permit conclusions about the comparative outcomes of local nonsurgical therapies for stage I NSCLC. The evidence for Key Questions 1 and 2 does not reach that level, so we have primarily limited comments to relevance of the PICOTS (Population, Intervention, Comparator, Outcomes, Timing, Setting) elements.[46] The PICOTS format comprises a practical and useful structure to review applicability in a systematic manner. These factors are summarized in Table 31 for Key Questions 1 and 2.

The degree to which the data presented in this report are applicable to clinical practice is a function of the similarity between populations in the included studies and the patient population that receives clinical care in diverse settings. It also is related to the relative availability of the interventions. The literature base is observational, lacking comparative evidence. Case series are descriptive studies that are limited in their ability to control for biases. Selection bias is of particular concern as patients receive treatment based on clinician preferences, center resources, patient characteristics and preference rather than random allocation. This evidence base is therefore insufficient to support any attempt to draw comparative conclusions.

Table 31. Summary of applicability of evidence for Key Questions 1 and 2

Domain	Applicability of Evidence
Populations	• Overall, the patients included in the single-arm studies were not suitable for surgery, or were suitable for surgery but declined it. • The patients with stage I NSCLC in the studies included in this report appear representative of cases that would be considered for a local nonsurgical intervention. • Patients typically were in their late 60s to mid-70s, congruent with the incidence of stage I NSCLC that tends to rise with age. • The medically inoperable patients of KQ1 had compromised cardiopulmonary reserves or other comorbidities that preclude surgical resection. • The medically operable patients of KQ2 were often not substantially different from the inoperable population of KQ1, but neither are considered as healthy as the population that undergoes surgery.
Interventions	• 3DRT, IMRT and SBRT represent different technological approaches to the delivery of conformal photon radiotherapy. The major advantage of these interventions as compared to traditional wide-field 2DRT is the ability to deliver tightly focused cytotoxic radiation by delineating the shape and size of the tumor using a CT-based or other imaging planning system. • 3DRT represents a minimum technical standard for delivery of conformal radiotherapy. It involves static fields with a fixed shape, modified by compensators (wedges and segments). 3DRT is widely available. • IMRT offers beam strength attenuation through a multileaf collimator (tungsten), with dynamic field shapes for each beam angle. IMRT is not as widely available as 3DRT, and requires a higher level of inverse planning and quality assurance. • SBRT is a hypofractionated technique administered in 5 or fewer fractions; 3DRT and IMRT typically deliver radiation in many more fractions than SBRT. • SBRT is not as widely available as 3DRT or IMRT but its use is growing. It may soon supplant other technologies in the KQ1 and KQ2 settings. The institutional programmatic requirements for SBRT are similar to those of IMRT. • This CER did not allow for a rigorous and systematic comparison of the relative performance of local nonsurgical therapies stratified by technological factors. The impact of these factors factors on health outcomes remains unclear. • The applicability of the evidence for PBRT and RFA is unknown due to limited evidence.
Comparators	• See above for Intervention
Outcomes	• The major health outcomes in this CER are OS, CSS, and LCT, typically reported over a period of one to five years. • OS is the primary direct outcome for any cancer intervention study. • CSS reflects the absolute effect of a cancer intervention on the disease. CSS is a highly relevant direct outcome in the KQ1 practice setting in that such patients are generally fragile and susceptible to succumbing to underlying comorbidities. Its relevance in KQ2 patients may be slightly less than in KQ1 as the former may be relatively healthier than the latter, but still not as healthy as good surgical candidates. • LCT is of interest to patients because it measures the effectiveness of an intervention in disease control. Upon local failure, patients enter into a new category centered on systemic chemotherapy. This is a potentially perilous position for the medically frail patients considered in KQ1, and perhaps many of those in KQ2.
Timing	• The relevant periods occur at the time of treatment through followup over months (palliation) or years (overall survival).
Setting	• The evidence for KQ1 and KQ2 is international, primarily obtained in tertiary institutional settings. More sophisticated interventions such as IMRT and SBRT require an institutional commitment to quality assurance and on-going training that may be difficult to achieve in smaller community-based centers. • We did not collect or analyze information to examine these issues.

2DRT = two-dimensional radiotherapy; 3DRT = three-dimensional radiotherapy; CER = comparative effectiveness review; CSS = cancer-specific survival; CT = computer tomography; IMRT = intensity-modulated radiotherapy; KQ = Key Question; n = number; LCT = local control; NSCLC = non–small-cell lung cancer; OS = overall survival; PBRT = proton beam radiotherapy; RFA = radiofrequency ablation; SBRT = stereotactic body radiotherapy

Key Question 3

Multiple shortcomings with the current evidence base preclude interpretation about general applicability. Firstly, the comparative benefits and harms of various endobronchial treatments are still unknown because of lack of good quality RCTs. The available studies were all poor quality, often small and not powered to detect a prespecified clinically meaningful difference in a standardized outcome of interest. Secondly, patient characteristics were poorly defined. The majority of studies did not report performance status and therefore it is difficult to assess the relative health and activity level of these patients and to whom this limited evidence applies. Thirdly, there was a wide variation in the outcomes measures to report symptom relief in the current studies. Fourthly, many studies did not report the frequency, the process or the method of assessing severity of treatment-related toxicities and therefore the true harms associated with these interventions are likely to be underrepresented in the current data. Factors that affect the applicability of the findings of this CER to practice are summarized in Table 32.

Table 32. Summary of applicability of evidence for Key Question 3

Domain	Applicability of Evidence
Populations	• The patients in the studies included in this report appear representative of cases that would be considered for a bronchoscopic intervention. All patients included in the 6 studies had histologically confirmed NSCLC with airway obstruction that required a bronchoscopic intervention. The mean age of patients included in these studies ranged from 61-68 years and this is congruent with the incidence of NSCLC that tends to rise with age.
Interventions	• The single modality interventions (brachytherapy, EBRT, electrocautery, laser, photodynamic, debridement, stenting) and 2 dual modality interventions (laser plus brachytherapy and brachytherapy plus EBRT) represent a general landscape of current treatments options for patients with endoluminal obstructive NSCLC and therefore are applicable.
Comparators	• See above for Intervention
Outcomes	• The major outcomes of interest were symptom relief, overall survival, disease specific survival, quality of life and treatment-related toxicity. • Although OS is the primary direct outcome for any cancer intervention study, it may not be the best measure of efficacy of a palliative intervention in symptomatic patients. Immediate relief of obstructive symptom and improvement in quality of life provide reasonable and pertinent justification for use of endobronchial intervention in such patients. • According to the structured review by the Patient Reported Outcome Measurement Group-Oxford on the use of PROMs (Patient Reported Outcomes Measures),[106] both generic and disease specific instruments exists that can be used in patients with lung cancer to assess the impact of interventions on QOL. These measures include generic measures such as SF-36 and EQ-5D and lung cancer specific measures such as EORTC QLQ-C30, EORTC QLQ-LC13 and FACT-L. However, QOL data was reported only by one small study of the six comparative studies. Therefore, applicability of the current evidence base on QOL cannot be determined.
Timing	• The relevant periods occur at the time of treatment through followup over months (palliation) or years (overall survival).
Setting	• The outcomes of local bronchoscopic therapies largely depend on the expertise of the provider and the center providing these services. We could not assess the impact of such operating characteristics on the treatment outcomes because these data were not available in the published papers.

EBRT = external-beam radiotherapy; EORTC QLQ = European Organization for Research and Treatment of Cancer Quality of Life Questionnaire; EQ-5D = EuroQOL 5 dimension; FACT-L = Functional Assessment of Cancer Therapy- Lung; NSCLC = non–small-cell lung cancer; QOL = quality of life; SF-36 = Short Form 36 Health Survey

Implications for Clinical and Policy Decisionmaking

Our results show no direct comparative evidence to support a decision among 3DRT, PBRT, RFA, or SBRT in stage I NSCLC patients. Comparative evidence is sparse among any of the interventions considered in Key Question 3.

In the absence of adequate direct comparative effectiveness data, other factors may be considered in making a treatment decision. Those could include relative convenience, and cost. The latter is outside the scope of this CER. Relative convenience would entail treatment duration and availability or access to a technology. Treatment duration can be substantially different for the interventions considered in Key Questions 1 and 2. It may reach 3 weeks or more for 3DRT or intensity-modulated radiation therapy (IMRT), compared with a week or less for SBRT or RFA. The availability of a technology locally, as opposed to a distant tertiary center, may be very relevant to NSCLC patients who are often elderly and perhaps debilitated by underlying comorbidities. According to the National Association for Proton Therapy (www.proton-therapy.org), PBRT is available for NSCLC therapy at 10 specialized centers in the United States, with seven under development. Thus, PBRT would be a limited choice for a large proportion of NSCLC patients.

Although we did not formally examine this issue, the body of published literature we identified for this CER suggests interest in SBRT has been growing over the past several years. It may be poised to supplant earlier conformal radiotherapy modalities in treating stage I NSCLC. This view is congruent with results of a recent survey of 1,600 radiation oncologists regarding SBRT use in the U.S.[107,108] The survey results indicated nearly 64 percent (95% confidence interval [CI], 60–68%) of radiation oncologists use SBRT in their practice, among whom about 50 percent adopted it in 2008 or later. Among SBRT users in this survey, 89 percent used it to treat lung cancer patients.

From the institutional perspective, decisionmakers may face pressures on acquisition that blend considerations of awareness and demand by referring physicians and patients with marketing and competition issues. These may lead to acquisition of one technology over another regardless of the availability of evidence of comparative effectiveness. Clinical uncertainties for all three Key Questions were a driver of development of this CER. Its findings ideally would provide a foundation for critically considering each technology in terms of the evidence available. However, it is unclear whether this CER will ultimately affect policy decisions.

Limitations of the Comparative Effectiveness Review Process

At the time of initiation of this CER, we expected that the total evidence base would be substantial. The volume of literature identified in the AHRQ Topic Development and Refinement process suggested the existence of a robust evidence base for all Key Questions. However, when we began to screen articles, it became evident that very few published comparative studies exist overall, none for Key Questions 1 and 2 and only six for Key Question 3.

Limitations of Evidence Base

Key Questions 1 and 2

The primary limitation is lack of comparative trials of any design for Key Questions 1 and 2. Percutaneous image-guided RFA has been investigated as an option for the treatment of stage I NSCLC. In our review, we found that RFA studies in lung primarily comprise heterogeneous case series that are complicated by several factors. First, many reports included metastatic and primary lesions from non-lung and lung sites, but did not stratify outcomes such as overall survival according to tumor stage or type. Second, the technical details of RFA, such as the type of equipment used, the power settings or wattage delivered, and details of followup assessment and subsequent therapy, were not consistent or consistently reported across studies. These factors conspired to severely limit RFA study selection in the report.

Although the body of evidence we included for the conformal radiotherapy techniques, particularly SBRT, was more substantial in quantity than for RFA, we have similar concerns about inter-study heterogeneity, with variability in radiotherapy dose, schedule of treatment, patient selection criteria, tumor size and location, and so forth. In a systematic review in general, heterogeneous, noncomparative evidence makes it very difficult to assess the benefits and harms of any intervention. In this CER, the type of evidence we identified for Key Questions 1 and 2 precludes comparative assessment among the interventions we investigated. We therefore believe further careful study of the interventions we considered in this CER is needed in the settings of Key Question 1 or 2 to identify optimal technical protocols and patient selection criteria, perhaps standardizing and comparing them across institutions. These data and methods could in theory be applied to the design and conduct of comparative studies of the local nonsurgical interventions for stage I NSCLC, as outlined in the Research Gaps section below.

Key Question 3

The body of evidence available for Key Question 3 comprised five RCTs, one nonrandomized comparative study and three relevant single arms from three otherwise comparative studies. We included the latter three study arms because we did not have higher level evidence for the interventions in question, debridement and stenting. Significant limitations in the quality and quantity of the evidence base led us to conclude that the evidence was insufficient to make conclusions about comparative effectiveness of local nonsurgical interventions to treat endobronchial obstructions in NSCLC patients. There was only one comparative study available per six unique treatment comparisons to draw inferences about comparative effectiveness. Therefore the consistency domain for SOE was unknown. All six studies received a low U.S. Preventive Services Task Force (USPSTF) study quality; often the studies were small and not powered to detect a prespecified clinically meaningful difference in a standardized outcome of interest thereby limiting their utility beyond hypothesis generation. Most studies lacked details about randomization and allocation concealment. The one nonrandomized comparative study available for Key Question 3 did not use statistical adjustment to reduce confounding; such adjustment for confounding should be consistently used in nonrandomized studies.

Research Gaps

Overview

Key Question 1 considers the relative clinical effectiveness of local nonsurgical interventions—3DRT, SBRT, PBRT and RFA—as sole therapy for patients with stage I NSCLC who are deemed to be medically inoperable. Key Question 2 addresses the same set of interventions in patients with stage I NSCLC who are deemed operable but who decline resection. The evidence base for Key Questions 1 and 2 comprises single-arm studies. The largest body of evidence is on SBRT, which suggests it may be gaining status among clinicians as a preferred treatment in patients with stage I disease. However, we did not identify evidence that supports one intervention relative to any other. Overall, the SOE is insufficient to draw conclusions on the comparative effectiveness of the interventions in terms of overall survival or cancer-specific survival.

Key Question 3 compared outcomes of available local endobronchial interventions used with curative or palliative intent to treat airway obstruction. There was only one comparative study available per six unique treatment comparisons to draw inferences about comparative effectiveness. Evidence on the patient outcomes was limited and, as such, is insufficient to make conclusions on the comparative effectiveness of the interventions in terms of symptom relief, overall survival or cancer-specific survival and harms of the treatment.

Key Questions 1 and 2

The primary research gap we identified in preparing this CER is the lack of evidence from comparative studies to draw conclusions as to the relative clinical benefits and harms of the local nonsurgical interventions used in the stage I NSCLC setting of medically inoperable or operable patients. We have also identified some feasibility issues associated with the interventions that are potential impediments to the type of rigorous comparative studies we suggest are necessary to determine their comparative effectiveness. In this section, we first describe characteristics of ideal comparative studies we believe are needed to compare these technologies. The potential impediments to such studies are discussed subsequently in this section.

Lack of Clinical Trial Evidence on Local Nonsurgical Interventions for Stage I NSCLC

We found no direct comparative evidence in this CER on the relative clinical effectiveness among any of the local nonsurgical interventions we evaluated: RFA, SBRT, 3DRT, IMRT or PBRT. As part of this review, we searched for ongoing clinical trials of these technologies in stage I NSCLC. In the process, we identified two international randomized, phase 3 clinical trials of surgical resection versus SBRT that are recruiting patients (NCT01336894 and NCT 00840749). However, neither of these trials will reveal relative outcomes among local nonsurgical interventions in stage I NSCLC. Thus, we suggest prospective studies are needed to properly evaluate the relative clinical benefits and harms of the technologies evaluated in this CER, taking into account the potential impediments to study we discuss below. Ideally, comparative studies in medically inoperable or operable stage I NSCLC patients would incorporate the following:

- To assure comparability of patients and minimize bias, standardized patient selection criteria would be used that involve consultation including a thoracic surgeon, medical oncologist, and radiation oncology specialist. Key factors to consider include comorbidity status (particularly cardiopulmonary function and capacity), age, performance status, tumor size and tumor location.
- Standardized intervention protocols with training and quality assurance programs within and across participating institutions are necessary for the best study. For radiotherapy, key factors would include the imaging and planning method, immobilization method, dose and fractionation schedule, and the biologically effective dose (BED) for comparisons of different modalities (e.g., SBRT, 3DRT, IMRT, PBRT). For RFA, issues would include treatment power and duration in the context of tumor size and location.
- Prespecified followup criteria and methods, in particular notation of subsequent systemic therapy administered at recurrence, are key considerations. Subsequent systemic therapy

is a key concern because it is impossible to discern the effect of an intervention followed by systemic therapy at progression from that achieved with the intervention alone. Is the effectiveness a function of the systemic therapy, the intervention, or the combination?

- Rigorous and standardized reporting is needed to account for all patients and treatments received. Data for operable and inoperable patients would be reported separately. Rigorous methods for conduct of RCTs is urged, particularly intent-to-treat analysis and adjustment of survival data to account for patients who develop recurrent disease and subsequently receive systemic chemotherapy as part of their treatment plan.
- Primary outcomes would include overall survival, cancer-specific survival, and local control. Prespecified, systematic collection of adverse events (AEs) using validated criteria (e.g., CTCAE criteria) is necessary to permit accurate assessment of relative benefits and risks of the interventions.

Potential Impediments to Comparative Studies of Local Nonsurgical Interventions for Stage I NSCLC

The general dissemination of conformal radiotherapy technologies into community clinical practice, most lately and specifically SBRT [107,108] is a potential impediment to comparative study of those technologies. Published survey results show that nearly 40 percent of solo practitioners treat patients with SBRT, which suggests that this technology is now accessible and its efficacy accepted in the broader radiation oncology community.[107,108] In addition, the shorter hypofractionated SBRT course is more "patient friendly" than those associated with conventionally fractionated conformal radiotherapy methods. This patient-specific advantage may represent an additional reason why SBRT has rapidly disseminated into clinical practice in the absence of direct comparative clinical trial evidence to support its reputation of clinical superiority over conventionally fractionated conformal techniques. We also recognize a number of other significant – perhaps insurmountable – technical impediments to conducting adequate comparative studies among the most widely available conformal radiotherapy-based modalities and other interventions such as RFA. These are outlined below.

Practical limitations exist to complicate comparative study of RFA and the conformal radiotherapy modalities in the stage I NSCLC setting. Although we did not evaluate these issues in this CER, it is generally thought that a tumor size greater than 4 cm, or a tumor location less than 1 cm from the hilum or large vessels, preclude the use of RFA.[28,109] Current clinical wisdom suggests RFA is best suited for patients with peripherally located, smaller lesions, due to the "heat sink" effect of large blood vessels that dissipates heat from the tumor and reduces its efficacy.[109-111] By contrast, although we didn't investigate any relationship in our systematic review, conformal radiotherapy-based modalities, particularly SBRT, have been used in patients with either peripheral or central tumors, as well as tumors > 4 and up to 7 cm in diameter, the latter corresponding to stage IB (T2N0M0).[4] Furthermore, radiotherapy effectiveness is not subject to a "heat sink" effect, as is RFA. Given those caveats, recruitment and accrual of sufficient numbers of similar stage I NSCLC patients to make clinically meaningful, relevant comparisons between RFA or conformal radiotherapy-based treatments would be difficult.

A key technical issue in comparing the radiotherapy interventions likely is the significant difference in the BED of radiation that can be safely delivered by SBRT, compared to IMRT or 3DRT delivered with conventional fractionation protocols. In brief, radiation therapy for NSCLC typically is delivered to a total dose of 60-70 Gray (Gy); SBRT delivers that dose in three to five fractions of 20 Gy each (estimated BED = 180 Gy_{10} using standard principles) whereas conventionally fractionated IMRT or 3DRT delivers 60-70 Gy in 30 fractions of 2 Gy each in 4 to 5 weeks, yielding an estimated BED of 72 Gy_{10}. The difference in the attainable BED is considered to have potential efficacy implications.[112] The higher BED causes tumor ablation, rather than tumor cell kill, allowing for little to no tumor cell repopulation between doses of radiation.

In this CER, we did not systematically investigate whether a higher BED delivered by any conformal radiotherapy modality can be associated with better clinical outcomes - such as overall survival - compared to a lower BED. This has been reported in published single-arm studies reviewed in this CER, for example the large, multicenter, retrospective series on SBRT in Japan by Onishi and colleagues.[84] However, we are not aware of any direct comparative evidence on this topic among any of the conformal radiotherapy technologies, so it is not possible to make even indirect comparisons between the delivered BED and clinical outcomes in any case. Furthermore, we are aware of no published clinical trial evidence to ascertain whether a higher BED delivered by SBRT is associated with differences in patient outcomes compared to a lower BED delivered either by SBRT or by a conventionally fractionated conformal radiotherapy modality. We acknowledge the difference in delivered BED has biologically plausible clinical implications, and perhaps ethical implications, that would need to be addressed in designing a study of any type to compare conformal radiotherapy-based technologies. But, it is not clear to us that the BED issue under discussion here is settled.

In summary, we acknowledge the views of some members of the radiation oncology and interventional radiology communities - that clinical trials of local nonsurgical modalities, including RFA, SBRT and other conformal radiotherapy modalities (e.g., 3DRT, IMRT, PBRT) in stage I NSCLC patients may be very difficult to recruit and conduct, based on technical and potential ethical issues related to perceptions of unequal clinical benefit among the interventions. However, we maintain that current evidence is insufficient to support a view that clinical outcomes achieved with one technology are superior or inferior to those achieved with other modalities. Clinical evidence from comparative studies is needed to establish the standard of care for local nonsurgical treatment of stage I NSCLC patients.

Key Question 3

Lack of Clinical Trial Evidence on Local Nonsurgical Interventions for Endoluminal Obstructive NSCLC

Key Question 3 compared outcomes of available local endobronchial interventions used with curative or palliative intent to treat airway obstruction as a result of NSCLC. Evidence on the patient outcomes is limited and, as such, is insufficient to make conclusions. We identified a number of research gaps during the course of review:

- Lack of comparative evidence generated from adequately powered RCTs regarding the benefits and harms of various bronchoscopic interventions used for treating endoluminal obstructions in patients with NSCLC.
- Lack of comparative evidence generated from good quality RCTs regarding the QOL data from patients who receive various bronchoscopic interventions used for treating endoluminal obstructions in patients with NSCLC.
- Need for systematic collection of treatment-related toxicities data from various bronchoscopic interventions used for treating endoluminal obstructions from actual clinical practice setting.

During our review, we identified two RCTs that aimed to compare local endobronchial interventions in patients with endobronchial NSCLC. However, both these trials were not completed due to lack of patient accrual. Among these two RCTs, the trial by Moghissi et al.,[102] is most notable. The objective of this trial was to compare two treatment policies in terms of symptom relief, respiratory function, performance status, QOL and survival. This study planned to recruit 400 patients in 3 years at 24 clinical centers in the UK. Even though the study organizers had successfully conducted many RCTs in the past, they failed to recruit patients in this clinical setting. Moreover, 20 percent of those randomized did not receive the assigned treatment. Another study by Langendijk[86] that randomized patients to brachytherapy plus EBRT or EBRT alone arm was discontinued due to lack of patient accrual before completing the planned enrollment of 160 patients.

Potential Impediments to Comparative Studies of Local Nonsurgical Interventions for Endoluminal Obstructive NSCLC

NSCLC patients with endoluminal obstructions are particularly difficult to randomize in trials because of many reasons particularly ethical issues. Most of these bronchoscopic interventions are considered complementary and are used sequentially in a clinical setting[113] and therefore randomizing critically ill patients to either therapy alone has ethical implications. Further, many of these patients present with an impending obstruction and immediate symptom relief is foremost. Obtaining informed consent in such a situation is a barrier in patient recruitment. These reasons are likely to obviate successful conduct of a future RCT.

Thus, a prospective cohort study may be able to answer the questions about relative harms and benefits of local endobronchial interventions. Though concerns of selection bias and unknown confounders always exist in this study design, addressing and collecting data about most relevant confounders *a priori* can provide much needed informative answers about comparative benefits (including QOL data) and harms of these therapies in population of interest. We recommend that the research team for conducting such a study be multi-disciplinary including oncologists experienced in treating NSCLC patients with endobronchial obstruction, methodologist with expertise in quality of life measurement, clinical researchers with expertise in planning and conduct of large cohort multicentric studies and ethicists. Relevant outcomes that would be measured in such a study would include symptom control, QOL, survival and treatment-related AEs. Data related to symptom control would be captured using a standardized validated tool applied uniformly across all interventions. In the current evidence base, Speiser Index was used commonly to assess symptomatic control but the validity and sensitivity of such a tool to capture treatment effect is unknown. Therefore, it is crucial to address and resolve the shortcomings of current tools that are used to asses symptom control to allow objective and uniform measurements of symptom control. Generic instruments such as Short Form 36 Health Survey (SF-36) and EuroQOL 5 dimension (EQ-5D) would be used in conjunction with lung cancer specific measures such as European Organization for Research and Treatment of Cancer Quality of Life Questionnaire (EORTC QLQ) modules C30 and LC13 and Functional Assessment of Cancer Therapy- Lung (FACT-L) to measure QOL data.

Treatment-related AEs would be assessed from the date of the procedure extending to a reasonable time preferably until death using standardized and well-defined criteria with an independent causality analysis. A process to capture AEs that occur when patients are not under direct medical supervision (such as home or long term care facility) would also be prespecified in the study protocol. Data on all potential prognostic covariates would include but not be limited to patient characteristics (age, sex, race, performance status, comorbidities), disease characteristics (tumor stage, histopathology, location, size, blockage) and technical attributes of the procedure (technical success, technical variables related to use of procedures, type of instrument used) as well data on the operator (expertise, years of experience, size of the facility).

Secondly, we propose setting up a registry to systematically collect treatment-related toxicity data for patients undergoing such procedures. According to the AHRQ publication on registries[114] for evaluating patient outcomes, registries need to be created with a question in mind which guides the identification of the target population, the exposures and outcomes of interest, number of patients and length of followup. Registries can be designed as an active surveillance system for identifying harms and may be particularly useful for assessing AEs.

Conclusion

We conducted a systematic review of the literature to evaluate the comparative effectiveness of local nonsurgical therapies in patients with NSCLC. Our review addressed three Key Questions with three distinct categories of patients: those with stage I NSCLC who were deemed medically inoperable (Key Question 1); those with stage I NSCLC who were deemed medically operable (Key Question 2); and those with symptoms secondary to the presence of endoluminal NSCLC (Key Question 3). For Key Questions 1 and 2 we included only single local nonsurgical interventions: 3DRT, PBRT, RFA, and SBRT. For Key Question 3 we allowed combinations of local nonsurgical therapies including neodymium-doped yttrium aluminum garnet (Nd-YAG) laser, PDT, endobronchial debridement with stenting, and EBRT, as well as systemic chemotherapy.

Evidence for both Key Questions 1 and 2 consists only of single-arm studies, with no direct comparisons among interventions. The best evidence for Key Question 3 consists of RCTs of one comparison only, precluding indirect comparisons. Evidence from single-arm studies also is available for several interventions relevant to Key Question 3. For all Key Questions, the evidence was insufficient to reach conclusions about the relative effectiveness and safety of the interventions in terms of overall survival, cancer-specific survival, local control, QOL, symptomatic relief and toxicities.

References

1. Goldstraw P, Ball D, Jett JR, et al. Non-small-cell lung cancer. Lancet. 2011 Nov 12;378(9804):1727-40. PMID: 21565398.

2. Jemal A, Siegel R, Xu J, et al. Cancer statistics, 2010. CA Cancer J Clin. 2010 Sep-Oct;60(5):277-300. PMID: 20610543.

3. Pfister DG, Johnson DH, Azzoli CG, et al. American Society of Clinical Oncology treatment of unresectable non-small-cell lung cancer guideline: update 2003. J Clin Oncol. 2004 Jan 15;22(2):330-53. PMID: 14691125.

4. Detterbeck FC, Boffa DJ, Tanoue LT. The new lung cancer staging system. Chest. 2009 Jul;136(1):260-71. PMID: 19584208.

5. Rankin SC. Staging of non-small cell lung cancer (NSCLC). Cancer Imaging. 2006;6:1-3. PMID: 16478697.

6. Goldstraw P, Crowley J, Chansky K, et al. The IASLC Lung Cancer Staging Project: proposals for the revision of the TNM stage groupings in the forthcoming (seventh) edition of the TNM Classification of malignant tumours. J Thorac Oncol. 2007 Aug;2(8):706-14. PMID: 17762336.

7. Robinson CG, Bradley JD. The treatment of early-stage disease. Semin Radiat Oncol. 2010 Jul;20(3):178-85. PMID: 20685580.

8. Rami-Porta R, Ball D, Crowley J, et al. The IASLC Lung Cancer Staging Project: proposals for the revision of the T descriptors in the forthcoming (seventh) edition of the TNM classification for lung cancer. J Thorac Oncol. 2007 Jul;2(7):593-602. PMID: 17607114.

9. Cerfolio RJ, Bryant AS. Survival of patients with true pathologic stage I non-small cell lung cancer. Ann Thorac Surg. 2009 Sep;88(3):917-22; discussion 22-3. PMID: 19699920.

10. Colice GL, Shafazand S, Griffin JP, et al. Physiologic evaluation of the patient with lung cancer being considered for resectional surgery: ACCP evidenced-based clinical practice guidelines (2nd edition). Chest. 2007 Sep;132(3 Suppl):161S-77S. PMID: 17873167.

11. Myrdal G, Gustafsson G, Lambe M, et al. Outcome after lung cancer surgery. Factors predicting early mortality and major morbidity. Eur J Cardiothorac Surg. 2001 Oct;20(4):694-9. PMID: 11574210.

12. Christie NA, Pennathur A, Burton SA, et al. Stereotactic radiosurgery for early stage non-small cell lung cancer: rationale, patient selection, results, and complications. Semin Thorac Cardiovasc Surg. 2008 Winter;20(4):290-7. PMID: 19251167.

13. Crino L, Weder W, van Meerbeeck J, et al. Early stage and locally advanced (non-metastatic) non-small-cell lung cancer: ESMO Clinical Practice Guidelines for diagnosis, treatment and follow-up. Ann Oncol. 2010 May;21 Suppl 5:v103-15. PMID: 20555058.

14. Decker RH, Tanoue LT, Colasanto JM, et al. Evaluation and definitive management of medically inoperable early-stage non-small-cell lung cancer. Part 1: Assessment and conventional radiotherapy. Oncology (Williston Park). 2006 Jun;20(7):727-36. PMID: 16841796.

15. McGarry RC, Song G, des Rosiers P, et al. Observation-only management of early stage, medically inoperable lung cancer: poor outcome. Chest. 2002 Apr;121(4):1155-8. PMID: 11948046.

16. Raz DJ, Zell JA, Ou SH, et al. Natural history of stage I non-small cell lung cancer: implications for early detection. Chest. 2007 Jul;132(1):193-9. PMID: 17505036.

17. Palma D, Lagerwaard F, Rodrigues G, et al. Curative Treatment of Stage I Non-small-cell Lung Cancer in Patients with Severe COPD: Stereotactic Radiotherapy Outcomes and Systematic Review. Int J Radiat Oncol Biol Phys. 2011 Jun 1PMID: 21640513.

18. Mohiuddin MM, Choi NC. The role of radiation therapy in non-small cell lung cancer. Semin Respir Crit Care Med. 2005 Jun;26(3):278-88. PMID: 16052429.

19. Patel RR, Mehta M. Three-dimensional conformal radiotherapy for lung cancer: promises and pitfalls. Curr Oncol Rep. 2002 Jul;4(4):347-53. PMID: 12044245.

20. Powell JW, Dexter E, Scalzetti EM, et al. Treatment advances for medically inoperable non-small-cell lung cancer: emphasis on prospective trials. Lancet Oncol. 2009 Sep;10(9):885-94. PMID: 19717090.

21. Widesott L, Amichetti M, Schwarz M. Proton therapy in lung cancer: clinical outcomes and technical issues. A systematic review. Radiother Oncol. 2008 Feb;86(2):154-64. PMID: 18241945.

22. Heinzerling JH, Kavanagh B, Timmerman RD. Stereotactic ablative radiation therapy for primary lung tumors. Cancer J. 2011 Jan-Feb;17(1):28-32. PMID: 21263264.

23. Martel MK. Advanced radiation treatment planning and delivery approaches for treatment of lung cancer. Hematol Oncol Clin North Am. 2004 Feb;18(1):231-43. PMID: 15005291.

24. Low DA, Moran JM, Dempsey JF, et al. Dosimetry tools and techniques for IMRT. Med Phys. 2011 Mar;38(3):1313-38. PMID: 21520843.

25. Santos RS, Raftopoulos Y, Keenan RJ, et al. Bronchoscopic palliation of primary lung cancer: single or multimodality therapy? Surg Endosc. 2004 Jun;18(6):931-6. PMID: 15108108.

26. Zhu JC, Yan TD, Morris DL. A systematic review of radiofrequency ablation for lung tumors. Ann Surg Oncol. 2008 Jun;15(6):1765-74. PMID: 18368456.

27. Haasbeek CJ, Senan S, Smit EF, et al. Critical review of nonsurgical treatment options for stage I non-small cell lung cancer. Oncologist. 2008 Mar;13(3):309-19. PMID: 18378542.

28. Das M, Abdelmaksoud MH, Loo BW, Jr., et al. Alternatives to surgery for early stage non-small cell lung cancer-ready for prime time? Curr Treat Options Oncol. 2010 Jun;11(1-2):24-35. PMID: 20577833.

29. Stewart AJ, Mutyala S, Holloway CL, et al. Intraoperative seed placement for thoracic malignancy-A review of technique, indications, and published literature. Brachytherapy. 2009 Jan-Mar;8(1):63-9. PMID: 19056322.

30. Dagnault A, Ebacher A, Vigneault E, et al. Retrospective study of 81 patients treated with brachytherapy for endobronchial primary tumor or metastasis. Brachytherapy. 2010 Jul-Sep;9(3):243-7. PMID: 20122873.

31. Ernst A, Feller-Kopman D, Becker HD, et al. Central airway obstruction. Am J Respir Crit Care Med. 2004 Jun 15;169(12):1278-97. PMID: 15187010.

32. Amjadi K, Voduc N, Cruysberghs Y, et al. Impact of interventional bronchoscopy on quality of life in malignant airway obstruction. Respiration. 2008;76(4):421-8. PMID: 18758153.

33. Morris CD, Budde JM, Godette KD, et al. Palliative management of malignant airway obstruction. Ann Thorac Surg. 2002 Dec;74(6):1928-32; discussion 32-3. PMID: 12643375.

34. Cardona AF, Reveiz L, Ospina EG, et al. Palliative endobronchial brachytherapy for non-small cell lung cancer. Cochrane Database Syst Rev. 2008(2):CD004284. PMID: 18425900.

35. Yerushalmi R, Fenig E, Shitrit D, et al. Endobronchial stent for malignant airway obstructions. Isr Med Assoc J. 2006 Sep;8(9):615-7. PMID: 17058411.

36. Maiwand MO, Asimakopoulos G. Cryosurgery for lung cancer: clinical results and technical aspects. Technol Cancer Res Treat. 2004 Apr;3(2):143-50. PMID: 15059020.

37. Helfand M, Balshem H. Methods Guide for Effectiveness and Comparative Effectiveness Reviews. August 2009. Rockville, MD. www.effectivehealthcare.ahrq.gov/index.cfm/search-for-guides-reviews-and-reports/?pageaction=displayProduct&productID=318.

38. Moher D, Liberati A, Tetzlaff J, et al. Preferred reporting items for systematic reviews and meta-analyses: the PRISMA statement. PLoS Med. 2009 Jul 21;6(7):e1000097. PMID: 19621072.

39. Pham B, Klassen TP, Lawson ML, et al. Language of publication restrictions in systematic reviews gave different results depending on whether the intervention was conventional or complementary. J Clin Epidemiol. 2005 Aug;58(8):769-76. PMID: 16086467.

40. Harris RP, Helfand M, Woolf SH, et al. Current methods of the US Preventive Services Task Force: a review of the process. Am J Prev Med. 2001 Apr;20(3 Suppl):21-35. PMID: 11306229.

41. Deeks JJ, Dinnes J, D'Amico R, et al. Evaluating non-randomised intervention studies. Health Technol Assess. 2003;7(27):iii-x, 1-173. PMID: 14499048.

42. Carey TS, Boden SD. A critical guide to case series reports. Spine (Phila Pa 1976). 2003 Aug 1;28(15):1631-4. PMID: 12897483.

43. Owens DK, Lohr KN, Atkins D, et al. AHRQ series paper 5: grading the strength of a body of evidence when comparing medical interventions--agency for healthcare research and quality and the effective health-care program. J Clin Epidemiol. 2010 May;63(5):513-23. PMID: 19595577.

44. Guyatt GH, Oxman AD, Vist G, et al. GRADE guidelines: 4. Rating the quality of evidence—study limitations (risk of bias). J Clin Epidemiol. 2011;64(4):407-15.

45. Brown P, Brunnhuber K, Chalkidou K, et al. How to formulate research recommendations. BMJ. 2006 Oct 14;333(7572):804-6. PMID: 17038740.

46. Atkins D, Chang SM, Gartlehner G, et al. Assessing applicability when comparing medical interventions: AHRQ and the Effective Health Care Program. J Clin Epidemiol. 2011 Nov;64(11):1198-207. PMID: 21463926.

47. Iwata H, Murakami M, Demizu Y, et al. High-dose proton therapy and carbon-ion therapy for stage I nonsmall cell lung cancer. Cancer. 2010 May 15;116(10):2476-85. PMID: 20225229.

48. Takeda A, Sanuki N, Kunieda E, et al. Stereotactic Body Radiotherapy for Primary Lung Cancer at a Dose of 50 Gy Total in Five Fractions to the Periphery of the Planning Target Volume Calculated Using a Superposition Algorithm. International Journal of Radiation Oncology Biology Physics. 2009;73(2):442-8.

49. Shibamoto Y, Hashizume C, Baba F, et al. Stereotactic body radiotherapy using a radiobiology-based regimen for stage I nonsmall cell lung cancer: a multicenter study. Cancer. 2012 Apr 15;118(8):2078-84. PMID: 22009495.

50. Bogart JA. Fractionated radiotherapy for high-risk patients with early-stage non-small cell lung cancer. Semin Thorac Cardiovasc Surg. 2010 Spring;22(1):44-52. PMID: 20813316.

51. Bradley JD, Wahab S, Lockett MA, et al. Elective nodal failures are uncommon in medically inoperable patients with Stage I non-small-cell lung carcinoma treated with limited radiotherapy fields. Int J Radiat Oncol Biol Phys. 2003 Jun 1;56(2):342-7. PMID: 12738307.

52. Bush DA, Slater JD, Shin BB, et al. Hypofractionated proton beam radiotherapy for stage I lung cancer. Chest. 2004 Oct;126(4):1198-203. PMID: 15486383.

53. Kopek N, Paludan M, Petersen J, et al. Co-morbidity index predicts for mortality after stereotactic body radiotherapy for medically inoperable early-stage non-small cell lung cancer. Radiother Oncol. 2009 Dec;93(3):402-7. PMID: 19559492.

54. Mirri MA, Arcangeli G, Benassi M, et al. Hypofractionated Conformal Radiotherapy (HCRT) for primary and metastatic lung cancers with small dimension : efficacy and toxicity. Strahlenther Onkol. 2009 Jan;185(1):27-33. PMID: 19224144.

55. Narayan S, Henning GT, Ten Haken RK, et al. Results following treatment to doses of 92.4 or 102.9 Gy on a phase I dose escalation study for non-small cell lung cancer. Lung Cancer. 2004 Apr;44(1):79-88. PMID: 15013586.

56. Nyman J, Johansson KA, Hulten U. Stereotactic hypofractionated radiotherapy for stage I non-small cell lung cancer--mature results for medically inoperable patients. Lung Cancer. 2006 Jan;51(1):97-103. PMID: 16213059.

57. Ricardi U, Filippi AR, Guarneri A, et al. Stereotactic body radiation therapy for early stage non-small cell lung cancer: results of a prospective trial. Lung Cancer. 2010 Apr;68(1):72-7. PMID: 19556022.

58. Taremi M, Hope A, Dahele M, et al. Stereotactic Body Radiotherapy for Medically Inoperable Lung Cancer: Prospective, Single-Center Study of 108 Consecutive Patients. Int J Radiat Oncol Biol Phys. 2011 Mar 4PMID: 21377293.

59. Vahdat S, Oermann EK, Collins SP, et al. CyberKnife radiosurgery for inoperable stage IA non-small cell lung cancer: 18F-fluorodeoxyglucose positron emission tomography/computed tomography serial tumor response assessment. J Hematol Oncol. 2010;3:6. PMID: 20132557.

60. Andratschke N, Zimmermann F, Boehm E, et al. Stereotactic radiotherapy of histologically proven inoperable stage I non-small cell lung cancer: Patterns of failure. Radiother Oncol. 2011 Nov;101(2):245-9. PMID: 21724287.

61. Baumann P, Nyman J, Hoyer M, et al. Outcome in a prospective phase II trial of medically inoperable stage I non-small-cell lung cancer patients treated with stereotactic body radiotherapy. J Clin Oncol. 2009 Jul 10;27(20):3290-6. PMID: 19414667.

62. Baumann P, Nyman J, Lax I, et al. Factors important for efficacy of stereotactic body radiotherapy of medically inoperable stage I lung cancer. A retrospective analysis of patients treated in the Nordic countries. Acta Oncol. 2006;45(7):787-95. PMID: 16982541.

63. Burdick MJ, Stephans KL, Reddy CA, et al. Maximum standardized uptake value from staging FDG-PET/CT does not predict treatment outcome for early-stage non-small-cell lung cancer treated with stereotactic body radiotherapy. Int J Radiat Oncol Biol Phys. 2010 Nov 15;78(4):1033-9. PMID: 20472359.

64. Coon D, Gokhale AS, Burton SA, et al. Fractionated stereotactic body radiation therapy in the treatment of primary, recurrent, and metastatic lung tumors: the role of positron emission tomography/computed tomography-based treatment planning. Clin Lung Cancer. 2008 Jul;9(4):217-21. PMID: 18650169.

65. Dunlap NE, Larner JM, Read PW, et al. Size matters: a comparison of T1 and T2 peripheral non-small-cell lung cancers treated with stereotactic body radiation therapy (SBRT). J Thorac Cardiovasc Surg. 2010 Sep;140(3):583-9. PMID: 20478576.

66. Fritz P, Kraus HJ, Blaschke T, et al. Stereotactic, high single-dose irradiation of stage I non-small cell lung cancer (NSCLC) using four-dimensional CT scans for treatment planning. Lung Cancer. 2008 May;60(2):193-9. PMID: 18045732.

67. Olsen JR, Robinson CG, El Naqa I, et al. Dose-response for stereotactic body radiotherapy in early-stage non-small-cell lung cancer. Int J Radiat Oncol Biol Phys. 2011 Nov 15;81(4):e299-303. PMID: 21477948.

68. Pennathur A, Luketich JD, Heron DE, et al. Stereotactic radiosurgery for the treatment of stage I non-small cell lung cancer in high-risk patients. J Thorac Cardiovasc Surg. 2009 Mar;137(3):597-604. PMID: 19258073.

69. Scorsetti M, Navarria P, Facoetti A, et al. Effectiveness of stereotactic body radiotherapy in the treatment of inoperable early-stage lung cancer. Anticancer Res. 2007 Sep-Oct;27(5B):3615-9. PMID: 17972525.

70. Song SY, Choi W, Shin SS, et al. Fractionated stereotactic body radiation therapy for medically inoperable stage I lung cancer adjacent to central large bronchus. Lung Cancer. 2009;66(1):89-93.

71. Stephans KL, Djemil T, Reddy CA, et al. A comparison of two stereotactic body radiation fractionation schedules for medically inoperable stage I non-small cell lung cancer: the Cleveland Clinic experience. J Thorac Oncol. 2009 Aug;4(8):976-82. PMID: 19633473.

72. Turzer M, Brustugun OT, Waldeland E, et al. Stereotactic body radiation therapy is effective and safe in patients with early-stage non-small cell lung cancer with low performance status and severe comorbidity. Case Rep Oncol. 2011;4(1):25-34. PMID: 21526003.

73. van der Voort van Zyp NC, Prevost JB, Hoogeman MS, et al. Stereotactic radiotherapy with real-time tumor tracking for non-small cell lung cancer: clinical outcome. Radiother Oncol. 2009 Jun;91(3):296-300. PMID: 19297048.

74. Videtic GMM, Stephans K, Reddy C, et al. Intensity-Modulated Radiotherapy-Based Stereotactic Body Radiotherapy for Medically Inoperable Early-Stage Lung Cancer: Excellent Local Control. International Journal of Radiation Oncology Biology Physics. 2010;77(2):344-9.

75. Bollineni VR, Widder J, Pruim J, et al. Residual (18)F-FDG-PET Uptake 12 Weeks After Stereotactic Ablative Radiotherapy for Stage I Non-Small-Cell Lung Cancer Predicts Local Control. Int J Radiat Oncol Biol Phys. 2012 Jul 15;83(4):e551-5. PMID: 22417800.

76. Campeau MP, Herschtal A, Wheeler G, et al. Local control and survival following concomitant chemoradiotherapy in inoperable stage I non-small-cell lung cancer. Int J Radiat Oncol Biol Phys. 2009 Aug 1;74(5):1371-5. PMID: 19250769.

77. Graham PH, Vinod SK, Hui AC. Stage I non-small cell lung cancer: results for surgery in a patterns-of-care study in Sydney and for high-dose concurrent end-phase boost accelerated radiotherapy. J Thorac Oncol. 2006 Oct;1(8):796-801. PMID: 17409962.

78. Jimenez MF, van Baardwijk A, Aerts HJ, et al. Effectiveness of surgery and individualized high-dose hyperfractionated accelerated radiotherapy on survival in clinical stage I non-small cell lung cancer. A propensity score matched analysis. Radiother Oncol. 2010 Dec;97(3):413-7. PMID: 20851487.

79. Nakayama H, Sugahara S, Tokita M, et al. Proton beam therapy for patients with medically inoperable stage I non-small-cell lung cancer at the university of tsukuba. Int J Radiat Oncol Biol Phys. 2010 Oct 1;78(2):467-71. PMID: 20056349.

80. Pennathur A, Luketich JD, Abbas G, et al. Radiofrequency ablation for the treatment of stage I non-small cell lung cancer in high-risk patients. J Thorac Cardiovasc Surg. 2007 Oct;134(4):857-64. PMID: 17903496.

81. Chen VJ, Oermann E, Vahdat S, et al. CyberKnife with Tumor Tracking: An Effective Treatment for High-Risk Surgical Patients with Stage I Non-Small Cell Lung Cancer. Front Oncol. 2012;2:9. PMID: 22655258.

82. Lagerwaard FJ, Verstegen NE, Haasbeek CJ, et al. Outcomes of Stereotactic Ablative Radiotherapy in Patients with Potentially Operable Stage I Non-Small-Cell Lung Cancer. Int J Radiat Oncol Biol Phys. 2011 Nov 19PMID: 22104360.

83. Onishi H, Shirato H, Nagata Y, et al. Stereotactic body radiotherapy (SBRT) for operable stage I non-small-cell lung cancer: can SBRT be comparable to surgery? Int J Radiat Oncol Biol Phys. 2011 Dec 1;81(5):1352-8. PMID: 20638194.

84. Onishi H, Shirato H, Nagata Y, et al. Hypofractionated stereotactic radiotherapy (HypoFXSRT) for stage I non-small cell lung cancer: updated results of 257 patients in a Japanese multi-institutional study. J Thorac Oncol. 2007 Jul;2(7 Suppl 3):S94-100. PMID: 17603311.

85. Mallick I, Sharma SC, Behera D, et al. Optimization of dose and fractionation of endobronchial brachytherapy with or without external radiation in the palliative management of non-small cell lung cancer: a prospective randomized study. J Cancer Res Ther. 2006 Jul-Sep;2(3):119-25. PMID: 17998689.

86. Langendijk H, de Jong J, Tjwa M, et al. External irradiation versus external irradiation plus endobronchial brachytherapy in inoperable non-small cell lung cancer: a prospective randomized study. Radiother Oncol. 2001 Mar;58(3):257-68. PMID: 11230886.

87. Stout R, Barber P, Burt P, et al. Clinical and quality of life outcomes in the first United Kingdom randomized trial of endobronchial brachytherapy (intraluminal radiotherapy) vs. external beam radiotherapy in the palliative treatment of inoperable non-small cell lung cancer. Radiother Oncol. 2000 Sep;56(3):323-7. PMID: 10974381.

88. Chella A, Ambrogi MC, Ribechini A, et al. Combined Nd-YAG laser/HDR brachytherapy versus Nd-YAG laser only in malignant central airway involvement: a prospective randomized study. Lung Cancer. 2000 Mar;27(3):169-75. PMID: 10699690.

89. Diaz-Jimenez JP, Martinez-Ballarin JE, Llunell A, et al. Efficacy and safety of photodynamic therapy versus Nd-YAG laser resection in NSCLC with airway obstruction. Eur Respir J. 1999 Oct;14(4):800-5. PMID: 10573224.

90. Boxem T, Muller M, Venmans B, et al. Nd-YAG laser vs bronchoscopic electrocautery for palliation of symptomatic airway obstruction: a cost-effectiveness study. Chest. 1999 Oct;116(4):1108-12. PMID: 10531180.

91. Lencioni R, Crocetti L, Cioni R, et al. Response to radiofrequency ablation of pulmonary tumours: a prospective, intention-to-treat, multicentre clinical trial (the RAPTURE study). Lancet Oncol. 2008 Jul;9(7):621-8. PMID: 18565793.

92. Allison R, Sibata C, Sarma K, et al. High-dose-rate brachytherapy in combination with stenting offers a rapid and statistically significant improvement in quality of life for patients with endobronchial recurrence. Cancer J. 2004 Nov-Dec;10(6):368-73. PMID: 15701268.

93. Chhajed PN, Baty F, Pless M, et al. Outcome of treated advanced non-small cell lung cancer with and without central airway obstruction. Chest. 2006 Dec;130(6):1803-7. PMID: 17167000.

94. Celebioglu B, Gurkan OU, Erdogan S, et al. High dose rate endobronchial brachytherapy effectively palliates symptoms due to inoperable lung cancer. Jpn J Clin Oncol. 2002 Nov;32(11):443-8. PMID: 12499415.

95. Aumont-le Guilcher M, Prevost B, Sunyach MP, et al. High-dose-rate brachytherapy for non-small-cell lung carcinoma: a retrospective study of 226 patients. Int J Radiat Oncol Biol Phys. 2011 Mar 15;79(4):1112-6. PMID: 20510543.

96. Petera J, Spasova I, Neumanova R, et al. High dose rate intraluminal brachytherapy in the treatment of malignant airway obstructions. Neoplasma. 2001;48(2):148-53. PMID: 11478697.

97. Jones BU, Helmy M, Brenner M, et al. Photodynamic therapy for patients with advanced non-small-cell carcinoma of the lung. Clinical Lung Cancer. 2001;3(1):37-41.

98. Muto P, Ravo V, Panelli G, et al. High-dose rate brachytherapy of bronchial cancer: treatment optimization using three schemes of therapy. Oncologist. 2000;5(3):209-14. PMID: 10884499.

99. Vucicevic S, Stankovic J, Jovanovic N, et al. Combined high-dose rate brachytherapy and external beam irradiation for non-small cell lung carcinoma. Journal of B.U.ON. 1999;4(4):377-82.

100. Celikoglu F, Celikoglu SI, York AM, et al. Intratumoral administration of cisplatin through a bronchoscope followed by irradiation for treatment of inoperable non-small cell obstructive lung cancer. Lung Cancer. 2006 Feb;51(2):225-36. PMID: 16359751.

101. Weinberg BD, Allison RR, Sibata C, et al. Results of combined photodynamic therapy (PDT) and high dose rate brachytherapy (HDR) in treatment of obstructive endobronchial non-small cell lung cancer (NSCLC). Photodiagnosis Photodyn Ther. 2010 Mar;7(1):50-8. PMID: 20230994.

102. Moghissi K, Bond MG, Sambrook RJ, et al. Treatment of endotracheal or endobronchial obstruction by non-small cell lung cancer: lack of patients in an MRC randomized trial leaves key questions unanswered. Medical Research Council Lung Cancer Working Party. 1999. www.mrw.interscience.wiley.com/cochrane/clcentral/articles/873/CN-00166873/frame.html.

103. Chou R, Aronson N, Atkins D, et al. AHRQ series paper 4: assessing harms when comparing medical interventions: AHRQ and the effective health-care program. J Clin Epidemiol. 2010 May;63(5):502-12. PMID: 18823754.

104. Tipton KN, Sullivan N, Bruening W, et al. Stereotactic Body Radiation Therapy. Rockville (MD); 2011.

105. Kvale PA, Selecky PA, Prakash UB. Palliative care in lung cancer: ACCP evidence-based clinical practice guidelines (2nd edition). Chest. 2007 Sep;132(3 Suppl):368S-403S. PMID: 17873181.

106. Comabella CCi, Gibbons E, Fitzpatrick R. A Structured Review of Patient-Reported Outcome Measures for Patients With Lung Cancer, 2010- Report to the Department of Health, 2010. University of Oxford, UK; 2010.

107. Pan H, Rose BS, Simpson DR, et al. Clinical Practice Patterns of Lung Stereotactic Body Radiation Therapy in the United States: A Secondary Analysis. Am J Clin Oncol. 2012 Apr 6PMID: 22495454.

108. Pan H, Simpson DR, Mell LK, et al. A survey of stereotactic body radiotherapy use in the United States. Cancer. 2011 Oct 1;117(19):4566-72. PMID: 21412761.

109. Dupuy DE. Image-guided thermal ablation of lung malignancies. Radiology. 2011 Sep;260(3):633-55. PMID: 21846760.

110. Goldberg SN, Hahn PF, Tanabe KK, et al. Percutaneous radiofrequency tissue ablation: does perfusion-mediated tissue cooling limit coagulation necrosis? J Vasc Interv Radiol. 1998 Jan-Feb;9(1 Pt 1):101-11. PMID: 9468403.

111. Gomez FM, Palussiere J, Santos E, et al. Radiofrequency thermocoagulation of lung tumours. Where we are, where we are headed. Clin Transl Oncol. 2009 Jan;11(1):28-34. PMID: 19155201.

112. Nguyen NP, Garland L, Welsh J, et al. Can stereotactic fractionated radiation therapy become the standard of care for early stage non-small cell lung carcinoma. Cancer Treat Rev. 2008 Dec;34(8):719-27. PMID: 18657910.

113. Lee P, Kupeli E, Mehta AC. Therapeutic bronchoscopy in lung cancer. Laser therapy, electrocautery, brachytherapy, stents, and photodynamic therapy. Clin Chest Med. 2002 Mar;23(1):241-56. PMID: 11901914.

114. Gliklich RE DN, eds. Registries for Evaluating Patient Outcomes: A User's Guide. (Prepared by Outcome DEcIDE Center [Outcome Sciences, Inc. dba Outcome] under Contract No. 290-2005-0035-I AHRQ Publication No. 07-EHC001-1. Rockville, MD: Agency for Healthcare Research and Quality; April, 2007. www.effectivehealthcare.ahrq.gov/repFiles/PatOutcomes.pdf.

Abbreviations

3DRT	Three-dimensional radiation therapy
ACE-27	Adult Co-Morbidity Evaluation-27 scoring system
BED	Biologically Effective Dose
CGE	Cobalt Gray equivalent
CI	Confidence interval
CSS	Cancer-specific survival
CT	Computed Tomography
CTC	Common Toxicity Criteria
CTCAE	Common Terminology Criteria for Adverse Events
DSS	Disease-specific survival
ECOG	Eastern Cooperative Oncology Group
EORTC	European Organization for Research and Treatment of Cancer
FACT-G	Functional Assessment of Cancer Therapy- General
FACT-L	Functional Assessment of Cancer Therapy- Lung
FDG	Fluorodeoxyglucose
FEV	Forced expiratory volume
FRS	Fractions
GY	Gray
IMRT	Intensity-modulated radiotherapy
KPS	Karnofsky performance status
LCS	Lung Cancer Subscale
LCT	Local control
LENT-SOMA	Late Effects Normal Tissue Task Force -Subjective, Objective, Management, Analytic scales
MeV	Million electron volts
mos	Months
N	Number
NA	Not applicable
NOS	Not otherwise specified Non–small-cell Lung Cancer
NR	Not reported
NSCLC	Non–small-cell lung cancer
OS	Overall Survival
PCS	Physical Component Summary
PDT	Photodynamic therapy
PS	Performance status
Pts	Patients
QLQ	Quality of life Questionnaire
QOL	Quality of life
RFA	Radiofrequency ablation
RT	Radiation Therapy
RTOG	Radiation Therapy Oncology Group
Rx	Treatment

SAS	Single arm study
SBRT	Stereotactic body radiotherapy
UICC	Union Internationale Contre le Cancer
WHO	World Health Organization
YAGL	Yttrium aluminum garnet laser

Appendix A. Search Strategy

The following electronic databases were searched by a medical librarian for citations:
- MEDLINE® (January 1995 to December 12, 2011) yielded 2883 records
- EMBASE® (January 1995 to December 13, 2011) yielded 1318 records
- Cochrane Controlled Trials Register (through December 13, 2011) yielded 99 records
- Search update of all three databases during peer review: (December 14, 2011-July 25, 2012) yielded 348 records

MEDLINE

Stage I

"Carcinoma, Non-Small-Cell Lung"[Mesh] OR ("Lung Neoplasms"[Mesh] OR "lung cancer")
AND ("non-small-cell" OR "non-small cell" OR "non small cell")
AND
"stage I" OR "stage one" OR "stage 1" OR T1N0M0 OR T2N0M0 OR early OR inoperable OR
unoperable OR nonoperable OR decline* OR refuse*
AND
"Brachytherapy"[Mesh] OR "Protons"[Mesh] OR "Radiotherapy, Intensity-Modulated"[Mesh]
OR "Radiotherapy, Conformal"[Mesh] OR "Ablation Techniques"[Mesh] OR
"Radiotherapy"[Mesh] OR "radiotherapy "[Subheading] OR "radiofrequency ablation" OR
(radiofrequency AND ablation) OR RFA OR radiotherapy OR radiation OR "external beam" OR
"3D conformal" OR "3-D Conformal" OR "intensity modulated radiotherapy" OR IMRT OR
brachytherapy OR "stereotactic radiotherapy" OR "stereotactic body radiotherapy" OR ("proton
beam" AND (radiation OR therapy OR radiotherapy))
AND
English language/Humans as limits

Advanced

"Carcinoma, Non-Small-Cell Lung"[Mesh] OR ("Lung Neoplasms"[Mesh] OR "lung cancer")
AND ("non-small-cell" OR "non-small cell" OR "non small cell")
AND
"stage III" OR "stage 3" OR "stage three" OR "stage IIIa" OR "stage IIIb" OR "stage IV" OR
"stage 4" OR "stage four" OR advanced
AND
"Brachytherapy"[Mesh] OR "Protons"[Mesh] OR "Radiotherapy, Intensity-Modulated"[Mesh]
OR "Radiotherapy, Conformal"[Mesh] OR "Ablation Techniques"[Mesh] OR
"Radiotherapy"[Mesh] OR "radiotherapy "[Subheading] OR "radiofrequency ablation" OR
(radiofrequency AND ablation) OR RFA OR radiotherapy OR radiation OR "external beam" OR
"intensity modulated radiotherapy" OR IMRT OR brachytherapy OR "stereotactic radiotherapy"
OR "stereotactic body radiotherapy" OR ("proton beam" AND (radiation OR therapy OR
radiotherapy)) OR "Stents"[Mesh] OR stent* OR (("Debridement"[Mesh] OR debridement)
AND (endoscopy OR endoscopic OR endobronchial))
AND
English language/Humans as limits

EMBASE

Stage I

'non-small-cell lung cancer'/exp OR ('lung neoplasms'/exp OR 'lung cancer'/exp AND ('non-small-cell' OR 'non-small cell' OR 'non small cell' OR nsclc))
AND
"stage I" OR "stage one" OR "stage 1" OR T1N0M0 OR T2N0M0 OR early OR inoperable OR unoperable OR nonoperable OR decline* OR refuse*
AND
"radiofrequency ablation" OR (radiofrequency AND ablation) OR RFA OR radiotherapy OR radiation OR "external beam" OR "3D conformal" OR "3-D Conformal" OR "intensity modulated radiotherapy" OR IMRT OR brachytherapy OR "stereotactic radiotherapy" OR "stereotactic body radiotherapy" OR ("proton beam" AND (radiation OR therapy OR radiotherapy))
AND
English language/Humans as limits
AND NOT MEDLINE

Advanced

'non-small-cell lung cancer'/exp OR ('lung neoplasms'/exp OR 'lung cancer'/exp AND ('non-small-cell' OR 'non-small cell' OR 'non small cell' OR nsclc))
AND
'stage iii' OR 'stage 3' OR 'stage three' OR 'stage iiia' OR 'stage iiib' OR 'stage iv' OR 'stage 4' OR 'stage four' OR advanced
AND
'radiofrequency ablation'/exp OR ('radiofrequency'/exp AND ablation) OR rfa OR 'radiotherapy'/exp OR 'radiation'/exp OR 'external beam' OR 'intensity modulated radiotherapy'/exp OR 'imrt'/exp OR 'brachytherapy'/exp OR 'stereotactic radiotherapy' OR 'stereotactic body radiotherapy'/exp OR ('proton beam'/exp AND ('radiation'/exp OR 'therapy'/exp OR 'radiotherapy'/exp)) OR stent* OR ('debridement'/exp AND ('endoscopy'/exp OR endoscopic OR endobronchial))
AND
English language/Humans as limits
AND NOT MEDLINE

COCHRANE

1. MeSH descriptor Carcinoma, Non-Small-Cell Lung explode all trees
2. (brachytherapy):ti,ab,kw or (radiotherapy):ti,ab,kw or (ablation):ti,ab,kw or (radiation):ti,ab,kw or (stereotactic):ti,ab,kw
3. (#1 AND #2)
4. (stent*):ti,ab,kw or (proton):ti,ab,kw or (radiofrequency):ti,ab,kw or (debridement):ti,ab,kw
5. ((#1 AND #4)
6. (#3 OR #5)

Search Strategy For Gray Literature

Regulatory Information

FDA (Drugs@FDA)

Source: http://www.accessdata.fda.gov/scripts/cdrh/cfdocs/cfpmn/pmn.cfm
Date searched: 5/30/12
Search strategy: "RF 3000," RF 3000 Radiofrequency Ablation System (Boston Scientific); "RITA StarBurst," RITA StarBurst Radiofrequency Ablation System (Angiodynamics (formerly RITA)); "Elektrotom 106," Berchtold Elektrotom 106 HFTT (Berchtold Corp.); "OncoSeed," OncoSeed(Oncura), "Best Iodine 125," Best Iodine-125 (Best Medical International, Inc); "Best Palladium 103 Seeds" Best Palladium-103 Seeds(Best Medical International, Inc.); "VariSource HDR afterloader," VariSource HDR afterloader (Varian Medical Systems); "GammaMedplus afterloader," GammaMedplus (Varian Medical Systems); "Clinac Linear Accelerator," Clinac Linear Accelerator(Varian Medical Systems); "Varian Trilogy system," Trilogy system (Varian Medical Systems); "Varian TrueBeam," TrueBeam (Varian Medical Systems); "Novalis," Novalis Tx (Varian Medical Systems); "ONCOR," ONCOR Impression & ONCOR Expression (Siemens Medical Solutions USA, Inc); "Primatom," Primatom (Siemens Medical Solutions USA, Inc); "Optivus PBTS," Proton Beam Therapy System (PBTS) (Optivus); "PT2 Varian Proton Therapy System," PT2 Varian Proton Therapy System (Varian Medical Systems); "Proteus One," Proteus One (IBA Particle Therapy); "Hood stent," Hood stent with rings (Hood Laboratories); "Plyflex stent, Ultraflex Metallic stents," Plyflex stent & Ultraflex Metallic stents (Boston Scientific); "Bryan Dumon," Bryan-Dumon Series II (Bryan Corporation); "Nd-YAG Laser," Nd-YAG Laser (Lee Laser Inc., Crystal Laser, & PowerTechnology Inc.)
Records: 0

Clinical Trial Registries

ClinicalTrials.gov

Source: http://clinicaltrials.gov/
Date searched: 5/30/12
Search strategy: ("NSCLC" OR "non-small cell") AND (("stage I") OR ("stage III" OR "stage IV")) | Closed Studies | Exclude Unknown | Phase 3, 4
Records: 81
Unpublished records: 1: NCT00687986

Conference Papers and Abstracts

- American Society of Clinical Oncology
- American Society for Radiation Oncology

Date searched: 5/30/12
Search strategy: ("NSCLC" OR "non-small cell") AND ("stage I" OR "stage III" OR "stage IV")
Records: 493

Manufacturer Database

Source: Covidien
Date posted: 5/24/12
Search strategy: Not applicable
Records: 95

Source: Accuray
Date posted: 5/24/12
Search strategy: Not applicable
Records: 74

Source: Elekta
Date posted: 5/24/12
Search strategy: Not applicable
Records: 11

Source: Loma Linda
Date posted: 5/24/12
Search strategy: Not applicable
Records: 5

Appendix B. Excluded Studies

Appendix Table B1. Key to study exclusion coding system

Code	Definition
FLA	Foreign language article
NRD	Not relevant design
NRP	Not relevant population
NRI	Not relevant intervention
NRO	Not relevant outcome
OPP	Overlapping patient population
USD	Unclear study description
UTO	Unable to obtain full text

Abacioglu, P. F. Yumuk, H. Caglar, M. Sengoz and N. S. Turhal. Concurrent chemoradiotherapy with low dose weekly gemcitabine in stage III non-small cell lung cancer. BMC Cancer 2005 5(): 71. NRP

Abe, J. Takahashi, H. Fukuda, S. Ono, S. Yoshioka, T. Akaizawa, K. Kubota, K. Yamada, T. Takahashi, K. Ohkuda, N. Asoh, M. Yonechi, N. Maehira, Y. Mariya and M. Aoki. A phase II study of cisplatin, oral administration of etoposide, OK-432 and radiation therapy for inoperable stage III non-small cell lung cancer. International Journal of Clinical Oncology 1998 3(6): 365-369. NRP

Abratt, L. J. Shepherd and D. G. Salton. Palliative radiation for stage 3 non-small cell lung cancer--a prospective study of two moderately high dose regimens. Lung Cancer 1995 13(2): 137-43. NRP

Adelstein, T. W. Rice, L. A. Rybicki, J. F. Greskovich, Jr., J. P. Ciezki, M. A. Carroll and M. M. DeCamp. Accelerated hyperfractionated radiation, concurrent paclitaxel/cisplatin chemotherapy and surgery for stage III non-small cell lung cancer. Lung Cancer 2002 36(2): 167-74. NRP

Adkison, D. Khuntia, S. M. Bentzen, G. M. Cannon, W. A. Tome, H. Jaradat, W. Walker, A. M. Traynor, T. Weigel and M. P. Mehta. Dose escalated, hypofractionated radiotherapy using helical tomotherapy for inoperable non-small cell lung cancer: preliminary results of a risk-stratified phase I dose escalation study. Technol Cancer Res Treat 2008 7(6): 441-7. NRI

Aerts, A. A. van Baardwijk, S. F. Petit, C. Offermann, J. Loon, R. Houben, A. M. Dingemans, R. Wanders, L. Boersma, J. Borger, G. Bootsma, W. Geraedts, C. Pitz, J. Simons, B. G. Wouters, M. Oellers, P. Lambin, G. Bosmans, A. L. Dekker and D. De Ruysscher. Identification of residual metabolic-active areas within individual NSCLC tumours using a pre-radiotherapy (18)Fluorodeoxyglucose-PET-CT scan. Radiother Oncol 2009 91(3): 386-92. NRO

Aerts, V. Surmont, R. J. van Klaveren, K. Y. Tan, S. Senan, G. van Wijhe, R. Vernhout, G. T. Verhoeven, H. C. Hoogsteden and J. P. van Meerbeeck. A phase II study of induction therapy with carboplatin and gemcitabine among patients with locally advanced non-small cell lung cancer. J Thorac Oncol 2006 1(6): 532-6. NRP

Ahmad, A. P. Sandhu, M. M. Fuster, K. Messer, M. Pu, P. Nobiensky, L. Bazhenova and S. Seagren. Hypofractionated radiotherapy as definitive treatment of stage I non-small cell lung cancer in older patients. Am J Clin Oncol 2011 34(3): 254-8. NRI

Ahmed, J. Bedford, J. Warrington and M. Hawkins. Volumetric modulated arc radiotherapy (VMAT) of tumours in the thorax-acute toxicity results from a single centre. Radiotherapy and Oncology 2011 99(): S499. NRD

Ahn, K. Park, D. Y. Kim, K. M. Kim, J. Kim, Y. M. Shim, K. S. Lee, J. Han, H. J. Kim, J. Kwon, D. H. Lim, Y. J. Noh, J. E. Lee and S. J. Huh. Preoperative concurrent chemoradiotherapy for stage IIIA non-small cell lung cancer. Acta Oncol 2001 40(5): 588-92. NRP

Ahn, M. S. Han, J. H. Yoon, S. Y. Jeon, C. H. Kim, H. J. Yoo and J. C. Lee. Treatment of stage I non-small cell lung cancer with CyberKnife, image-guided robotic stereotactic radiosurgery. Oncol Rep 2009 21(3): 693-6. NRO

Ahn, Y. C. Kim, K. S. Kim, K. O. Park, W. K. Chung, T. K. Nam, B. S. Nah, J. Y. Song and M. S. Yoon. Results of curative radiation therapy with or without chemotherapy for stage III unresectable non-small cell lung cancer. Cancer Res Treat 2005 37(5): 268-72. NRP

Aich, K. Bhattacharaya, P. Gupta and P. K. Sur. Hypofractionated radiotherapy (MRC trial) - A preferred schedule for locally advanced non-small cell lung cancers. Indian Journal of Radiology and Imaging 1998 8(3): 177-181. UTO

Aisner, C. P. Belani, C. Kearns, B. Conley, D. Hiponia, C. Engstrom, E. Zuhowski and M. J. Egorin. Feasibility and pharmacokinetics of paclitaxel, carboplatin, and concurrent radiotherapy for regionally advanced squamous cell carcinoma of the head and neck and for regionally advanced non-small cell lung cancer. Semin Oncol 1995 22(5 Suppl 12): 17-21. NRP

Ajlouni, R. Chapman and J. H. Kim. Accelerated-interrupted radiation therapy given concurrently with chemotherapy for locally advanced non-small cell lung cancer. Cancer J Sci Am 1996 2(6): 314-20. NRP

Akerley and H. Choy. Concurrent paclitaxel and thoracic radiation for advanced non-small cell lung cancer. Lung Cancer 1995 12 Suppl 2(): S107-15. NRP

Akerley and H. Choy. Single-agent paclitaxel and radiation for non-small cell lung cancer. Semin Radiat Oncol 1999 9(2 Suppl 1): 85-9. NRP

Akerley, J. E. Herndon, Jr., A. P. Lyss, H. Choy, A. Turrisi, S. Graziano, T. Williams, C. Zhang, E. E. Vokes and M. R. Green. Induction paclitaxel/carboplatin followed by concurrent chemoradiation therapy for unresectable stage III non-small-cell lung cancer: a limited-access study--CALGB 9534. Clin Lung Cancer 2005 7(1): 47-53. NRP

Albain, J. J. Crowley, A. T. Turrisi, 3rd, D. R. Gandara, W. B. Farrar, J. I. Clark, K. R. Beasley and R. B. Livingston. Concurrent cisplatin, etoposide, and chest radiotherapy in pathologic stage IIIB non-small-cell lung cancer: a Southwest Oncology Group phase II study, SWOG 9019. J Clin Oncol 2002 20(16): 3454-60. NRP

Albain, R. S. Swann, V. W. Rusch, A. T. Turrisi, 3rd, F. A. Shepherd, C. Smith, Y. Chen, R. B. Livingston, R. H. Feins, D. R. Gandara, W. A. Fry, G. Darling, D. H. Johnson, M. R. Green, R. C. Miller, J. Ley, W. T. Sause and J. D. Cox. Radiotherapy plus chemotherapy with or without surgical resection for stage III non-small-cell lung cancer: a phase III randomised controlled trial. Lancet 2009 374(9687): 379-86. NRP

Albain, V. W. Rusch, J. J. Crowley, T. W. Rice, A. T. Turrisi, 3rd, J. K. Weick, V. A. Lonchyna, C. A. Presant, R. J. McKenna, D. R. Gandara and et al.. Concurrent cisplatin/etoposide plus chest radiotherapy followed by surgery for stages IIIA (N2) and IIIB non-small-cell lung cancer: mature results of Southwest Oncology Group phase II study 8805. J Clin Oncol 1995 13(8): 1880-92. NRP

Alberto, R. O. Mirimanoff, B. Mermillod, S. Leyvraz, H. Nagy-Mignotte, M. Bolla, D. Wellmann, D. Moro and E. Brambilla. Rapidly alternating combination of cisplatin-based chemotherapy and hyperfractionated accelerated radiotherapy in split course for stage IIIA and stage IIIB non-small cell lung cancer: results of a phase I-II study by the GOTHA group. Group d'Oncologie Thoracique des Regions Alpines. Eur J Cancer 1995 31A(3): 342-8. NRP

Alexander, M. Othus, H. B. Caglar and A. M. Allen. Tumor volume is a prognostic factor in non-small-cell lung cancer treated with chemoradiotherapy. Int J Radiat Oncol Biol Phys 2011 79(5): 1381-7. NRP

Ali, M. J. Kraut, M. Valdivieso, A. J. Wozniak, G. Cummings and G. P. Kalemkerian. A phase II study of mitomycin C, etoposide, and cisplatin in advanced non-small cell lung cancer. Cancer Invest 2000 18(1): 1-5. NRP

Allison, A. Schulsinger, K. H. Shin and V. Vongtama. Chemoradiation enhances response in stage IIIB lung cancer. Radiation Oncology Investigations 1996 4(4): 171-175. NRP

Ambrogi, O. Fanucchi, R. Cioni, P. Dini, A. De Liperi, C. Cappelli, F. Davini, C. Bartolozzi and A. Mussi. Long-Term Results of Radiofrequency Ablation Treatment of Stage I Non-small Cell Lung Cancer: A Prospective Intention-to-Treat Study. J Thorac Oncol 2011 6(12): 2044-51. NRP

Ambrogi, P. Dini, F. Melfi and A. Mussi. Radiofrequency ablation of inoperable non-small cell lung cancer. J Thorac Oncol 2007 2(5 Suppl): S2-3. NRP

Ampil and S. V. Sanghani. Timing of radiotherapy in asymptomatic patients with inoperable non-small cell lung cancer: a survival analysis and literature review. Radiat Med 1996 14(4): 211-4. NRP

Anacak, N. Mogulkoc, S. Ozkok, T. Goksel, A. Haydaroglu and U. Bayindir. High dose rate endobronchial brachytherapy in combination with external beam radiotherapy for stage III non-small cell lung cancer. Lung Cancer 2001 34(2): 253-9. NRP

Anderson, J. J. McAleer, S. Stranex and G. Prescott. Radical radiotherapy for inoperable non-small cell lung cancer: what factors predict prognosis?. Clin Oncol (R Coll Radiol) 2000 12(1): 48-52. NRI

Anderson, P. Hopwood, R. J. Stephens, N. Thatcher, B. Cottier, M. Nicholson, R. Milroy, T. S. Maughan, S. J. Falk, M. G. Bond, P. A. Burt, C. K. Connolly, M. B. McIllmurray and J. Carmichael. Gemcitabine plus best supportive care (BSC) vs BSC in inoperable non-small cell lung cancer--a randomized trial with quality of life as the primary outcome. UK NSCLC Gemcitabine Group. Non-Small Cell Lung Cancer. Br J Cancer 2000 83(4): 447-53. NRP

Anku. Successful low-dose concurrent chemotherapy and radiation for locally advanced or inoperable non-small cell lung carcinoma: a report of six cases. J Natl Med Assoc 2000 92(3): 105-15. NRD

Anscher, J. Garst, L. B. Marks, N. Larrier, F. Dunphy, J. E. Herndon, 2nd, R. Clough, C. Marino, Z. Vujaskovic, S. Zhou, M. W. Dewhirst, T. D. Shafman and J. Crawford. Assessing the ability of the antiangiogenic and anticytokine agent thalidomide to modulate radiation-induced lung injury. Int J Radiat Oncol Biol Phys 2006 66(2): 477-82. NRP

Anscher, L. B. Marks, T. D. Shafman, R. Clough, H. Huang, A. Tisch, M. Munley, J. E. Herndon, J. Garst, J. Crawford and R. L. Jirtle. Risk of long-term complications after TFG-beta1-guided very-high-dose thoracic radiotherapy. Int J Radiat Oncol Biol Phys 2003 56(4): 988-95. NRP

Anton, N. Diaz-Fernandez, J. L. Gonzalez Larriba, C. Vadell, B. Masutti, J. Montalar, I. Barneto, A. Artal and R. Rosell. Phase II trial assessing the combination of gemcitabine and cisplatin in advanced non-small cell lung cancer (NSCLC). Lung Cancer 1998 22(2): 139-48. NRP

Antonadou, N. Throuvalas, A. Petridis, N. Bolanos, A. Sagriotis and M. Synodinou. Effect of amifostine on toxicities associated with radiochemotherapy in patients with locally advanced non-small-cell lung cancer. Int J Radiat Oncol Biol Phys 2003 57(2): 402-8. NRP

Antonadou. Radiotherapy or chemotherapy followed by radiotherapy with or without amifostine in locally advanced lung cancer. Semin Radiat Oncol 2002 12(1 Suppl 1): 50-8. NRP

Antonia, H. Wagner, C. Williams, M. Alberts, D. Hubbell, L. Robinson, J. Hilstro and J. C. Ruckdeschel. Concurrent paclitaxel/cisplatin with thoracic radiation in patients with stage IIIA/B non-small cell carcinoma of the lung. Semin Oncol 1995 22(4 Suppl 9): 34-7. NRP

Ardizzoni, F. Grossi, T. Scolaro, S. Giudici, F. Foppiano, L. Boni, L. Tixi, M. Cosso, C. Mereu, G. B. Ratto, V. Vitale and R. Rosso. Induction chemotherapy followed by concurrent standard radiotherapy and daily low-dose cisplatin in locally advanced non-small-cell lung cancer. Br J Cancer 1999 81(2): 310-5. NRP

Argiris, M. Liptay, M. LaCombe, M. Marymont, M. S. Kies, S. Sundaresan and G. Masters. A phase I/II trial of induction chemotherapy with carboplatin and gemcitabine followed by concurrent vinorelbine and paclitaxel with chest radiation in patients with stage III non-small cell lung cancer. Lung Cancer 2004 45(2): 243-53. NRP

Aristu, J. Rebollo, R. Martinez-Monge, J. M. Aramendia, J. C. Viera, I. Azinovic, J. Herreros and A. Brugarolas. Cisplatin, mitomycin, and vindesine followed by intraoperative and postoperative radiotherapy for stage III non-small cell lung cancer: final results of a phase II study. Am J Clin Oncol 1997 20(3): 276-81. NRP

Armstrong, A. Raben, M. Zelefsky, M. Burt, S. Leibel, C. Burman, G. Kutcher, L. Harrison, C. Hahn, R. Ginsberg, V. Rusch, M. Kris and Z. Fuks. Promising survival with three-dimensional conformal radiation therapy for non-small cell lung cancer. Radiother Oncol 1997 44(1): 17-22. NRP

Armstrong, M. J. Zelefsky, S. A. Leibel, C. Burman, C. Han, L. B. Harrison, G. J. Kutcher and Z. Y. Fuks. Strategy for dose escalation using 3-dimensional conformal radiation therapy for lung cancer. Ann Oncol 1995 6(7): 693-7. NRP

Arpin, D. Perol, J. Y. Blay, L. Falchero, L. Claude, S. Vuillermoz-Blas, I. Martel-Lafay, C. Ginestet, L. Alberti, D. Nosov, B. Etienne-Mastroianni, V. Cottin, M. Perol, J. C. Guerin, J. F. Cordier and C. Carrie. Early variations of circulating interleukin-6 and interleukin-10 levels during thoracic radiotherapy are predictive for radiation pneumonitis. J Clin Oncol 2005 23(34): 8748-56. NRP

Arrieta, D. Gallardo-Rincon, C. Villarreal-Garza, R. M. Michel, A. M. Astorga-Ramos, L. Martinez-Barrera and J. de la Garza. High frequency of radiation pneumonitis in patients with locally advanced non-small cell lung cancer treated with concurrent radiotherapy and gemcitabine after induction with gemcitabine and carboplatin. J Thorac Oncol 2009 4(7): 845-52. NRP

Atagi, M. Kawahara, A. Yokoyama, H. Okamoto, N. Yamamoto, Y. Ohe, S. Ishikura, H. Fukuda, N. Saijo and T. Tamura. Standard thoracic radiotherapy with or without concurrent daily low-dose carboplatin in elderly patients with locally advanced non-small cell lung cancer - A phase III trial of the Japan clinical oncology group (JCOG0301). European Journal of Cancer 2011 47(): S273. NRD

Atagi, M. Kawahara, M. Ogawara, K. Matsui, N. Masuda, S. Kudoh, S. Negoro and K. Furuse. Phase II trial of daily low-dose carboplatin and thoracic radiotherapy in elderly patients with locally advanced non-small cell lung cancer. Jpn J Clin Oncol 2000 30(2): 59-64. NRI

Atagi, M. Kawahara, S. Hosoe, M. Ogawara, T. Kawaguchi, K. Okishio, N. Naka, T. Sunami, S. Mitsuoka and M. Akira. A phase II study of continuous concurrent thoracic radiotherapy in combination with mitomycin, vindesine and cisplatin in unresectable stage III non-small cell lung cancer. Lung Cancer 2002 36(1): 105-11. NRP

Atagi, M. Kawahara, T. Tamura, K. Noda, K. Watanabe, A. Yokoyama, T. Sugiura, H. Senba, S. Ishikura, H. Ikeda, N. Ishizuka and N. Saijo. Standard thoracic radiotherapy with or without concurrent daily low-dose carboplatin in elderly patients with locally advanced non-small cell lung cancer: a phase III trial of the Japan Clinical Oncology Group (JCOG9812). Jpn J Clin Oncol 2005 35(4): 195-201. NRP

Auchter, D. Scholtens, S. Adak, H. Wagner, D. F. Cella and M. P. Mehta. Quality of life assessment in advanced non-small-cell lung cancer patients undergoing an accelerated radiotherapy regimen: report of ECOG study 4593. Eastern Cooperative Oncology Group. Int J Radiat Oncol Biol Phys 2001 50(5): 1199-206. NRP

Aviram, E. Yu, P. Tai and M. S. Lefcoe. Computed tomography to assess pulmonary injury associated with concurrent chemo-radiotherapy for inoperable non-small cell lung cancer. Can Assoc Radiol J 2001 52(6): 385-91. NRP

Aydiner, F. Sen, E. K. Saglam, E. N. Oral, Y. Eralp, F. Tas, A. Toker and S. Dilege. Induction chemotherapy with triweekly docetaxel and cisplatin followed by concomitant chemoradiotherapy with or without surgery in stage III non-small-cell lung cancer: a phase II study. Clin Lung Cancer 2011 12(5): 286-92. NRP

Baba, Y. Shibamoto, H. Ogino, R. Murata, C. Sugie, H. Iwata, S. Otsuka, K. Kosaki, A. Nagai, T. Murai and A. Miyakawa. Clinical outcomes of stereotactic body radiotherapy for stage I non-small cell lung cancer using different doses depending on tumor size. Radiat Oncol 2010 5(): 81. USD

Baba, Y. Shibamoto, N. Tomita, C. Ikeya-Hashizume, K. Oda, S. Ayakawa, H. Ogino and C. Sugie. Stereotactic body radiotherapy for stage I lung cancer and small lung metastasis: evaluation of an immobilization system for suppression of respiratory tumor movement and preliminary results. Radiat Oncol 2009 4(): 15. OPP

Bahri, J. C. Flickinger, A. M. Kalend, M. Deutsch, C. P. Belani, F. C. Sciurba, J. D. Luketich and J. S. Greenberger. Results of multifield conformal radiation therapy of nonsmall-cell lung carcinoma using multileaf collimation beams. Radiat Oncol Investig 1999 7(5): 297-308. NRP

Bailey, M. K. Parmar and R. J. Stephens. Patient-reported short-term and long-term physical and psychologic symptoms: results of the continuous hyperfractionated accelerated correction of acclerated radiotherapy (CHART) randomized trial in non-small-cell lung cancer. CHART Steering Committee. 1998 16(): 3082-93. NRP

Baisden, D. A. Romney, A. G. Reish, J. Cai, K. Sheng, D. R. Jones, S. H. Benedict, P. W. Read and J. M. Larner. Dose as a function of lung volume and planned treatment volume in helical tomotherapy intensity-modulated radiation therapy-based stereotactic body radiation therapy for small lung tumors. Int J Radiat Oncol Biol Phys 2007 68(4): 1229-37. NRP

Baka, C. Faivre-Finn, P. Papakotoulas, F. Blackhall, H. Anderson, P. Lorigan and N. Thatcher. Platinum-based chemotherapy with thoracic radiotherapy in stage III good performance status non-small cell lung cancer patients. European Journal of Cancer, Supplement 2005 3(3): 41-50. NRD

Bakitas, K. D. Lyons, M. T. Hegel, S. Balan, F. C. Brokaw, J. Seville, J. G. Hull, Z. Li, T. D. Tosteson, I. R. Byock and T. A. Ahles. Effects of a palliative care intervention on clinical outcomes in patients with advanced cancer: The project ENABLE II randomized controlled trial. JAMA - Journal of the American Medical Association 2009 302(7): 741-749. NRP

Baldini, G. Silvano, C. Tibaldi, S. Campoccia, L. Cionini and P. Conte. Sequential chemoradiation therapy with vinorelbine, ifosfamide, and cisplatin in stage IIIB non-small cell lung cancer: a phase II study. Semin Oncol 2000 27(1 Suppl 1): 28-32. NRP

Ball, J. Bishop, J. Smith, E. Crennan, P. O'Brien, S. Davis, G. Ryan, D. Joseph and Q. Walker. A phase III study of accelerated radiotherapy with and without carboplatin in nonsmall cell lung cancer: an interim toxicity analysis of the first 100 patients. 1995 31(): 267-72. NRI

Ball, J. Bishop, J. Smith, P. O'Brien, S. Davis, G. Ryan, I. Olver, G. Toner, Q. Walker and D. Joseph. A randomised phase III study of accelerated or standard fraction radiotherapy with or without concurrent carboplatin in inoperable non-small cell lung cancer: final report of an Australian multi-centre trial. Radiother Oncol 1999 52(2): 129-36. NRI

Ball, J. Smith, A. Wirth and M. Mac Manus. Failure of T stage to predict survival in patients with non-small-cell lung cancer treated by radiotherapy with or without concomitant chemotherapy. 2002 54(): 1007-13. NRI

Ball, J. Smith, J. Bishop, I. Olver, S. Davis, P. O'Brien, D. Bernshaw, G. Ryan and M. Millward. A phase III study of radiotherapy with and without continuous-infusion fluorouracil as palliation for non-small-cell lung cancer. Br J Cancer 1997 75(5): 690-7. NRP

Ball, M. Y. Lin, M. Wu, R. Fisher, S. Brennan, M. P. Campeau, D. Binns, M. P. MacManus, B. Solomon and R. J. Hicks. Absence of a relationship between 18F-fluoro-deoxglucose (FDG) uptake and survival in non-small cell lung cancer patients treated with radical radiotherapy or concomitatnt chemoradiotherapy. Journal of Thoracic Oncology 2011 6(3): S15-S16. NRD

Bardet, A. Riviere, A. Charloux, D. Spaeth, A. Ducolone, A. Le Groumellec, B. Pellae-Cosset, M. Henry-Amar and J. Y. Douillard. A phase II trial of radiochemotherapy with daily carboplatin, after induction chemotherapy (carboplatin and etoposide), in locally advanced nonsmall-cell lung cancer: final analysis. Int J Radiat Oncol Biol Phys 1997 38(1): 163-8. NRP

Barone, D. C. Corsi, C. Pozzo, A. Cassano, G. Alvaro, G. Colloca, M. Landriscina and A. Astone. Vinorelbine and alternating cisplatin and ifosfamide in the treatment of non-small cell lung cancer. Oncology 2000 58(1): 25-30. NRP

Barriger, A. J. Fakiris, N. Hanna, M. Yu, P. Mantravadi and R. C. McGarry. Dose-volume analysis of radiation pneumonitis in non-small-cell lung cancer patients treated with concurrent cisplatinum and etoposide with or without consolidation docetaxel. Int J Radiat Oncol Biol Phys 2010 78(5): 1381-6. NRP

Barriger, J. A. Forquer, J. G. Brabham, D. L. Andolino, R. H. Shapiro, M. A. Henderson, P. A. Johnstone and A. J. Fakiris. A Dose-Volume Analysis of Radiation Pneumonitis in Non-Small Cell Lung Cancer Patients Treated with Stereotactic Body Radiation Therapy. Int J Radiat Oncol Biol Phys 2010 82(1):457-63. NRI, USD

Basaki, Y. Abe, M. Aoki, H. Kondo, Y. Hatayama and S. Nakaji. Prognostic factors for survival in stage III non-small-cell lung cancer treated with definitive radiation therapy: impact of tumor volume. Int J Radiat Oncol Biol Phys 2006 64(2): 449-54. NRP

Bastos, G. F. Hatoum, G. R. Walker, K. Tolba, C. Takita, J. Gomez, E. S. Santos, G. Lopes and L. E. Raez. Efficacy and toxicity of chemoradiotherapy with carboplatin and irinotecan followed by consolidation docetaxel for unresectable stage III non-small cell lung cancer. J Thorac Oncol 2010 5(4): 533-9. NRP

Baumann, J. Nyman, M. Hoyer, G. Gagliardi, I. Lax, B. Wennberg, N. Drugge, L. Ekberg, S. Friesland, K. A. Johansson, J. S. Lund, E. Morhed, K. Nilsson, N. Levin, M. Paludan, C. Sederholm, A. Traberg, L. Wittgren and R. Lewensohn. Stereotactic body radiotherapy for medically inoperable patients with stage I non-small cell lung cancer - a first report of toxicity related to COPD/CVD in a non-randomized prospective phase II study. Radiother Oncol 2008 88(3): 359-67. OPP

Baumann, T. Herrmann, R. Koch, W. Matthiessen, S. Appold, B. Wahlers, L. Kepka, G. Marschke, D. Feltl, R. Fietkau, V. Budach, J. Dunst, R. Dziadziuszko, M. Krause and D. Zips. Final results of the randomized phase III CHARTWEL-trial (ARO 97-1) comparing hyperfractionated-accelerated versus conventionally fractionated radiotherapy in non-small cell lung cancer (NSCLC). Radiother Oncol 2011 100(1): 76-85. USD

Bebb, C. Smith, S. Rorke, W. Boland, L. Nicacio, R. Sukhoo and A. Brade. Phase I clinical trial of the anti-EGFR monoclonal antibody nimotuzumab with concurrent external thoracic radiotherapy in Canadian patients diagnosed with stage IIb, III or IV non-small cell lung cancer unsuitable for radical therapy. Cancer Chemother Pharmacol 2011 67(4): 837-45. NRP

Beckmann, R. Fietkau, R. M. Huber, P. Kleine, M. Schmidt, S. Semrau, D. Aubert, A. Fittipaldo and M. Flentje. Oral vinorelbine and cisplatin with concomitant radiotherapy in stage III non-small cell lung cancer (NSCLC): a feasibility study. Onkologie 2006 29(4): 137-42. NRP

Bedini, L. Tavecchio, A. Gramaglia, S. Villa and M. Palazzi. Radiotherapy and concurrent continuous infusion of cisplatin with adjuvant surgery in nonresectable Stage III lung carcinoma: short- and long-term results of a Phase II study. Int J Radiat Oncol Biol Phys 1999 45(3): 613-21. NRP

Beitler, E. A. Badine, D. El-Sayah, D. Makara, P. Friscia, P. Silverman and T. Terjanian. Stereotactic body radiation therapy for nonmetastatic lung cancer: an analysis of 75 patients treated over 5 years. Int J Radiat Oncol Biol Phys 2006 65(1): 100-6. NRP

Belani and R. K. Ramanathan. Combined-modality treatment of locally advanced non-small cell lung cancer: incorporation of novel chemotherapeutic agents. Chest 1998 113(1 Suppl): 53S-60S. NRD

Belani, H. Choy, P. Bonomi, C. Scott, P. Travis, J. Haluschak and W. J. Curran, Jr.. Combined chemoradiotherapy regimens of paclitaxel and carboplatin for locally advanced non-small-cell lung cancer: a randomized phase II locally advanced multi-modality protocol. J Clin Oncol 2005 23(25): 5883-91. NRP

Belani, J. Aisner, R. Ramanathan, J. Jett, J. Greenberger, R. Day, M. J. Capazolli, D. Hiponia and C. Engstrom. Paclitaxel and carboplatin with simultaneous thoracic irradiation in regionally advanced non-small cell lung cancer. Seminars in Radiation Oncology 1997 7(2 SUPPL. 1): S1-11-S1-14. NRP

Belani, W. Wang, D. H. Johnson, H. Wagner, J. Schiller, M. Veeder and M. Mehta. Phase III study of the Eastern Cooperative Oncology Group (ECOG 2597): induction chemotherapy followed by either standard thoracic radiotherapy or hyperfractionated accelerated radiotherapy for patients with unresectable stage IIIA and B non-small-cell lung cancer. J Clin Oncol 2005 23(16): 3760-7. NRP

Belderbos, K. De Jaeger, W. D. Heemsbergen, Y. Seppenwoolde, P. Baas, L. J. Boersma and J. V. Lebesque. First results of a phase I/II dose escalation trial in non-small cell lung cancer using three-dimensional conformal radiotherapy. Radiother Oncol 2003 66(2): 119-26. USD

Belderbos, L. Uitterhoeve, N. van Zandwijk, H. Belderbos, P. Rodrigus, P. van de Vaart, A. Price, N. van Walree, C. Legrand, S. Dussenne, H. Bartelink, G. Giaccone and C. Koning. Randomised trial of sequential versus concurrent chemo-radiotherapy in patients with inoperable non-small cell lung cancer (EORTC 08972-22973). Eur J Cancer 2007 43(1): 114-21. NRI

Belderbos, W. D. Heemsbergen, K. De Jaeger, P. Baas and J. V. Lebesque. Final results of a Phase I/II dose escalation trial in non-small-cell lung cancer using three-dimensional conformal radiotherapy. Int J Radiat Oncol Biol Phys 2006 66(1): 126-34. USD

Belderbos, W. Heemsbergen, M. Hoogeman, K. Pengel, M. Rossi and J. Lebesque. Acute esophageal toxicity in non-small cell lung cancer patients after high dose conformal radiotherapy. Radiother Oncol 2005 75(2): 157-64. USD

Belliere, N. Girard, O. Chapet, M. Khodri, A. Kubas, P. J. Souquet and F. Mornex. Feasibility of high-dose three-dimensional radiation therapy in the treatment of localised non-small-cell lung cancer. Cancer Radiother 2009 13(4): 298-304. NRP

Beltramo, A. Bergantin, A. Martinotti, P. Bonfanti and L. C. Bianchi. Stereotactic body ablative radiotherapy for stage I non small cell lung cancer. Radiotherapy and Oncology 2011 99(): S570-S571. NRD

Bepler, T. J. Dilling, H. Wagner, T. Hazelton, C. Williams, D. T. Chen, H. Greenberg, F. Walsh, G. Simon, T. Tanvetyanon, A. Chiappori, E. Haura and C. Stevens. Phase II trial of induction gemcitabine and carboplatin followed by conformal thoracic radiation to 74 Gy with weekly paclitaxel and carboplatin in unresectable stage III non-small cell lung cancer. J Thorac Oncol 2011 6(3): 553-8. NRP

Berghmans, P. Van Houtte, M. Paesmans, V. Giner, J. Lecomte, G. Koumakis, M. Richez, S. Holbrechts, M. Roelandts, A. P. Meert, S. Alard, N. Leclercq and J. P. Sculier. A phase III randomised study comparing concomitant radiochemotherapy as induction versus consolidation treatment in patients with locally advanced unresectable non-small cell lung cancer. Lung Cancer 2009 64(2): 187-93. NRP

Bernier, J. Denekamp, A. Rojas, M. Trovo, J. C. Horiot, H. Hamers, P. Antognoni, O. Dahl, P. Richaud, J. Kaanders, M. van Glabbeke and M. Pierart. ARCON: accelerated radiotherapy with carbogen and nicotinamide in non small cell lung cancer: a phase I/II study by the EORTC. Radiother Oncol 1999 52(2): 149-56. NRP

Beslija, Z. Dizdarevic, J. Lomigoric, H. Zutic, M. Musanovic, B. Mehic, A. Cardjic, B. Paralija and N. Obralic. Randomized phase II study of induction chemotherapy with gemcitabine plus cisplatin followed by sequential radiotherapy versus radiotherapy alone in patients with stage III non-small cell lung cancer. J BUON 2005 10(3): 347-55. NRP

Bezjak, P. Dixon, M. Brundage, D. Tu, M. J. Palmer, P. Blood, C. Grafton, C. Lochrin, C. Leong, L. Mulroy, C. Smith, J. Wright and J. L. Pater. Randomized phase III trial of single versus fractionated thoracic radiation in the palliation of patients with lung cancer (NCIC CTG SC.15). Int J Radiat Oncol Biol Phys 2002 54(3): 719-28. NRP

Bhatia, N. Hanna, R. Ansari, L. Einhorn and A. Sandler. Carboplatin plus paclitaxel and sequential radiation followed by consolidation carboplatin and paclitaxel in patients with previously untreated locally advanced NSCLC. A Hoosier Oncology Group (HOG) phase II study. Lung Cancer 2002 38(1): 85-9. NRP

Bhatnagar, J. C. Flickinger, S. Bahri, M. Deutsch, C. Belani, J. D. Luketich and J. S. Greenberger. Update on results of multifield conformal radiation therapy of non-small-cell lung cancer using multileaf collimated beams. Clin Lung Cancer 2002 3(4): 259-64. NRP

Bhatt, B. K. Mohani, L. Kumar, S. Chawla, D. N. Sharma and G. K. Rath. Palliative treatment of advanced non small cell lung cancer with weekly fraction radiotherapy. Indian J Cancer 2000 37(4): 148-52. NRP

Bi, M. Yang, L. Zhang, X. Chen, W. Ji, G. Ou, D. Lin and L. Wang. Cyclooxygenase-2 genetic variants are associated with survival in unresectable locally advanced non-small cell lung cancer. Clin Cancer Res 2010 16(8): 2383-90. NRP

Biedermann, C. Landmann, R. Kann, J. Passweg, M. Soler, A. Lohri, C. Rochlitz, R. Herrmann and M. Pless. Combined chemoradiotherapy with daily low-dose cisplatin in locally advanced inoperable non-small cell lung cancer. Radiother Oncol 2000 56(2): 169-73. NRI

Birim, A. P. Kappetein, T. Goorden, R. J. van Klaveren and A. J. Bogers. Proper treatment selection may improve survival in patients with clinical early-stage nonsmall cell lung cancer. Ann Thorac Surg 2005 80(3): 1021-6. NRI

Bishawi, B. Kim, W. H. Moore and T. V. Bilfinger. Pulmonary Function Testing After Stereotactic Body Radiotherapy to the Lung. Int J Radiat Oncol Biol Phys 2011 (): . NRO

Blackstock, C. Ho, J. Butler, J. Fletcher-Steede, L. D. Case, W. Hinson and A. A. Miller. Phase Ia/Ib chemo-radiation trial of gemcitabine and dose-escalated thoracic radiation in patients with stage III A/B non-small cell lung cancer. J Thorac Oncol 2006 1(5): 434-40. NRP

Blackstock, G. J. Lesser, J. Fletcher-Steede, L. D. Case, R. W. Tucker, S. M. Russo, D. R. White and A. Miller. Phase I study of twice-weekly gemcitabine and concurrent thoracic radiation for patients with locally advanced non-small-cell lung cancer. Int J Radiat Oncol Biol Phys 2001 51(5): 1281-9. NRP

Blanco, J. Sole, J. Montesinos, C. Mesia, M. Algara, J. Terrassa, M. Gay, M. Domenech, R. Bastus, I. Bover, M. Nogue and C. Vadell. Induction chemotherapy with cisplatin and gemcitabine followed by concurrent chemoradiation with twice-weekly gemcitabine in unresectable stage III non-small cell lung cancer: final results of a phase II study. Lung Cancer 2008 62(1): 62-71. NRP

Blanke, R. Ansari, R. Mantravadi, R. Gonin, R. Tokars, W. Fisher, K. Pennington, T. O'Connor, S. Rynard, M. Miller and et al.. Phase III trial of thoracic irradiation with or without cisplatin for locally advanced unresectable non-small-cell lung cancer: a Hoosier Oncology Group protocol. J Clin Oncol 1995 13(6): 1425-9. NRI

Blanke, R. DeVore, Y. Shyr, B. Epstein, M. Murray, K. Hande, S. Stewart and D. Johnson. A pilot study of protracted low dose cisplatin and etoposide with concurrent thoracic radiotherapy in unresectable stage III nonsmall cell lung cancer. Int J Radiat Oncol Biol Phys 1997 37(1): 111-6. NRP

Blumenschein, Jr., R. Paulus, W. J. Curran, F. Robert, F. Fossella, M. Werner-Wasik, R. S. Herbst, P. O. Doescher, H. Choy and R. Komaki. Phase II study of cetuximab in combination with chemoradiation in patients with stage IIIA/B non-small-cell lung cancer: RTOG 0324. J Clin Oncol 2011 29(17): 2312-8. NRP

Bogart and R. Govindan. A randomized phase II study of radiation therapy, pemetrexed, and carboplatin with or without cetuximab in stage III non-small-cell lung cancer. Clin Lung Cancer 2006 7(4): 285-7. NRP

Bogart, T. E. Alpert, M. C. Kilpatrick, B. L. Keshler, S. S. Pohar, H. Shah, E. Dexter and J. N. Aronowitz. Dose-intensive thoracic radiation therapy for patients at high risk with early-stage non-small-cell lung cancer. Clin Lung Cancer 2005 6(6): 350-4. NRI

Bollineni, E. M. Wiegman, J. Pruim, J. A. Langendijk and J. Widder. 18F-FDG-PET 12 weeks after stereotactic body radiotherapy for stage I non-small-cell lung cancer predicts outcome. European Journal of Cancer 2011 47(): S595. NRD

Bonfili, M. Di Staso, G. L. Gravina, P. Franzese, S. Buonopane, F. Solda, C. Festuccia and V. Tombolini. Hypofractionated radical radiotherapy in elderly patients with medically inoperable stage I-II non-small-cell lung cancer. Lung Cancer 2010 67(1): 81-5. NRP

Bongers, C. J. Haasbeek, F. J. Lagerwaard, B. J. Slotman and S. Senan. Incidence and risk factors for chest wall toxicity after risk-adapted stereotactic radiotherapy for early-stage lung cancer. J Thorac Oncol 2011 6(12): 2052-7. USD

Bonner, W. L. McGinnis, P. J. Stella, R. F. Marschke, Jr., J. A. Sloan, E. G. Shaw, J. A. Mailliard, E. T. Creagan, R. K. Ahuja and P. A. Johnson. The possible advantage of hyperfractionated thoracic radiotherapy in the treatment of locally advanced nonsmall cell lung carcinoma: results of a North Central Cancer Treatment Group Phase III Study. Cancer 1998 82(6): 1037-48. NRP

Bonnet, D. Bush, G. A. Cheek, J. D. Slater, D. Panossian, C. Franke and J. M. Slater. Effects of proton and combined proton/photon beam radiation on pulmonary function in patients with resectable but medically inoperable non-small cell lung cancer. Chest 2001 120(6): 1803-10. NRP

Bonomi, A. Blanco-Savorio, L. Cerchietti, A. Navigante, M. Castro, B. Roth and J. P. Wisnivesky. Continuous hyperfractionated accelerated radiation therapy week-end less in combination with neoadjuvant chemotherapy for the treatment of stage III non-small-cell lung cancer. Lung Cancer 2008 60(1): 75-82. NRP

Borst, K. De Jaeger, J. S. Belderbos, S. A. Burgers and J. V. Lebesque. Pulmonary function changes after radiotherapy in non-small-cell lung cancer patients with long-term disease-free survival. Int J Radiat Oncol Biol Phys 2005 62(3): 639-44. USD

Bouillet, J. F. MorÃ¨re, J. J. Mazeron, S. Piperno-Neuman, C. Boaziz, E. Haddad and J. L. Breau. Induction chemotherapy followed by concomitant combined radiotherapy and chemotherapy in stage III non-small cell bronchial carcinoma. 1997 1(): 121-31. FLA

Brade, A. Bezjak, R. MacRae, S. Laurie, A. Sun, J. Cho, N. Leighl, S. Pearson, B. Southwood, L. Wang, S. McGill, N. Iscoe and F. A. Shepherd. Phase I trial of radiation with concurrent and consolidation pemetrexed and cisplatin in patients with unresectable stage IIIA/B non-small-cell lung cancer. Int J Radiat Oncol Biol Phys 2011 79(5): 1395-401. NRP

Bradley, C. B. Scott, K. J. Paris, W. F. Demas, M. Machtay, R. Komaki, B. Movsas, P. Rubin and W. T. Sause. A phase III comparison of radiation therapy with or without recombinant beta-interferon for poor-risk patients with locally advanced non-small-cell lung cancer (RTOG 93-04). Int J Radiat Oncol Biol Phys 2002 52(5): 1173-9. NRP

Bradley, I. El Naqa, R. E. Drzymala, M. Trovo, G. Jones and M. D. Denning. Stereotactic body radiation therapy for early-stage non-small-cell lung cancer: the pattern of failure is distant. Int J Radiat Oncol Biol Phys 2010 77(4): 1146-50. NRP

Bradley, J. Moughan, M. V. Graham, R. Byhardt, R. Govindan, J. Fowler, J. A. Purdy, J. M. Michalski, E. Gore and H. Choy. A phase I/II radiation dose escalation study with concurrent chemotherapy for patients with inoperable stages I to III non-small-cell lung cancer: phase I results of RTOG 0117. Int J Radiat Oncol Biol Phys 2010 77(2): 367-72. NRP

Bradley, J. O. Deasy, S. Bentzen and I. El-Naqa. Dosimetric correlates for acute esophagitis in patients treated with radiotherapy for lung carcinoma. Int J Radiat Oncol Biol Phys 2004 58(4): 1106-13. NRI

Bradley, K. Bae, M. V. Graham, R. Byhardt, R. Govindan, J. Fowler, J. A. Purdy, J. M. Michalski, E. Gore and H. Choy. Primary analysis of the phase II component of a phase I/II dose intensification study using three-dimensional conformal radiation therapy and concurrent chemotherapy for patients with inoperable non-small-cell lung cancer: RTOG 0117. J Clin Oncol 2010 28(14): 2475-80. NRI

Bradley, M. V. Graham, K. Winter, J. A. Purdy, R. Komaki, W. H. Roa, J. K. Ryu, W. Bosch and B. Emami. Toxicity and outcome results of RTOG 9311: a phase I-II dose-escalation study using three-dimensional conformal radiotherapy in patients with inoperable non-small-cell lung carcinoma. Int J Radiat Oncol Biol Phys 2005 61(2): 318-28. USD

Bradley, N. Ieumwananonthachai, J. A. Purdy, T. H. Wasserman, M. A. Lockett, M. V. Graham and C. A. Perez. Gross tumor volume, critical prognostic factor in patients treated with three-dimensional conformal radiation therapy for non-small-cell lung carcinoma. Int J Radiat Oncol Biol Phys 2002 52(1): 49-57. USD

Bral, H. Van Parijs, G. Soete, N. Linthout, L. Van Moorter, D. Verellen and G. Storme. A feasibility study of image-guided hypofractionated conformal arc therapy for inoperable patients with localized non-small cell lung cancer. Radiother Oncol 2007 84(3): 252-6. NRP

Bral, M. Duchateau, H. Versmessen, B. Engels, K. Tournel, V. Vinh-Hung, M. De Ridder, D. Schallier and G. Storme. Toxicity and outcome results of a class solution with moderately hypofractionated radiotherapy in inoperable Stage III non-small cell lung cancer using helical tomotherapy. Int J Radiat Oncol Biol Phys 2010 77(5): 1352-9. NRP

Bral, M. Duchateau, H. Versmessen, D. Verdries, B. Engels, M. De Ridder, K. Tournel, C. Collen, H. Everaert, D. Schallier, J. De Greve and G. Storme. Toxicity report of a phase 1/2 dose-escalation study in patients with inoperable, locally advanced nonsmall cell lung cancer with helical tomotherapy and concurrent chemotherapy. Cancer 2010 116(1): 241-50. NRP

Bral, M. Duchateau, M. De Ridder, H. Everaert, K. Tournel, D. Schallier, D. Verellen and G. Storme. Volumetric response analysis during chemoradiation as predictive tool for optimizing treatment strategy in locally advanced unresectable NSCLC. Radiother Oncol 2009 91(3): 438-42. NRP

Bral, T. Gevaert, N. Linthout, H. Versmessen, C. Collen, B. Engels, D. Verdries, H. Everaert, N. Christian, M. De Ridder and G. Storme. Prospective, risk-adapted strategy of stereotactic body radiotherapy for early-stage non-small-cell lung cancer: results of a Phase II trial. Int J Radiat Oncol Biol Phys 2011 80(5): 1343-9. NRP

Brattstrom, M. Bergqvist, P. Hesselius, G. Wagenius and O. Brodin. Different fraction schedules and combinations with chemotherapy in radiation treatment of non-small cell lung cancer. Anticancer Res 2000 20(3B): 2087-90. NRP

Breathnach, V. Kasturi, F. Kaye, L. Herscher, M. S. Georgiadis, M. Edison, B. S. Schuler, P. Pizzella, S. M. Steinberg, K. O'Neil and B. E. Johnson. Phase II neoadjuvant trial of paclitaxel by 96-hour continuous infusion (CIVI) in combination with cisplatin followed by chest radiotherapy for patients with stage III non-small-cell lung cancer. Am J Clin Oncol 2002 25(3): 269-73. NRP

Bretel, R. Arriagada, T. Le Chevalier, P. Baldeyrou, D. Grunenwald, C. Le PÃ©choux, B. Pellae-Cosset and P. RuffiÃ©. Optimization of combined radiotherapy and chemotherapy in treatment of non-small cell lung carcinoma. 1997 1(): 148-53. FLA

Brown, F. Fayad, J. Hevezi, J. Fowler, M. I. Monterroso, S. Garcia, A. Medina and J. Schwade. Individualized higher dose of 70-75 Gy using five-fraction robotic stereotactic radiotherapy for non-small-cell lung cancer: a feasibility study. Comput Aided Surg 2011 16(1): 1-10. NRI

Brown, X. Wu, B. Amendola, M. Perman, H. Han, F. Fayad, S. Garcia, A. Lewin, A. Abitbol, A. de la Zerda and J. G. Schwade. Treatment of early non-small cell lung cancer, stage IA, by image-guided robotic stereotactic radioablation--CyberKnife. Cancer J 2007 13(2): 87-94. NRI

Brown, X. Wu, B. C. Wen, J. F. Fowler, F. Fayad, B. E. Amendola, S. Garcia, A. De La Zerda, Z. Huang and J. G. Schwade. Early results of CyberKnife image-guided robotic stereotactic radiosurgery for treatment of lung tumors. Comput Aided Surg 2007 12(5): 253-61. NRI

Brown, X. Wu, F. Fayad, J. F. Fowler, B. E. Amendola, S. Garcia, H. Han, A. de la Zerda, E. Bossart, Z. Huang and J. G. Schwade. CyberKnife radiosurgery for stage I lung cancer: results at 36 months. Clin Lung Cancer 2007 8(8): 488-92. NRI

Brown, X. Wu, F. Fayad, J. F. Fowler, S. Garcia, M. I. Monterroso, A. de la Zerda and J. G. Schwade. Application of robotic stereotactic radiotherapy to peripheral stage I non-small cell lung cancer with curative intent. Clin Oncol (R Coll Radiol) 2009 21(8): 623-31. NRI

Brundage, A. Bezjak, P. Dixon, L. Grimard, M. Larochelle, P. Warde and D. Warr. The role of palliative thoracic radiotherapy in non-small cell lung cancer. Can J Oncol 1996 6 Suppl 1(): 25-32. NRD

Brunsvig, R. Hatlevoll, R. Berg, G. Lauvvang, K. Owre, M. Wang and S. Aamdal. Weekly docetaxel with concurrent radiotherapy in locally advanced non-small cell lung cancer: a phase I/II study with 5 years' follow-up. Lung Cancer 2005 50(1): 97-105. NRP

Burfeind Jr, T. A. D'Amico, E. M. Toloza, W. G. Wolfe, D. H. Harpole, D. L. Miller, M. M. Decamp and R. J. Cerfolio. Low morbidity and mortality for bronchoplastic procedures with and without induction therapy. Annals of Thoracic Surgery 2005 80(2): 418-422. NRP

Burmeister, D. I. Fielding, J. R. Ramsay, K. C. Baumann, M. Dauth and E. T. Walpole. A phase I study of moderate-dose radiation therapy and weekly gemcitabine in patients with locally advanced non-small cell lung cancer not suitable for radical chemoradiation therapy. Clin Oncol (R Coll Radiol) 2005 17(5): 332-6. NRP

Burmeister, M. Michael, E. Burmeister, S. Cox, M. Lehman, A. Wirth, K. Horwood, G. Sasso, B. Forouzesh and D. Ball. A Randomized Phase II Trial of Two Regimens of Moderate Dose Chemoradiation Therapy for Patients with Non-small Cell Lung Cancer Not Suitable for Curative Therapy: Trans Tasman Radiation Oncology Study TROG 03.07. J Thorac Oncol 2011 6(12): 2076-82. NRP

Burmeister, N. K. Gogna, G. P. Bryant, J. Armstrong, W. Kelly, J. Mackintosh, E. Walpole and K. Morton. Chemoradiation for inoperable non small cell lung cancer: a phase II study using a regimen with acceptable toxicity. Lung Cancer 1999 23(3): 233-40. NRI

Bush, J. D. Slater, R. Bonnet, G. A. Cheek, R. D. Dunbar, M. Moyers and J. M. Slater. Proton-beam radiotherapy for early-stage lung cancer. Chest 1999 116(5): 1313-9. USD

Bush, R. D. Dunbar, R. Bonnet, J. D. Slater, G. A. Cheek and J. M. Slater. Pulmonary injury from proton and conventional radiotherapy as revealed by CT. AJR Am J Roentgenol 1999 172(3): 735-9. NRO

Bush, S. Y. Do and J. D. Slater. Comorbidity-adjusted survival in early stage lung cancer patients treated with hypofractionated proton therapy. Journal of Oncology 2010 (): . OPP

Byhardt and C. Scott. A palliative accelerated irradiation regimen for advanced non-small-cell lung cancer vs. conventionally fractionated 60 Gy: results of a randomized equivalence study: regarding Nestle et al. IJROBP 2000; 48:95-103. Int J Radiat Oncol Biol Phys 2001 50(3): 837. NRD

Byhardt, C. B. Scott, D. S. Ettinger, W. J. Curran, R. L. Doggett, C. Coughlin, C. Scarantino, M. Rotman and B. Emami. Concurrent hyperfractionated irradiation and chemotherapy for unresectable nonsmall cell lung cancer. Results of Radiation Therapy Oncology Group 90-15. Cancer 1995 75(9): 2337-44. NRP

Byhardt, C. Scott, W. T. Sause, B. Emami, R. Komaki, B. Fisher, J. S. Lee and C. Lawton. Response, toxicity, failure patterns, and survival in five Radiation Therapy Oncology Group (RTOG) trials of sequential and/or concurrent chemotherapy and radiotherapy for locally advanced non-small-cell carcinoma of the lung. Int J Radiat Oncol Biol Phys 1998 42(3): 469-78. NRP

Byhardt, L. Vaickus, P. L. Witt, A. Y. Chang, T. McAuliffe, J. F. Wilson, C. A. Lawton, J. Breitmeyer, M. E. Alger and E. C. Borden. Recombinant human interferon-beta (rHuIFN-beta) and radiation therapy for inoperable non-small cell lung cancer. J Interferon Cytokine Res 1996 16(11): 891-902. NRP

Byrne, M. Phillips, A. Powell, F. Cameron, D. Joseph, N. Spry, J. Dewar, G. Van Hazel, M. Buck, H. Lund, Y. De Melker and M. Newman. Cisplatin and gemcitabine induction chemotherapy followed by concurrent chemoradiotherapy or surgery for locally advanced non-small cell lung cancer. Intern Med J 2005 35(6): 336-42. NRP

Caglar, E. H. Baldini, M. Othus, M. S. Rabin, R. Bueno, D. J. Sugarbaker, S. J. Mentzer, P. A. Janne, B. E. Johnson and A. M. Allen. Outcomes of patients with stage III nonsmall cell lung cancer treated with chemotherapy and radiation with and without surgery. Cancer 2009 115(18): 4156-66. NRP

Caglayan, A. Fidan, B. Salepci, N. Kiral, E. Torun, T. Salepci and A. Mayadagli. Effects of prognostic factors and treatment on survival in advanced non-small cell lung cancer. Tuberk Toraks 2004 52(4): 323-32. NRP

Cai, F. G. Dai, Q. F. Min, M. Shi, J. X. Miao and R. C. Luo. Clinical study of the effects of radiotherapy in combination with traditional Chinese medicine on non-small cell lung cancer. 2002 22(): 1112-3. FLA

Cai, L. Y. Xu, L. Wang, J. A. Hayman, A. C. Chang, A. Pickens, K. B. Cease, M. B. Orringer and F. M. Kong. Comparative survival in patients with postresection recurrent versus newly diagnosed non-small-cell lung cancer treated with radiotherapy. Int J Radiat Oncol Biol Phys 2010 76(4): 1100-5. NRP

Cakir and I. Egehan. A randomised clinical trial of radiotherapy plus cisplatin versus radiotherapy alone in stage III non-small cell lung cancer. Lung Cancer 2004 43(3): 309-16. NRP

Call, R. Rami-Porta, C. Obiols, M. Serra-Mitjans, G. Gonzalez-Pont, R. Bastus-Piulats, S. Quintana and J. Belda-Sanchis. Repeat mediastinoscopy in all its indications: Experience with 96 patients and 101 procedures. European Journal of Cardio-thoracic Surgery 2011 39(6): 1022-1027. NRP

Camilleri, A. Lewis and H. Eldeeb. Concurrent chemoradiotherapy for NSCLC with cisplatin and etoposide - A single centre experience. Clinical Oncology 2011 23(3): S32. NRD

Cappuzzo, F. De Marinis, F. Nelli, C. Calandri, A. Maestri, G. Benedetti, M. R. Migliorino, E. Cortesi, F. Rastelli, O. Martelli, M. Andruccetti, S. Bartolini and L. Crino. Phase II study of gemcitabine-cisplatin-paclitaxel triplet as induction chemotherapy in inoperable, locally-advanced non-small cell lung cancer. Lung Cancer 2003 42(3): 355-61. NRP

Cappuzzo, G. Selvaggi, V. Gregorc, F. Mazzoni, M. Betti, M. Rita Migliorino, S. Novello, A. Maestri, F. De Marinis, S. Darwish, V. De Angelis, F. Nelli, S. Bartolini, G. V. Scagliotti, M. Tonato and L. Crino. Gemcitabine and cisplatin as induction chemotherapy for patients with unresectable Stage IIIA-bulky N2 and Stage IIIB nonsmall cell lung carcinoma: an Italian Lung Cancer Project Observational Study. Cancer 2003 98(1): 128-34. NRP

Cardenal, M. D. Arnaiz, T. Moran, J. Jove, E. Nadal, R. Porta, J. M. Sole, I. Brao, R. Palmero, R. Fuentes, I. Nunez, E. Caveda and A. Cassinello. Phase I study of concurrent chemoradiation with pemetrexed and cisplatin followed by consolidation pemetrexed for patients with unresectable stage III non-small cell lung cancer. Lung Cancer 2011 74(1): 69-74. NRP

Carter, D. Garfield, J. Hathorn, R. Mundis, K. A. Boehm, D. Ilegbodu, L. Asmar and C. Reynolds. A Randomized Phase III Trial of Combined Paclitaxel, Carboplatin, and Radiation Therapy Followed by Weekly Paclitaxel or Observation for Patients With Locally Advanced Inoperable Non-Small-Cell Lung Cancer. Clin Lung Cancer 2011 (): . NRP

Casal, S. Varela, U. Anido, M. Lazaro, J. L. Firvida, S. Vazquez, M. Caeiro, P. Calvo, G. Huidobro and M. Amenedo. Induction chemotherapy with docetaxel (D) and cisplatin (C) followed by concurrent thoracic radiotherapy with biweekly d and C for stage III non-small cell lung cancer (NSCLC) - A galician lung cancer group study. European Journal of Cancer 2011 47(): S603. NRD

Casas, N. Vinolas, F. Ferrer, C. Agusti, M. Sanchez, J. Maria Gimferrer, F. Lomena, M. Campayo and B. Jeremic. Long-term results of a phase II trial of induction paclitaxel-carboplatin followed by concurrent radiation therapy and weekly paclitaxel and consolidation paclitaxel-carboplatin in stage III non-small cell lung cancer. J Thorac Oncol 2011 6(1): 79-85. NRP

Casas, P. Arguis, N. Vinolas, P. Lomena, R. Marrades and M. Catalan. Radiofrequency ablation combined with conventional radiotherapy - A treatment option for patients with medically inoperable lung cancer. European Journal of Cancer 2011 47(): S603. NRD

Catalano, B. A. Jereczek-Fossa, T. De Pas, M. E. Leon, F. Cattani, L. Spaggiari, G. Veronesi, F. de Braud and R. Orecchia. Three-times-daily radiotherapy with induction chemotherapy in locally advanced non-small cell lung cancer. Feasibility and toxicity study. Strahlenther Onkol 2005 181(6): 363-71. NRP

Catalano, T. De Pas, L. Spaggiari, S. Gandini, B. A. Jereczek-Fossa, F. De Braud, F. Leo, G. Veronesi and R. Orecchia. Three-times daily radiotherapy after chemotherapy in stage III non-small cell lung cancer. Single-institution prospective study. Anticancer Res 2008 28(6B): 4121-7. NRP

Center, W. J. Petty, D. Ayala, W. H. Hinson, J. Lovato, J. Capellari, T. Oaks, A. A. Miller and A. W. Blackstock. A phase I study of gefitinib with concurrent dose-escalated weekly docetaxel and conformal three-dimensional thoracic radiation followed by consolidative docetaxel and maintenance gefitinib for patients with stage III non-small cell lung cancer. J Thorac Oncol 2010 5(1): 69-74. NRP

Ceresoli, V. Gregorc, S. Cordio, K. B. Bencardino, S. Schipani, C. Cozzarini, R. Bordonaro and E. Villa. Phase II study of weekly paclitaxel as second-line therapy in patients with advanced non-small cell lung cancer. Lung Cancer 2004 44(2): 231-9. NRP

Cerfolio, A. S. Bryant, E. Scott, M. Sharma, F. Robert, S. A. Spencer and R. I. Garver. Women with pathologic stage I, II, and III non-small cell lung cancer have better survival than men. Chest 2006 130(6): 1796-1802. NRP

Cesario, S. Margaritora, L. Trodella, S. Valente, G. M. Corbo, G. Macis, D. Galetta, R. M. d'Angelillo, V. Porziella, S. Ramella, M. G. Mangiacotti and P. Granone. Incidental surgical findings of a phase I trial of weekly gemcitabine and concurrent radiotherapy in patients with unresectable non-small cell lung cancer. Lung Cancer 2002 37(2): 207-12. NRP

Cetingoz, S. Kentli, O. U. Ataman and M. Kinay. Is hypofractionated reirradiation effective after symptomatic local recurrence in non-small cell lung cancer?. Journal of B.U.ON. 2000 5(4): 421-425. NRP

Cetingoz, S. Kentli, O. Uruk, E. Demirtas, M. Sen and M. Kinay. The role of palliative radiotherapy in locally advanced non-small cell lung cancer. Neoplasma 2001 48(6): 506-10. NRP

Chakravarthy and H. Choy. A phase I trial of outpatient weekly irinotecan/carboplatin and concurrent radiation for stage III unresectable non small-cell lung cancer: a Vanderbilt-Ingram Cancer Center Affiliate Network Trial. Clin Lung Cancer 2000 1(4): 310-1. NRP

Chan, D. E. Dupuy, W. W. Mayo-Smith, T. Ng and T. A. DiPetrillo. Combined radiofrequency ablation and high-dose rate brachytherapy for early-stage non-small-cell lung cancer. Brachytherapy 2011 10(3): 253-9. NRI

Chang, K. H. Chi, S. J. Kao, P. S. Hsu, Y. W. Tsang, H. J. Chang, Y. W. Yeh, Y. S. Hsieh and J. S. Jiang. Upfront gefitinib/erlotinib treatment followed by concomitant radiotherapy for advanced lung cancer: a mono-institutional experience. Lung Cancer 2011 73(2): 189-94. NRP

Chang, P. A. Balter, L. Dong, Q. Yang, Z. Liao, M. Jeter, M. K. Bucci, M. F. McAleer, R. J. Mehran, J. A. Roth and R. Komaki. Stereotactic body radiation therapy in centrally and superiorly located stage I or isolated recurrent non-small-cell lung cancer. Int J Radiat Oncol Biol Phys 2008 72(4): 967-71. NRP

Chang, R. Komaki, C. Lu, H. Y. Wen, P. K. Allen, A. Tsao, M. Gillin, R. Mohan and J. D. Cox. Phase 2 study of high-dose proton therapy with concurrent chemotherapy for unresectable stage III nonsmall cell lung cancer. Cancer 2011 117(20): 4707-4713. NRP

Chang, R. Komaki, H. Y. Wen, B. De Gracia, J. B. Bluett, M. F. McAleer, S. G. Swisher, M. Gillin, R. Mohan and J. D. Cox. Toxicity and patterns of failure of adaptive/ablative proton therapy for early-stage, medically inoperable non-small cell lung cancer. Int J Radiat Oncol Biol Phys 2011 80(5): 1350-7. NRP

Chang, R. Komaki, R. Sasaki, Z. Liao, C. W. Stevens, C. Lu, F. V. Fossella, P. K. Allen, J. D. Cox, M. R. Spitz and X. Wu. High mutagen sensitivity in peripheral blood lymphocytes predicts poor overall and disease-specific survival in patients with stage III non-small cell lung cancer treated with radiotherapy and chemotherapy. Clin Cancer Res 2005 11(8): 2894-8. NRP

Chapet, F. M. Kong, J. S. Lee, J. A. Hayman and R. K. Ten Haken. Normal tissue complication probability modeling for acute esophagitis in patients treated with conformal radiation therapy for non-small cell lung cancer. Radiother Oncol 2005 77(2): 176-81. NRP

Chen, B. A. Neville, D. J. Sher, K. Chen and D. Schrag. Survival outcomes after radiation therapy for stage III non-small-cell lung cancer after adoption of computed tomography-based simulation. J Clin Oncol 2011 29(17): 2305-11. NRP

Chen, G. L. Jiang, H. Qian, L. J. Wang, H. J. Yang, X. L. Fu, K. L. Wu, Z. Zang and S. Zhao. Escalated hyperfractionated accelerated radiation therapy for locally advanced non-small cell lung cancer: a clinical phase II trial. Radiother Oncol 2004 71(2): 157-62. NRP

Chen, G. L. Jiang, X. L. Fu, L. J. Wang, H. Qian, S. Zhao and T. F. Liu. Prognostic factors for local control in non-small-cell lung cancer treated with definitive radiation therapy. Am J Clin Oncol 2002 25(1): 76-80. NRP

Chen, J. A. Hayman, R. K. Ten Haken, D. Tatro, S. Fernando and F. M. Kong. Long-term results of high-dose conformal radiotherapy for patients with medically inoperable T1-3N0 non-small-cell lung cancer: is low incidence of regional failure due to incidental nodal irradiation?. Int J Radiat Oncol Biol Phys 2006 64(1): 120-6. NRP

Chen, J. H. Chen, J. Y. Shih, C. H. Yang, C. J. Yu and P. C. Yang. Octogenarians with advanced non-small cell lung cancer: treatment modalities, survival, and prognostic factors. J Thorac Oncol 2010 5(1): 82-9. NRP

Chen, J. Y. Chao, C. M. Tsai, C. Y. Shiau, M. J. Liang, S. H. Yen and R. P. Perng. Treatment of non-small-cell lung cancer: the Chinese experience in a general teaching hospital. Zhonghua Yi Xue Za Zhi (Taipei) 2000 63(6): 459-66. NRD

Chen, K. J. Pandya, O. Hyrien, P. C. Keng, T. Smudzin, J. Anderson, R. Qazi, B. Smith, T. J. Watson, R. H. Feins and D. W. Johnstone. Preclinical and pilot clinical studies of docetaxel chemoradiation for Stage III non-small-cell lung cancer. Int J Radiat Oncol Biol Phys 2011 80(5): 1358-64. NRP

Chen, L. Ignacio, R. Jacobs, M. Kozloff, M. Telfer, R. Elahi, R. Evans and S. Vijayakumar. Results of a phase II concurrent chemoradiotherapy study using three-dimensional conformal radiotherapy with cisplatin and oral etoposide in stage III nonsmall-cell lung cancer. Radiat Oncol Investig 1999 7(1): 49-53. NRP

Chen, Y. Matsuo, A. Yoshizawa, T. Sato, H. Sakai, T. Bando, K. Okubo, K. Shibuya and H. Date. Salvage lung resection for non-small cell lung cancer after stereotactic body radiotherapy in initially operable patients. J Thorac Oncol 2010 5(12): 1999-2002. NRI

Chen, Y. Y. Chen, Y. Bao, C. G. Xian, G. Z. Liu, L. Zhang, G. C. Xu, X. W. Deng, T. X. Lu, J. Y. Qian and N. J. Cui. Neoadjuvant chemotherapy followed by late-course accelerated hyperfractionated radiation therapy for locally advanced non-small-cell lung cancer: long-term results of a phase I/II clinical trial. Clin Lung Cancer 2005 6(5): 304-9. NRP

Cheruvu, S. K. Metcalfe, J. Metcalfe, Y. Chen, P. Okunieff and M. T. Milano. Comparison of outcomes in patients with stage III versus limited stage IV non-small cell lung cancer. Radiat Oncol 2011 6(): 80. NRP

Cheung, L. T. Yeung, V. Basrur, Y. C. Ung, J. Balogh and C. E. Danjoux. Accelerated hypofractionation for early-stage non-small-cell lung cancer. Int J Radiat Oncol Biol Phys 2002 54(4): 1014-23. NRI

Cheung, W. J. Mackillop, P. Dixon, M. D. Brundage, Y. M. Youssef and S. Zhou. Involved-field radiotherapy alone for early-stage non-small-cell lung cancer. Int J Radiat Oncol Biol Phys 2000 48(3): 703-10. NRI

Chidel, J. H. Suh, J. F. Greskovich, P. A. Kupelian and G. H. Barnett. Treatment outcome for patients with primary nonsmall-cell lung cancer and synchronous brain metastasis. Radiat Oncol Investig 1999 7(5): 313-9. NRP

Chien, S. W. Chen, C. Y. Hsieh, J. A. Liang, S. N. Yang, C. Y. Huang and F. J. Lin. Intra-thoracic failure pattern and survival status following 3D conformal radiotherapy for non-small cell lung cancer: a preliminary report. Jpn J Clin Oncol 2001 31(2): 55-60. NRP

Chien, Y. C. Hsu, Y. C. Wang and L. L. Ting. Clinical risk factors of radiation pneumonitis after 3D conformal radiotherapy for lung cancer. Chinese Journal of Radiology 2005 30(1): 25-29. NRP

Chikamori, D. Kishino, N. Takigawa, K. Hotta, N. Nogami, H. Kamei, S. Kuyama, K. Gemba, M. Takemoto, S. Kanazawa, H. Ueoka, Y. Segawa, S. Takata, M. Tabata, K. Kiura and M. Tanimoto. A phase I study of combination S-1 plus cisplatin chemotherapy with concurrent thoracic radiation for locally advanced non-small cell lung cancer. Lung Cancer 2009 65(1): 74-9. NRP

Cho, S. J. Ahn, H. R. Pyo, K. S. Kim, Y. C. Kim, S. H. Moon, J. Y. Han, H. T. Kim, W. S. Koom and J. S. Lee. A Phase II study of synchronous three-dimensional conformal boost to the gross tumor volume for patients with unresectable Stage III non-small-cell lung cancer: results of Korean Radiation Oncology Group 0301 study. Int J Radiat Oncol Biol Phys 2009 74(5): 1397-404. NRP

Choong, A. M. Mauer, D. J. Haraf, E. Lester, P. C. Hoffman, M. Kozloff, S. Lin, J. E. Dancey, L. Szeto, T. Grushko, O. I. Olopade, R. Salgia and E. E. Vokes. Phase I trial of erlotinib-based multimodality therapy for inoperable stage III non-small cell lung cancer. J Thorac Oncol 2008 3(9): 1003-11. NRP

Choong, E. E. Vokes, D. J. Haraf, P. K. Tothy, M. K. Ferguson, K. Kasza, C. M. Rudin, P. C. Hoffman, S. A. Krauss, L. Szeto and A. M. Mauer. Phase I study of induction chemotherapy and concomitant chemoradiotherapy with irinotecan, carboplatin, and paclitaxel for stage III non-small cell lung cancer. J Thorac Oncol 2008 3(1): 59-67. NRP

Choy, A. Chakravarthy, R. F. Devore, 3rd, M. Jagasia, K. R. Hande, J. R. Roberts, D. H. Johnson and F. Yunus. Weekly irinotecan and concurrent radiation therapy for stage III unresectable NSCLC. Oncology (Williston Park) 2000 14(7 Suppl 5): 43-6. NRP

Choy, A. K. Jain, J. Moughan, W. Curran, G. Whipple, W. F. Demas and D. S. Ettinger. RTOG 0017: a phase I trial of concurrent gemcitabine/carboplatin or gemcitabine/paclitaxel and radiation therapy ("ping-pong trial") followed by adjuvant chemotherapy for patients with favorable prognosis inoperable stage IIIA/B non-small cell lung cancer. J Thorac Oncol 2009 4(1): 80-6. NRP

Choy, A. Nabid, B. Stea, C. Scott, W. Roa, L. Kleinberg, J. Ayoub, C. Smith, L. Souhami, S. Hamburg, W. Spanos, H. Kreisman, A. P. Boyd, P. J. Cagnoni and W. J. Curran. Phase II multicenter study of induction chemotherapy followed by concurrent efaproxiral (RSR13) and thoracic radiotherapy for patients with locally advanced non-small-cell lung cancer. J Clin Oncol 2005 23(25): 5918-28. NRD

Choy, H. Safran, W. Akerley, S. L. Graziano, J. A. Bogart and B. F. Cole. Phase II trial of weekly paclitaxel and concurrent radiation therapy for locally advanced non-small cell lung cancer. Clin Cancer Res 1998 4(8): 1931-6. NRP

Choy, L. Yee and B. F. Cole. Combined-modality therapy for advanced non-small cell lung cancer: paclitaxel and thoracic irradiation. Semin Oncol 1995 22(6 Suppl 15): 38-44. NRP

Choy, R. F. Devore, 3rd, K. R. Hande, L. L. Porter, P. Rosenblatt, F. Yunus, L. Schlabach, C. Smith, Y. Shyr and D. H. Johnson. A phase II study of paclitaxel, carboplatin, and hyperfractionated radiation therapy for locally advanced inoperable non-small-cell lung cancer (a Vanderbilt Cancer Center Affiliate Network Study). Int J Radiat Oncol Biol Phys 2000 47(4): 931-7. NRP

Choy, R. F. DeVore, 3rd, K. R. Hande, L. L. Porter, P. Rosenblatt, F. Yunus, L. Schlabach, C. Smith, Y. Shyr, K. LaPorte and D. H. Johnson. Preliminary analysis of a phase II study of paclitaxel, carboplatin, and hyperfractionated radiation therapy for locally advanced inoperable non-small cell lung cancer. Semin Oncol 1997 24(4 Suppl 12): S12-21-S12-26. NRP

Choy, R. F. DeVore, K. R. Hande, L. L. Porter, P. A. Rosenblatt, B. Slovis, K. Laporte, Y. Shyr and D. H. Johnson. Phase I trial of outpatient weekly docetaxel, carboplatin and concurrent thoracic radiation therapy for stage III unresectable non-small-cell lung cancer: a Vanderbilt cancer center affiliate network (VCCAN) trial. Lung Cancer 2001 34(3): 441-9. NRP

Clamon, J. Herndon, R. Cooper, A. Y. Chang, J. Rosenman and M. R. Green. Radiosensitization with carboplatin for patients with unresectable stage III non-small-cell lung cancer: a phase III trial of the Cancer and Leukemia Group B and the Eastern Cooperative Oncology Group. J Clin Oncol 1999 17(1): 4-11. NRP

Coate, C. Massey, A. Hope, A. Sacher, K. Barrett, A. Pierre, N. Leighl, A. Brade, M. de Perrot, T. Waddell, G. Liu, R. Feld, R. Burkes, B. C. Cho, G. Darling, A. Sun, S. Keshavjee, A. Bezjak and F. A. Shepherd. Treatment of the elderly when cure is the goal: the influence of age on treatment selection and efficacy for stage III non-small cell lung cancer. J Thorac Oncol 2011 6(3): 537-44. NRP

Coen, M. Van Lancker, W. De Neve and G. Storme. Prognostic factors in locoregional non-small cell lung cancer treated with radiotherapy. Am J Clin Oncol 1995 18(2): 111-7. NRI

Collen, D. Van Brummelen, H. Versmessen, S. Bral, D. Schallier, J. De Greve and M. De Ridder. Concurrent chemoradiation in locally advanced, Unresectable non small-Cell lung cancer (LA-NSCLC): Comparison of efficacy and treatment tolerance in the elderly. European Journal of Cancer 2011 47(): S276. NRD

Collins, K. Erickson, C. A. Reichner, S. P. Collins, G. J. Gagnon, S. Dieterich, D. A. McRae, Y. Zhang, S. Yousefi, E. Levy, T. Chang, C. Jamis-Dow, F. Banovac and E. D. Anderson. Radical stereotactic radiosurgery with real-time tumor motion tracking in the treatment of small peripheral lung tumors. Radiat Oncol 2007 2(): 39. NRI

Collins, S. Vahdat, K. Erickson, S. P. Collins, S. Suy, X. Yu, Y. Zhang, D. Subramaniam, C. A. Reichner, I. Sarikaya, G. Esposito, S. Yousefi, C. Jamis-Dow, F. Banovac and E. D. Anderson. Radical cyberknife radiosurgery with tumor tracking: an effective treatment for inoperable small peripheral stage I non-small cell lung cancer. J Hematol Oncol 2009 2(): 1. NRI

Collins, S. Vahdat, S. P. Collins, E. K. Oermann, Y. Xia, C. Reichner, E. Anderson, F. Gharagozloo and M. Margolis. Cyberknife radiosurgery for inoperable patients with peripheral stage IA. International Journal of Medical Robotics and Computer Assisted Surgery 2011 7(): 1. NRD

Comella, G. Frasci, G. Scoppa, C. Guida, A. Gravina, F. Fiore, R. Casaretti, A. Daponte, P. Ruffolo and P. Comella. Weekly paclitaxel/cisplatin with concurrent radiotherapy in patients with locally advanced non-small cell lung cancer: a phase I study. Semin Oncol 1997 24(4 Suppl 12): S12-113-S12-116. NRP

Concurrent chemoradiotherapy followed by consolidation docetaxel in stage IIIB non-small-cell-lung cancer (SWOG 9504). Clinical Lung Cancer 2000 2(1): 25-26. NRP

Correa, V. Sharma, V. Rangarajan, S. Sunder and K. A. Dinshaw. Can 99mTc-DTPA aerosol scanning predict radiation pneumonitis?. Int J Radiat Oncol Biol Phys 2003 56(2): 367-74. NRP

Cortesi, L. Moscetti, F. Nelli, F. De Marinis, U. De Paula, C. Bangrazi, M. R. Migliorino and V. Donato. Induction therapy with paclitaxel and carboplatin followed by hyperfractionated radiotherapy plus weekly concurrent chemotherapy and subsequent consolidation therapy in unresectable locally advanced non-small-cell lung cancer. Tumori 2007 93(2): 133-7. NRP

Corti, L. Toniolo, C. Boso, F. Colaut, D. Fiore, P. C. Muzzio, M. I. Koukourakis, R. Mazzarotto, M. Pignataro, L. Loreggian and G. Sotti. Long-term survival of patients treated with photodynamic therapy for carcinoma in situ and early non-small-cell lung carcinoma. Lasers Surg Med 2007 39(5): 394-402. NRP

Crabtree, C. E. Denlinger, B. F. Meyers, I. El Naqa, J. Zoole, A. S. Krupnick, D. Kreisel, G. A. Patterson and J. D. Bradley. Stereotactic body radiation therapy versus surgical resection for stage I non-small cell lung cancer. J Thorac Cardiovasc Surg 2010 140(2): 377-86. USD

Cross, S. Berman, L. Buswell, B. Johnson and E. H. Baldini. Prospective study of palliative hypofractionated radiotherapy (8.5 Gy x 2) for patients with symptomatic non-small-cell lung cancer. Int J Radiat Oncol Biol Phys 2004 58(4): 1098-105. NRP

Cruciani, A. Vergnenegre, E. Blasco-Colmenares, M. Thomas, J. Medina and A. Carrato. Clinical management and treatment outcomes in patients receiving treatment for non-small cell lung cancer (NSCLC) across Europe - Epiclin-lung study. European Journal of Cancer 2011 47(): S609. NRD

Crvenkova and V. Krstevska. Sequential chemoradiotherapy compared with concurrent chemoradiotherapy in locally advanced non-small cell lung cancer: our experience. Prilozi 2009 30(2): 197-207. NRP

Cuneyt Ulutin and Y. Pak. Preliminary results of radiotherapy with or without weekly paclitaxel in locally advanced non-small cell lung cancer. J Cancer Res Clin Oncol 2003 129(1): 52-6. NRP

Curran, Jr. and H. Choy. Optimizing chemoradiation in locally advanced non-small-cell lung cancer. Oncology (Williston Park) 2001 15(3 Suppl 6): 43-5. NRP

Curran, Jr., R. Paulus, C. J. Langer, R. Komaki, J. S. Lee, S. Hauser, B. Movsas, T. Wasserman, S. A. Rosenthal, E. Gore, M. Machtay, W. Sause and J. D. Cox. Sequential vs. concurrent chemoradiation for stage III non-small cell lung cancer: randomized phase III trial RTOG 9410. J Natl Cancer Inst 2011 103(19): 1452-60. NRP

Cyjon, M. Nili, G. Fink, M. R. Kramer, E. Fenig, J. Sandbank, A. Sulkes and E. Rakowsky. Advanced non-small cell lung cancer: induction chemotherapy and chemoradiation before operation. Ann Thorac Surg 2002 74(2): 342-7. NRP

Dahele, A. Brade, S. Pearson and A. Bezjak. Stereotactic radiation therapy for inoperable, early-stage non-small-cell lung cancer. CMAJ 2009 180(13): 1326-8. NRD

Dahele, D. Palma, F. Lagerwaard, B. Slotman and S. Senan. Radiological changes after stereotactic radiotherapy for stage I lung cancer. J Thorac Oncol 2011 6(7): 1221-8. NRO

Dai, W. Jiang, J. Yuan and R. Wei. A randomized study on the effects of paclitaxel liposme and cisplatin induction chemotherapy followed concurrent chemoradiotherapy and sequential radiotherapy on locally advanced non-small cell lung cancer patients. 2011 14(): 137-40. FLA

Dale, V. Harsaker, D. T. Kristoffersen, O. Bruland and D. R. Olsen. CT density in lung cancer patients after radiotherapy sensitized by metoclopramide. A subgroup analysis of a randomized trial. Strahlenther Onkol 2010 186(3): 163-8. NRP

Dang, G. Li, X. Lu, L. Yao, S. Zhang and Z. Yu. Analysis of related factors associated with radiation pneumonitis in patients with locally advanced non-small-cell lung cancer treated with three-dimensional conformal radiotherapy. J Cancer Res Clin Oncol 2010 136(8): 1169-78. NRP

D'Angelillo, L. Trodella, M. Ciresa, F. Cellini, M. Fiore, C. Greco, E. Pompeo, T. C. Mineo, L. Paleari, P. Granone, S. Ramella and A. Cesario. Multimodality treatment of stage III non-small cell lung cancer: analysis of a phase II trial using preoperative cisplatin and gemcitabine with concurrent radiotherapy. J Thorac Oncol 2009 4(12): 1517-23. NRP

Dasgupta, C. Dasgupta, S. Basu and A. Majumdar. A prospective and randomized study of radiotherapy, sequential chemotherapy radiotherapy and concomitant chemotherapy-radiotherapy in unresectable non small cell carcinoma of the lung. J Cancer Res Ther 2006 2(2): 47-51. NRP

Davies, K. Chansky, D. H. Lau, B. R. Leigh, L. E. Gaspar, G. R. Weiss, A. J. Wozniak, J. J. Crowley and D. R. Gandara. Phase II study of consolidation paclitaxel after concurrent chemoradiation in poor-risk stage III non-small-cell lung cancer: SWOG S9712. J Clin Oncol 2006 24(33): 5242-6. NRP

De Candis, S. C. Stani, P. Bidoli, V. A. Bedini, P. Potepan, P. Navarria, S. Aglione and E. Bajetta. Induction chemotherapy with carboplatin/paclitaxel followed by surgery or standard radiotherapy and concurrent daily low-dose cisplatin for locally advanced non-small cell lung cancer (NSCLC). Am J Clin Oncol 2003 26(3): 265-9. NRP

De Giorgi, D. Blaise, A. Lange, P. Viens, M. Marangolo, A. Madroszyk, M. Brune, B. V. Afanassiev, G. Rosti and T. Demirer. High-dose chemotherapy with peripheral blood progenitor cell support for patients with non-small cell lung cancer: the experience of the European Group for Bone Marrow Transplantation (EBMT) Solid Tumours Working Party. Bone Marrow Transplant 2007 40(11): 1045-8. NRP

De Jaeger, Y. Seppenwoolde, L. J. Boersma, S. H. Muller, P. Baas, J. S. Belderbos and J. V. Lebesque. Pulmonary function following high-dose radiotherapy of non-small-cell lung cancer. Int J Radiat Oncol Biol Phys 2003 55(5): 1331-40. USD

De Leyn, J. Vansteenkiste, Y. Lievens, D. Van Raemdonck, P. Nafteux, G. Decker, W. Coosemans, H. Decaluwe, J. Moons and T. Lerut. Survival after trimodality treatment for superior sulcus and central T4 non-small cell lung cancer. J Thorac Oncol 2009 4(1): 62-8. NRP

De Marinis, F. Nelli, M. R. Migliorino, O. Martelli, E. Cortesi, S. Treggiari, L. Portalone, C. Crispino, L. Brancaccio and C. Gridelli. Gemcitabine, paclitaxel, and cisplatin as induction chemotherapy for patients with biopsy-proven Stage IIIA(N2) nonsmall cell lung carcinoma: a Phase II multicenter study. Cancer 2003 98(8): 1707-15. NRP

De Pas, G. Curigliano, G. Veronesi, G. Catalano, C. Catania, B. Jereczek-Fossa, R. Orecchia, L. Spaggiari and F. de Braud. Optimization of the schedule of gemcitabine-cisplatin combination as induction regimen for patients with biopsy-proven stage IIIa N2 - stage IIIb non-small-cell lung cancer: a prospective phase-II study. Bull Cancer 2004 91(9): E273-7. NRP

De Pauw and J. P. Van Meerbeeck. Resection vs radiotherapy following induction chemotherapy in stage IIIA-N2 non-small cell lung cancer: Randomized controlled trial. American Journal of Hematology/ Oncology 2007 6(9): 509-512. NRP

De Petris, I. Lax, F. Sirzen and S. Friesland. Role of gross tumor volume on outcome and of dose parameters on toxicity of patients undergoing chemoradiotherapy for locally advanced non-small cell lung cancer. Med Oncol 2005 22(4): 375-81. NRP

De Ruysscher, A. Houben, H. J. Aerts, C. Dehing, R. Wanders, M. Ollers, A. M. Dingemans, M. Hochstenbag, L. Boersma, J. Borger, A. Dekker and P. Lambin. Increased (18)F-deoxyglucose uptake in the lung during the first weeks of radiotherapy is correlated with subsequent Radiation-Induced Lung Toxicity (RILT): a prospective pilot study. Radiother Oncol 2009 91(3): 415-20. NRP

De Ruysscher, A. van Baardwijk, J. Steevens, A. Botterweck, G. Bosmans, B. Reymen, R. Wanders, J. Borger, A. M. C. Dingemans, G. Bootsma, C. Pitz, R. Lunde, W. Geraedts, M. Oellers, A. Dekker and P. Lambin. Individualised isotoxic accelerated radiotherapy and chemotherapy are associated with improved long-term survival of patients with stage III NSCLC: A prospective population-based study. Radiotherapy and Oncology 2011 (): . NRP

De Ruysscher, C. Dehing, S. Yu, R. Wanders, M. Ollers, A. M. Dingemans, G. Bootsma, M. Hochstenbag, W. Geraedts, C. Pitz, J. Simons, L. Boersma, J. Borger, A. Dekker and P. Lambin. Dyspnea evolution after high-dose radiotherapy in patients with non-small cell lung cancer. Radiother Oncol 2009 91(3): 353-9. USD

De Ruysscher, R. Wanders, E. van Haren, M. Hochstenbag, W. Geraedts, C. Pitz, J. Simons, L. Boersma, T. Verschueren, A. Minken, S. M. Bentzen and P. Lambin. HI-CHART: a phase I/II study on the feasibility of high-dose continuous hyperfractionated accelerated radiotherapy in patients with inoperable non-small-cell lung cancer. Int J Radiat Oncol Biol Phys 2008 71(1): 132-8. NRP

De Ruysscher, S. Wanders, E. van Haren, M. Hochstenbag, W. Geeraedts, I. Utama, J. Simons, J. Dohmen, A. Rhami, U. Buell, P. Thimister, G. Snoep, L. Boersma, T. Verschueren, A. van Baardwijk, A. Minken, S. M. Bentzen and P. Lambin. Selective mediastinal node irradiation based on FDG-PET scan data in patients with non-small-cell lung cancer: a prospective clinical study. Int J Radiat Oncol Biol Phys 2005 62(4): 988-94. NRP

De Ruysscher, Y. Lievens, P. Van den Brande, K. Nackaerts and J. Vansteenkiste. Dose-intensified accelerated vindesine-ifosfamide-cisplatin (VIP) chemotherapy followed by high-dose accelerated hyperfractionated radiotherapy in patients with pathologically proven stage IIIB non-small cell lung cancer: a feasibility study. Radiother Oncol 2002 64(1): 33-6. NRP

De Waele, M. Serra-Mitjans, J. Hendriks, P. Lauwers, J. Belda-Sanchis, P. Van Schil and R. Rami-Porta. Accuracy and survival of repeat mediastinoscopy after induction therapy for non-small cell lung cancer in a combined series of 104 patients. Eur J Cardiothorac Surg 2008 33(5): 824-8. NRP

DeArmond, A. Mahtabifard, C. B. Fuller and R. J. McKenna, Jr.. Photodynamic therapy followed by thoracoscopic sleeve lobectomy for locally advanced lung cancer. Ann Thorac Surg 2008 85(5): e24-6. NRD

Debevec, A. Debeljak, J. Erzen, V. Kovac and I. Kern. Characterization of lung cancer patients, their actual treatment and survival: Experience in Slovenia. Radiology and Oncology 2005 39(2): 115-121+161. NRP

DeCamp, T. W. Rice, D. J. Adelstein, M. A. Chidel, L. A. Rybicki, S. C. Murthy and E. H. Blackstone. Value of accelerated multimodality therapy in stage IIIA and IIIB non-small cell lung cancer. J Thorac Cardiovasc Surg 2003 126(1): 17-27. NRP

Decoster, D. Schallier, H. Everaert, K. Nieboer, M. Meysman, B. Neyns, J. De Mey and J. De Greve. Complete metabolic tumour response, assessed by 18-fluorodeoxyglucose positron emission tomography (18FDG-PET), after induction chemotherapy predicts a favourable outcome in patients with locally advanced non-small cell lung cancer (NSCLC). Lung Cancer 2008 62(1): 55-61. NRP

Dediu, A. Tarlea, P. Iorga, M. Radut, A. Alexandru, G. Miron, C. Cornila and P. Bailesteanu. Split course radiation with concurrent vinorelbine and cisplatin in locally advanced non-small cell lung cancer. A phase II study. J BUON 2004 9(2): 167-72. NRP

Dediu, E. Crisan, M. Radut, A. Tarlea, D. Median, A. Alexandru, G. Vremes and C. Gal. The favorable prognostic significance of atelectasis in patients with advanced non-small cell lung cancer: Results of a prospective observational study. Lung Cancer 2009 63(2): 271-276. NRP

Dehing-Oberije, D. De Ruysscher, H. van der Weide, M. Hochstenbag, G. Bootsma, W. Geraedts, C. Pitz, J. Simons, J. Teule, A. Rahmy, P. Thimister, H. Steck and P. Lambin. Tumor volume combined with number of positive lymph node stations is a more important prognostic factor than TNM stage for survival of non-small-cell lung cancer patients treated with (chemo)radiotherapy. Int J Radiat Oncol Biol Phys 2008 70(4): 1039-44. NRP

Dehing-Oberije, D. De Ruysscher, S. Petit, J. Van Meerbeeck, K. Vandecasteele, W. De Neve, A. M. Dingemans, I. El Naqa, J. Deasy, J. Bradley, E. Huang and P. Lambin. Development, external validation and clinical usefulness of a practical prediction model for radiation-induced dysphagia in lung cancer patients. Radiother Oncol 2010 97(3): 455-61. NRO

Dehing-Oberije, S. Yu, D. De Ruysscher, S. Meersschout, K. Van Beek, Y. Lievens, J. Van Meerbeeck, W. De Neve, B. Rao, H. van der Weide and P. Lambin. Development and external validation of prognostic model for 2-year survival of non-small-cell lung cancer patients treated with chemoradiotherapy. Int J Radiat Oncol Biol Phys 2009 74(2): 355-62. USD

Descourt, A. Vergnenegre, F. Barlesi, H. Lena, P. Fournel, L. Falchero, H. Berard, J. Hureaux, H. Le Caer, J. M. Chavaillon, L. Geriniere, I. Monnet, S. Chouabe and G. Robinet. Oral vinorelbine and cisplatin with concurrent radiotherapy after induction chemotherapy with cisplatin and docetaxel for patients with locally advanced non-small cell lung cancer: the GFPC 05-03 study. J Thorac Oncol 2011 6(2): 351-7. NRP

Dillman, J. Herndon, S. L. Seagren, W. L. Eaton, Jr. and M. R. Green. Improved survival in stage III non-small-cell lung cancer: seven-year follow-up of cancer and leukemia group B (CALGB) 8433 trial. J Natl Cancer Inst 1996 88(17): 1210-5. NRP

Din, J. Lester, A. Cameron, J. Ironside, A. Gee, S. Falk, S. A. Morgan, J. Worvill and M. Q. Hatton. Routine use of continuous, hyperfractionated, accelerated radiotherapy for non-small-cell lung cancer: a five-center experience. Int J Radiat Oncol Biol Phys 2008 72(3): 716-22. USD

Dingemans, G. Bootsma, A. Van Baardwijk, B. Reijmen, R. Wanders, M. Hochstenbag, A. Van Belle, R. Houben, P. Lambin and D. De Ruysscher. Determination of standard dose cetuximab together with concurrent individualised, isotoxic accelerated radiotherapy (RT) and cisplatin-vinorelbine for patients (pts) with stage III non-small cell lung cancer (NSCLC): A phase I study (NCT00522886). European Journal of Cancer 2011 47(): S602. NRD

Divers, S. A. Spencer, D. Carey, E. M. Busby, M. D. Hyatt and F. Robert. Phase I/IIa study of cisplatin and gemcitabine as induction chemotherapy followed by concurrent chemoradiotherapy with gemcitabine and paclitaxel for locally advanced non-small-cell lung cancer. J Clin Oncol 2005 23(27): 6664-73. NRP

Donato, A. Zurlo, P. Bonfili, M. Petrongari, M. Santarelli, A. Costa and R. M. Enrici. Hypofractionated radiation therapy for inoperable advanced stage non-small cell lung cancer. Tumori 1999 85(3): 174-6. NRP

Dowell, R. Sinard, D. A. Yardley, V. Aviles, M. Machtay, R. S. Weber, G. S. Weinstein, A. A. Chalian, D. P. Carbone and D. I. Rosenthal. Seven-week continuous-infusion paclitaxel concurrent with radiation therapy for locally advanced non-small cell lung and head and neck cancers. Semin Radiat Oncol 1999 9(2 Suppl 1): 97-101. NRP

Dupuy, T. DiPetrillo, S. Gandhi, N. Ready, T. Ng, W. Donat and W. W. Mayo-Smith. Radiofrequency ablation followed by conventional radiotherapy for medically inoperable stage I non-small cell lung cancer. Chest 2006 129(3): 738-45. NRI

Dworzecki, A. Idasiak, D. Sygula, U. Dworzecka and R. Suwinski. Stereotactic radiotherapy (SBRT) as asole or salvage therapy in non-small cell lung cancer patients. Neoplasma 2012 59(1): 114-20. USD

Eberhardt, G. Stamatis, M. Stuschke, H. Wilke, M. R. Muller, S. Kolks, M. Flasshove, J. Schutte, M. Stahl, L. Schlenger, V. Budach, D. Greschuchna, G. Stuben, H. Teschler, H. Sack and S. Seeber. Prognostically orientated multimodality treatment including surgery for selected patients of small-cell lung cancer patients stages IB to IIIB: long-term results of a phase II trial. Br J Cancer 1999 81(7): 1206-12. NRP

Eberhardt, H. Wilke, G. Stamatis, M. Stuschke, A. Harstrick, H. Menker, B. Krause, M. R. Mueller, M. Stahl, M. Flasshove, V. Budach, D. Greschuchna, N. Konietzko, H. Sack and S. Seeber. Preoperative chemotherapy followed by concurrent chemoradiation therapy based on hyperfractionated accelerated radiotherapy and definitive surgery in locally advanced non-small-cell lung cancer: mature results of a phase II trial. J Clin Oncol 1998 16(2): 622-34. NRP

Edelman, M. Suntharalingam, W. Burrows, K. F. Kwong, N. Mitra, Z. Gamliel, M. Riley, L. B. Cooper, N. L. Kennedy, S. Buskirk, P. Hausner, L. A. Doyle and M. J. Krasna. Phase I/II trial of hyperfractionated radiation and chemotherapy followed by surgery in stage III lung cancer. Ann Thorac Surg 2008 86(3): 903-10. NRP

El Sharouni, H. B. Kal and J. J. Battermann. Tumour control probability of stage III inoperable non-small cell lung tumours after sequential chemo-radiotherapy. Anticancer Res 2005 25(6C): 4655-61. NRP

Elias, A. T. Skarin, T. Leong, S. Mentzer, G. Strauss, T. Lynch, L. Shulman, C. Jacobs, A. Abner, E. H. Baldini, E. Frei, 3rd and D. J. Sugarbaker. Neoadjuvant therapy for surgically staged IIIA N2 non-small cell lung cancer (NSCLC). Lung Cancer 1997 17(1): 147-61. NRP

Endo, Y. Takada, K. Obayashi, Y. Kotani, M. Satouchi, T. Kado and K. Sugimura. Weekly paclitaxel and carboplatin with concurrent radiation therapy in locally advanced non-small cell lung cancer: phase I study. Radiat Med 2005 23(5): 331-5. NRP

Erridge, M. N. Gaze, A. Price, C. G. Kelly, G. R. Kerr, A. Cull, R. H. MacDougall, G. C. Howard, V. J. Cowie and A. Gregor. Symptom control and quality of life in people with lung cancer: a randomised trial of two palliative radiotherapy fractionation schedules. 2005 17(): 61-7. NRP

Eschmann, G. Friedel, F. Paulsen, M. Reimold, T. Hehr, W. Budach, J. Scheiderbauer, H. J. Machulla, H. Dittmann, R. Vonthein and R. Bares. Is standardised 18F-FDG uptake value an outcome predictor in patients with stage III non-small cell lung cancer?. European Journal of Nuclear Medicine and Molecular Imaging 2006 33(3): 263-269. NRP

Etiz, L. B. Marks, S. M. Zhou, G. C. Bentel, R. Clough, M. L. Hernando and P. A. Lind. Influence of tumor volume on survival in patients irradiated for non-small-cell lung cancer. Int J Radiat Oncol Biol Phys 2002 53(4): 835-46. USD

Fakiris, R. C. McGarry, C. T. Yiannoutsos, L. Papiez, M. Williams, M. A. Henderson and R. Timmerman. Stereotactic body radiation therapy for early-stage non-small-cell lung carcinoma: four-year results of a prospective phase II study. Int J Radiat Oncol Biol Phys 2009 75(3): 677-82. NRI, USD

Falk, D. J. Girling, R. J. White, P. Hopwood, A. Harvey, W. Qian and R. J. Stephens. Immediate versus delayed palliative thoracic radiotherapy in patients with unresectable locally advanced non-small cell lung cancer and minimal thoracic symptoms: randomised controlled trial. BMJ 2002 325(7362): 465. NRP

Fang, R. Komaki, P. Allen, T. Guerrero, R. Mohan and J. D. Cox. Comparison of outcomes for patients with medically inoperable Stage I non-small-cell lung cancer treated with two-dimensional vs. three-dimensional radiotherapy. Int J Radiat Oncol Biol Phys 2006 66(1): 108-16. NRP

Faria, L. Souhami, L. Portelance, M. Duclos, T. Vuong, D. Small and C. R. Freeman. Absence of toxicity with hypofractionated 3-dimensional radiation therapy for inoperable, early stage non-small cell lung cancer. Radiat Oncol 2006 1(): 42. NRP

Farr, A. Khalil, M. Knap and C. Grau. Radiation pneumonitis and treatment outcome in radical radiotherapy of stage III non small cell lung cancer. European Journal of Cancer 2011 47(): S605-S606. NRD

Favaretto, A. Paccagnella, L. Tomio, F. Sartori, A. Cipriani, R. Zuin, L. Reffosco, F. Calabro, F. Rea, C. Ghiotto, V. Chiarion-Sileni, F. Oniga, L. Loreggian and M. V. Fiorentino. Pre-operative chemoradiotherapy in non-small cell lung cancer stage III patients. Feasibility, toxicity and long-term results of a phase II study. Eur J Cancer 1996 32A(12): 2064-9. NRP

Felip, J. M. Del Campo, R. Bodi, R. Vera, S. Casado and D. Rubio. Cisplatin and vinorelbine followed by radiotherapy in the treatment of stage III-B non-small-cell lung cancer patients. Am J Clin Oncol 1997 20(4): 404-6. NRP

Fernandes, J. Shen, J. Finlay, N. Mitra, T. Evans, J. Stevenson, C. Langer, L. Lin, S. Hahn, E. Glatstein and R. Rengan. Elective nodal irradiation (ENI) vs. involved field radiotherapy (IFRT) for locally advanced non-small cell lung cancer (NSCLC): A comparative analysis of toxicities and clinical outcomes. Radiother Oncol 2010 95(2): 178-84. NRP

Fernandes, N. Mitra, E. Xanthopoulos, T. Evans, J. Stevenson, C. Langer, J. C. Kucharczuk, L. Lin and R. Rengan. The Impact of Extent and Location of Mediastinal Lymph Node Involvement on Survival in Stage III Non-Small-Cell Lung Cancer Patients Treated with Definitive Radiotherapy. Int J Radiat Oncol Biol Phys 2011 (): . NRP

Fernando, A. De Hoyos, R. J. Landreneau, S. Gilbert, W. E. Gooding, P. O. Buenaventura, N. A. Christie, C. Belani and J. D. Luketich. Radiofrequency ablation for the treatment of non-small cell lung cancer in marginal surgical candidates. J Thorac Cardiovasc Surg 2005 129(3): 639-44. OPP

Fiorica, F. Cartei, S. Ursino, A. Stefanelli, Y. Zagatti, S. Berretta, S. Figura, D. Maugeri, E. Zanet, D. Sparta, C. La Morella, U. Tirelli and M. Berretta. Safety and feasibility of radiotherapy treatment in elderly non-small-cell lung cancer (NSCLC) patients. Arch Gerontol Geriatr 2010 50(2): 185-91. NRP

Firat, A. Pleister, R. W. Byhardt and E. Gore. Age is independent of comorbidity influencing patient selection for combined modality therapy for treatment of stage III nonsmall cell lung cancer (NSCLC). Am J Clin Oncol 2006 29(3): 252-7. NRP

Firat, M. Bousamra, E. Gore and R. W. Byhardt. Comorbidity and KPS are independent prognostic factors in stage I non-small-cell lung cancer. Int J Radiat Oncol Biol Phys 2002 52(4): 1047-57. NRP

Firat, R. W. Byhardt and E. Gore. Comorbidity and Karnofksy performance score are independent prognostic factors in stage III non-small-cell lung cancer: an institutional analysis of patients treated on four RTOG studies. Radiation Therapy Oncology Group. Int J Radiat Oncol Biol Phys 2002 54(2): 357-64. NRP

Fischer, M. Soberman, P. Randolph, K. Crawford and D. J. Perry. Phase II trial of concurrent paclitaxel, carboplatin, and external-beam radiation followed by surgical resection in locally advanced non-small-cell lung cancer, protocol 99-444. Clin Lung Cancer 2006 8(1): 56-61. NRP

Forquer, A. J. Fakiris, R. D. Timmerman, S. S. Lo, S. M. Perkins, R. C. McGarry and P. A. Johnstone. Brachial plexopathy from stereotactic body radiotherapy in early-stage NSCLC: dose-limiting toxicity in apical tumor sites. Radiother Oncol 2009 93(3): 408-13. NRP

Fournel, G. Robinet, P. Thomas, P. J. Souquet, H. Lena, A. Vergnenegre, J. Y. Delhoume, J. Le Treut, J. A. Silvani, E. Dansin, M. C. Bozonnat, J. P. Daures, F. Mornex and M. Perol. Randomized phase III trial of sequential chemoradiotherapy compared with concurrent chemoradiotherapy in locally advanced non-small-cell lung cancer: Groupe Lyon-Saint-Etienne d'Oncologie Thoracique-Groupe Francais de Pneumo-Cancerologie NPC 95-01 Study. J Clin Oncol 2005 23(25): 5910-7. NRP

Frasci, P. Comella, G. Scoppa, C. Guida, A. Gravina, F. Fiore, R. Casaretti, A. Daponte, A. Parziale and G. Comella. Weekly paclitaxel and cisplatin with concurrent radiotherapy in locally advanced non-small-cell lung cancer: a phase I study. J Clin Oncol 1997 15(4): 1409-17. NRP

Friedel, D. Hruska, W. Budach, M. Wolf, T. Kyriss, M. Hurtgen, H. P. Eulenbruch, R. Dierkesmann and H. Toomes. Neoadjuvant chemoradiotherapy of stage III non-small-cell lung cancer. Lung Cancer 2000 30(3): 175-85. NRP

Friedel, W. Budach, J. Dippon, W. Spengler, S. M. Eschmann, C. Pfannenberg, F. Al-Kamash, T. Walles, H. Aebert, T. Kyriss, S. Veit, M. Kimmich, M. Bamberg, M. Kohlhaeufl, V. Steger and T. Hehr. Phase II trial of a trimodality regimen for stage III non-small-cell lung cancer using chemotherapy as induction treatment with concurrent hyperfractionated chemoradiation with carboplatin and paclitaxel followed by subsequent resection: a single-center study. J Clin Oncol 2010 28(6): 942-8. NRP

Fritz, H. J. Kraus, W. Muhlnickel, U. Hammer, W. Dolken, W. Engel-Riedel, A. Chemaissani and E. Stoelben. Stereotactic, single-dose irradiation of stage I non-small cell lung cancer and lung metastases. Radiat Oncol 2006 1(): 30. USD

Fromm, A. Rottenfusser, D. Berger, R. Pirker, R. Potter and B. Pokrajac. 3D-conformal radiotherapy for inoperable non-small-cell lung cancer - A single centre experience. Radiology and Oncology 2007 41(3): 133-143. USD

Fujii, H. Kunikane, H. Okamoto, K. Watanabe, H. Kunitoh, K. Mori, A. Yokoyama, H. Fukuda, T. Tamura and N. Saijo. A phase II study of cisplatin and irinotecan as induction chemotherapy followed by accelerated hyperfractionated thoracic radiotherapy with daily low-dose carboplatin in unresectable stage III non-small cell lung cancer: JCOG 9510. Jpn J Clin Oncol 2009 39(12): 784-90. NRP

Fujino, H. Shirato, H. Onishi, H. Kawamura, K. Takayama, M. Koto, R. Onimaru, Y. Nagata and M. Hiraoka. Characteristics of patients who developed radiation pneumonitis requiring steroid therapy after stereotactic irradiation for lung tumors. Cancer J 2006 12(1): 41-6. NRP

Fukuda, H. Soda, A. Kinoshita, Y. Nakamura, S. Nagashima, H. Takatani, K. Tsukamoto, S. Kohno and M. Oka. Irinotecan and cisplatin with concurrent split-course radiotherapy in locally advanced nonsmall-cell lung cancer: a multiinstitutional phase 2 study. Cancer 2007 110(3): 606-13. NRP

Fukumoto, H. Shirato, S. Shimzu, S. Ogura, R. Onimaru, K. Kitamura, K. Yamazaki, K. Miyasaka, M. Nishimura and H. Dosaka-Akita. Small-volume image-guided radiotherapy using hypofractionated, coplanar, and noncoplanar multiple fields for patients with inoperable Stage I nonsmall cell lung carcinomas. Cancer 2002 95(7): 1546-53. USD

Furuse, K. Kubota, M. Kawahara, N. Kodama, M. Ogawara, M. Akira, S. Nakajima, M. Takada, Y. Kusunoki, S. Negoro and et al.. Phase II study of concurrent radiotherapy and chemotherapy for unresectable stage III non-small-cell lung cancer. Southern Osaka Lung Cancer Study Group. J Clin Oncol 1995 13(4): 869-75. NRP

Furuse, M. Fukuoka, M. Kawahara, H. Nishikawa, Y. Takada, S. Kudoh, N. Katagami and Y. Ariyoshi. Phase III study of concurrent versus sequential thoracic radiotherapy in combination with mitomycin, vindesine, and cisplatin in unresectable stage III non-small-cell lung cancer. J Clin Oncol 1999 17(9): 2692-9. NRP

Furuta, K. Hayakawa, S. Katano, Y. Saito, Y. Nakayama, T. Takahashi, R. Imai, T. Ebara, N. Mitsuhashi and H. Niibe. Radiation therapy for stage I-II non-small cell lung cancer in patients aged 75 years and older. Jpn J Clin Oncol 1996 26(2): 95-8. NRI

Gadaleta, A. Catino and V. Mattioli. Radiofrequency thermal ablation in the treatment of lung malignancies. In Vivo 2006 20(6A): 765-7. NRP

Gadgeel, J. C. Ruckdeschel, B. B. Patel, A. Wozniak, A. Konski, M. Valdivieso, D. Hackstock, W. Chen, K. Belzer, A. M. Burger, L. Marquette and A. Turrisi. Phase II study of pemetrexed and cisplatin, with chest radiotherapy followed by docetaxel in patients with stage III non-small cell lung cancer. J Thorac Oncol 2011 6(5): 927-33. NRP

Gagel, M. Piroth, M. Pinkawa, P. Reinartz, M. Zimny, K. Fischedik, S. Stanzel, C. Breuer, E. Skobel, B. Asadpour, A. Schmachtenberg, U. Buell and M. J. Eble. Gemcitabine concurrent with thoracic radiotherapy after induction chemotherapy with gemcitabine/vinorelbine in locally advanced non-small cell lung cancer: a phase I study. Strahlenther Onkol 2006 182(5): 263-9. NRP

Gagel, M. Piroth, M. Pinkawa, P. Reinartz, T. Krohn, H. J. Kaiser, S. Stanzel, C. Breuer, B. Asadpour, A. Schmachtenberg and M. J. Eble. Sequential (gemcitabine/vinorelbine) and concurrent (gemcitabine) radiochemotherapy with FDG-PET-based target volume definition in locally advanced non-small cell lung cancer: first results of a phase I/II study. BMC Cancer 2007 7(): 112. NRP

Galetta, A. Cesario, S. Margaritora, V. Porziella, A. Piraino, R. M. D'Angelillo, M. A. Gambacorta, S. Ramella, L. Trodella, S. Valente, G. M. Corbo, G. Macis, A. Mule, V. Cardaci, S. Sterzi, P. Granone and P. Russo. Multimodality treatment of unresectable stage III non-small cell lung cancer: interim analysis of a phase II trial with preoperative gemcitabine and concurrent radiotherapy. J Thorac Cardiovasc Surg 2006 131(2): 314-21. NRP

Galetta, A. Cesario, S. Margaritora, V. Porziella, G. Macis, R. M. D'Angelillo, L. Trodella, S. Sterzi and P. Granone. Enduring challenge in the treatment of nonsmall cell lung cancer with clinical stage IIIB: results of a trimodality approach. Ann Thorac Surg 2003 76(6): 1802-8; discussion 1808-9. NRP

Gandara, K. Chansky, K. S. Albain, B. R. Leigh, L. E. Gaspar, P. N. Lara, Jr., H. Burris, P. Gumerlock, J. P. Kuebler, J. D. Bearden, 3rd, J. Crowley and R. Livingston. Consolidation docetaxel after concurrent chemoradiotherapy in stage IIIB non-small-cell lung cancer: phase II Southwest Oncology Group Study S9504. J Clin Oncol 2003 21(10): 2004-10. NRP

Gandara, K. Chansky, K. S. Albain, L. E. Gaspar, P. N. Lara, Jr., K. Kelly, J. Crowley and R. Livingston. Long-term survival with concurrent chemoradiation therapy followed by consolidation docetaxel in stage IIIB non-small-cell lung cancer: a phase II Southwest Oncology Group Study (S9504). Clin Lung Cancer 2006 8(2): 116-21. NRP

Garrido, R. Rosell, B. Massuti, F. Cardenal, V. Alberola, M. Domine, I. Maeztu, A. Ramos and A. Arellano. Predictors of long-term survival in patients with lung cancer included in the randomized Spanish Lung Cancer Group 0008 phase II trial using concomitant chemoradiation with docetaxel and carboplatin plus induction or consolidation chemotherapy. Clin Lung Cancer 2009 10(3): 180-6. NRP

Gaspar, E. Teixeira, R. Sotto-Mayor, M. Ortiz and R. Susano. Sequential chemo-radiation in non-small cell lung cancer: A retrospective study of 100 patients. Revista Portuguesa de Pneumologia 2003 9(3): 215-223. FLA

Gauden and L. Tripcony. The curative treatment by radiation therapy alone of Stage I non-small cell lung cancer in a geriatric population. Lung Cancer 2001 32(1): 71-9. NRI

Gauden, J. Ramsay and L. Tripcony. The curative treatment by radiotherapy alone of stage I non-small cell carcinoma of the lung. Chest 1995 108(5): 1278-82. NRI

Ghosh, V. Sujendran, C. Alexiou, L. Beggs and D. Beggs. Long term results of surgery versus continuous hyperfractionated accelerated radiotherapy (CHART) in patients aged >70 years with stage 1 non-small cell lung cancer. Eur J Cardiothorac Surg 2003 24(6): 1002-7. NRI

Giannitto, D. Giuffrida, A. Pappalardo, A. Russo, B. Vincenzi, S. Saita, E. Potenza, F. Marletta, G. La Venia, S. Castorina and R. Bordonaro. Paclitaxel, carboplatin and gemcitabine combination as induction chemotherapy for stage IIIA N2 bulky non-small cell lung cancer. Oncology 2005 69(4): 295-300. NRP

Gielda, J. C. Marsh, T. W. Zusag, L. P. Faber, M. Liptay, S. Basu, W. H. Warren, M. J. Fidler, M. Batus, R. A. Abrams and P. Bonomi. Split-course chemoradiotherapy for locally advanced non-small cell lung cancer: a single-institution experience of 144 patients. J Thorac Oncol 2011 6(6): 1079-86. NRP

Gielda, P. Mehta, A. Khan, J. C. Marsh, T. W. Zusag, W. H. Warren, M. J. Fidler, R. A. Abrams, P. Bonomi, M. Liptay and L. P. Faber. Weight gain in advanced non-small-cell lung cancer patients during treatment with split-course concurrent chemoradiotherapy is associated with superior survival. Int J Radiat Oncol Biol Phys 2011 81(4): 985-91. NRP

Giorgio, A. Pappalardo, A. Russo, D. Santini, C. Di Rosa, C. Di Salvo, S. Castorina, F. Marletta, G. Bellissima, N. Palermo, C. Scuderi and R. Bordonaro. A phase II study of induction chemotherapy followed by concurrent chemoradiotherapy in elderly patients with locally advanced non-small-cell lung cancer. Anticancer Drugs 2007 18(6): 713-9. NRP

Girard, F. Mornex, J. Y. Douillard, N. Bossard, E. Quoix, V. Beckendorf, D. Grunenwald, E. Amour and B. Milleron. Is neoadjuvant chemoradiotherapy a feasible strategy for stage IIIA-N2 non-small cell lung cancer? Mature results of the randomized IFCT-0101 phase II trial. Lung Cancer 2010 69(1): 86-93. NRP

Gobitti, G. Franchin, E. Minatel, M. Gigante, B. Basso, L. Bujor and M. G. Trovo. Thoracic radiation therapy and concomitant low-dose daily paclitaxel in non-small cell lung cancer: a phase I study. Oncol Rep 2005 14(6): 1647-53. NRP

Goldsmith, J. Cesaretti and J. P. Wisnivesky. Radiotherapy Planning Complexity and Survival after Treatment of Advanced Stage Lung Cancer in the Elderly. Cancer 2009 115(20): 4865-4873. NRP

Gollins, W. D. Ryder, P. A. Burt, P. V. Barber and R. Stout. Massive haemoptysis death and other morbidity associated with high dose rate intraluminal radiotherapy for carcinoma of the bronchus. Radiother Oncol 1996 39(2): 105-16. USD

Gomez. Predictive dosimetric factors for high-grade esophagitis in patients treated for non-small cell lung cancer (NSCLC) with definitive 3D conformal therapy (3D-CRT), intensity modulated radiation therapy (IMRT), or proton beam therapy (PBT). Radiotherapy and Oncology 2011 99(): S210. NRD

Gopal, G. Starkschall, S. L. Tucker, J. D. Cox, Z. Liao, M. Hanus, J. F. Kelly, C. W. Stevens and R. Komaki. Effects of radiotherapy and chemotherapy on lung function in patients with non-small-cell lung cancer. International Journal of Radiation Oncology Biology Physics 2003 56(1): 114-120. NRP

Gore, K. Bae, C. Langer, M. Extermann, B. Movsas, P. Okunieff, G. Videtic and H. Choy. Phase I/II trial of a COX-2 inhibitor with limited field radiation for intermediate prognosis patients who have locally advanced non-small-cell lung cancer: radiation therapy oncology group 0213. Clin Lung Cancer 2011 12(2): 125-30. NRP

Gore, K. Bae, S. J. Wong, A. Sun, J. A. Bonner, S. E. Schild, L. E. Gaspar, J. A. Bogart, M. Werner-Wasik and H. Choy. Phase III comparison of prophylactic cranial irradiation versus observation in patients with locally advanced non-small-cell lung cancer: primary analysis of radiation therapy oncology group study RTOG 0214. J Clin Oncol 2011 29(3): 272-8. NRP

Gouda, H. M. Kohail, N. A. Eldeeb, A. M. Omar, M. M. El-Geneidy and Y. M. Elkerm. Randomized study of concurrent carboplatin, paclitaxel, and radiotherapy with or without prior induction chemotherapy in patients with locally advanced non-small cell lung cancer. J Egypt Natl Canc Inst 2006 18(1): 73-81. NRP

Gouders, P. Maingon, M. Paesmans, P. Rodrigus, B. Hahn, M. D. Arnaiz, T. Nguyen, C. Landmann, J. F. Bosset, S. Danhier and P. Van Houtte. Exclusive radiotherapy for non small cell lung cancer. A retrospective multicentric study. Reports of Practical Oncology and Radiotherapy 2003 8(1): 7-14. NRI

Govindan, J. Bogart, T. Stinchcombe, X. Wang, L. Hodgson, R. Kratzke, J. Garst, T. Brotherton and E. E. Vokes. Randomized phase II study of pemetrexed, carboplatin, and thoracic radiation with or without cetuximab in patients with locally advanced unresectable non-small-cell lung cancer: Cancer and Leukemia Group B trial 30407. J Clin Oncol 2011 29(23): 3120-5. NRP

Graham, C. Clark, F. Abell, L. Browne, A. Capp, P. Clingan, P. De Sousa, C. Fox and M. Links. Concurrent end-phase boost high-dose radiation therapy for non-small-cell lung cancer with or without cisplatin chemotherapy. Australas Radiol 2006 50(4): 342-8. NRP

Graham, J. A. Purdy, B. Emami, J. W. Matthews and W. B. Harms. Preliminary results of a prospective trial using three dimensional radiotherapy for lung cancer. Int J Radiat Oncol Biol Phys 1995 33(5): 993-1000. NRP

Graham, M. Jahanzeb, C. M. Dresler, J. D. Cooper, B. Emami and J. E. Mortimer. Results of a trial with topotecan dose escalation and concurrent thoracic radiation therapy for locally advanced, inoperable nonsmall cell lung cancer. Int J Radiat Oncol Biol Phys 1996 36(5): 1215-20. NRP

Graham, T. E. Pajak, A. M. Herskovic, B. Emami and C. A. Perez. Phase I/II study of treatment of locally advanced (T3/T4) non-oat cell lung cancer with concomitant boost radiotherapy by the Radiation Therapy Oncology Group (RTOG 83-12): long-term results. Int J Radiat Oncol Biol Phys 1995 31(4): 819-25. NRP

Graham, V. J. Gebski and A. O. Langlands. Radical radiotherapy for early nonsmall cell lung cancer. Int J Radiat Oncol Biol Phys 1995 31(2): 261-6. NRI

Granone, S. Margaritora, A. Cesario, P. Bonatti, D. Galetta and A. Picciocchi. Concurrent radio-chemotherapy in N2 non small cell lung cancer: Interim analysis. European Journal of Cardio-thoracic Surgery 1997 12(3): 366-371. NRP

Greco, S. L. Stroup and J. D. Hainsworth. Paclitaxel by 1-hour infusion in combination chemotherapy of stage III non-small cell lung cancer. Semin Oncol 1995 22(4 Suppl 9): 75-7. NRP

Greco, S. L. Stroup, J. R. Gray and J. D. Hainsworth. Paclitaxel in combination chemotherapy with radiotherapy in patients with unresectable stage III non-small-cell lung cancer. J Clin Oncol 1996 14(5): 1642-8. NRP

Greenberger, C. P. Belani, J. D. Leuketich, A. Argiris, S. S. Ramalingam, W. Gooding, A. Pennathur, D. Petro, M. W. Epperly and A. A. Tarhini. A phase I study demonstrating manganese superoxide dismutase plasmid liposome complex (MNSOD-Pl) reduction of esophagitis following standard chemoradiation in surgically unresectable stage III NSCLC. International Journal of Radiation Oncology Biology Physics 2010 78(3): S201. NRD

Greillier, F. Barlesi, C. Doddoli, O. Durieux, J. P. Torre, C. Gimenez and J. P. Kleisbauer. Vascular stenting for palliation of superior vena cava obstruction in non-small-cell lung cancer patients: a future 'standard' procedure?. Respiration 2004 71(2): 178-83. NRP

Gridelli, C. Guida, E. Barletta, T. Gatani, F. Fiore, M. L. Barzelloni, A. Rossi, M. de Bellis, R. D'Aniello and F. Scognamiglio. Thoracic radiotherapy and daily vinorelbine as radiosensitizer in locally advanced non small cell lung cancer: a phase I study. Lung Cancer 2000 29(2): 131-7. NRP

Grieco, C. J. Simon, W. W. Mayo-Smith, T. A. DiPetrillo, N. E. Ready and D. E. Dupuy. Percutaneous image-guided thermal ablation and radiation therapy: outcomes of combined treatment for 41 patients with inoperable stage I/II non-small-cell lung cancer. J Vasc Interv Radiol 2006 17(7): 1117-24. NRI

Grills, V. S. Mangona, R. Welsh, G. Chmielewski, E. McInerney, S. Martin, J. Wloch, H. Ye and L. L. Kestin. Outcomes after stereotactic lung radiotherapy or wedge resection for stage I non-small-cell lung cancer. J Clin Oncol 2010 28(6): 928-35. NRI

Groen, A. H. van der Leest, E. G. de Vries, D. R. Uges, B. G. Szabo and N. H. Mulder. Continuous carboplatin infusion during 6 weeks' radiotherapy in locally inoperable non-small-cell lung cancer: a phase I and pharmacokinetic study. Br J Cancer 1995 72(4): 992-7. NRP

Groen, A. H. W. van der Leest, E. Fokkema, P. R. Timmer, G. D. Nossent, W. J. G. Smit, J. Nabers, H. J. Hoekstra, J. Hermans, R. Otter, J. W. G. van Putten, E. G. E. de Vries and N. H. Mulder. Continuously infused carboplatin used as radiosensitizer in locally unresectable non-small-cell lung cancer: A multicenter phase III study. Annals of Oncology 2004 15(3): 427-432. NRP

Groen, T. W. van der Mark, A. H. van der Leest, E. G. de Vries and N. H. Mulder. Pulmonary function changes in lung-cancer patients treated with radiation with or without carboplatin. Am J Respir Crit Care Med 1995 152(6 Pt 1): 2044-8. NRP

Grossi, M. Millward, R. Fisher, S. Porceddu, M. Mac Manus, G. Ryan, A. Wirth and D. Ball. Combined modality treatment using concurrent radiotherapy and pharmacologically-guided carboplatin for inoperable and incompletely resected non-small cell lung cancer. Lung Cancer 2001 31(1): 73-82. NRP

Grunenwald, F. Andre, C. Le Pechoux, P. Girard, C. Lamer, A. Laplanche, M. Tarayre, R. Arriagada and T. Le Chevalier. Benefit of surgery after chemoradiotherapy in stage IIIB (T4 and/or N3) non-small cell lung cancer. J Thorac Cardiovasc Surg 2001 122(4): 796-802. NRP

Guckenberger, J. Wulf, G. Mueller, T. Krieger, K. Baier, M. Gabor, A. Richter, J. Wilbert and M. Flentje. Dose-response relationship for image-guided stereotactic body radiotherapy of pulmonary tumors: relevance of 4D dose calculation. Int J Radiat Oncol Biol Phys 2009 74(1): 47-54. NRP

Guckenberger, K. Heilman, J. Wulf, G. Mueller, G. Beckmann and M. Flentje. Pulmonary injury and tumor response after stereotactic body radiotherapy (SBRT): results of a serial follow-up CT study. Radiother Oncol 2007 85(3): 435-42. NRP

Haasbeek, F. J. Lagerwaard, K. de Jaeger, B. J. Slotman and S. Senan. Outcomes of stereotactic radiotherapy for a new clinical stage I lung cancer arising postpneumonectomy. Cancer 2009 115(3): 587-94. NRP

Haasbeek, F. J. Lagerwaard, M. E. Antonisse, B. J. Slotman and S. Senan. Stage I nonsmall cell lung cancer in patients aged > or =75 years: outcomes after stereotactic radiotherapy. Cancer 2010 116(2): 406-14. NRP

Hainsworth and E. E. Vokes. Docetaxel (Taxotere) in combination with radiation therapy and the potential of weekly administration in elderly and/or poor performance status patients with advanced non-small cell lung cancer. Semin Oncol 2001 28(1 Suppl 2): 22-7. NRD

Hainsworth, J. R. Gray, S. Litchy, J. D. Bearden, D. W. Shaffer, G. A. Houston and F. A. Greco. A phase II trial of preoperative concurrent radiation therapy and weekly paclitaxel/carboplatin for patients with locally advanced non-small-cell lung cancer. Clin Lung Cancer 2004 6(1): 33-42. NRP

Hallqvist, G. Wagenius, H. Rylander, O. Brodin, E. Holmberg, B. Loden, S. B. Ewers, S. Bergstrom, G. Wichardt-Johansson, K. Nilsson, L. Ekberg, C. Sederholm and J. Nyman. Concurrent cetuximab and radiotherapy after docetaxel-cisplatin induction chemotherapy in stage III NSCLC: Satellite-A phase II study from the Swedish Lung Cancer Study Group. Lung Cancer 2011 71(2): 166-172. NRP

Hamamoto, Y. Sugawara, T. Inoue, M. Kataoka, T. Ochi, T. Takahashi and S. Sakai. Relationship between pretreatment FDG uptake and local control after stereotactic body radiotherapy in stage I non-small-cell lung cancer: the preliminary results. Jpn J Clin Oncol 2011 41(4): 543-7. USD

Hamouda, Y. Dorgham, A. Yosry and M. Abdel Wahab. Neoadjuvant chemotherapy in locally advanced non-small cell lung cancer. Gulf J Oncolog 2007 (2): 55-64. NRP

Han, D. Prasetyo and G. M. Wright. Endobronchial palliation using Nd:YAG laser is associated with improved survival when combined with multimodal adjuvant treatments. Journal of Thoracic Oncology 2007 2(1): 59-64. USD

Hanna, M. Neubauer, C. Yiannoutsos, R. McGarry, J. Arseneau, R. Ansari, C. Reynolds, R. Govindan, A. Melnyk, W. Fisher, D. Richards, D. Bruetman, T. Anderson, N. Chowhan, S. Nattam, P. Mantravadi, C. Johnson, T. Breen, A. White and L. Einhorn. Phase III study of cisplatin, etoposide, and concurrent chest radiation with or without consolidation docetaxel in patients with inoperable stage III non-small-cell lung cancer: the Hoosier Oncology Group and U.S. Oncology. J Clin Oncol 2008 26(35): 5755-60. NRP

Harada, N. Yamamoto, T. Takahashi, M. Endo, H. Murakami, A. Tsuya, Y. Nakamura, A. Ono, S. Igawa, T. Shukuya, A. Tamiya and T. Nishimura. Comparison of chemotherapy regimens for concurrent chemoradiotherapy in unresectable stage III non-small cell lung cancer. Int J Clin Oncol 2009 14(6): 507-12. NRP

Harada, T. Seto, S. Igawa, A. Tsuya, M. Wada, K. Kaira, T. Naito, K. Hayakawa, T. Nishimura, N. Masuda and N. Yamamoto. Phase I Results of Vinorelbine with Concurrent Radiotherapy in Elderly Patients with Unresectable, Locally Advanced Non-Small-Cell Lung Cancer: West Japan Thoracic Oncology Group (WJTOG3005-DI). Int J Radiat Oncol Biol Phys 2011 (): . NRP

Harms, P. Schraube, H. Becker, D. Latz, F. Herth, P. Fritz and M. Wannenmacher. Effect and toxicity of endoluminal high-dose-rate (HDR) brachytherapy in centrally located tumors of the upper respiratory tract. Strahlenther Onkol 2000 176(2): 60-6. USD

Hartsell, C. B. Scott, G. S. Dundas, M. Mohiuddin, R. F. Meredith, P. Rubin and I. J. Weigensberg. Can serum markers be used to predict acute and late toxicity in patients with lung cancer? Analysis of RTOG 91-03. Am J Clin Oncol 2007 30(4): 368-76. NRP

Hasegawa, S. Takanashi, K. Okudera, M. Aoki, K. Basaki, H. Kondo, T. Takahata, N. Yasui-Furukori, T. Tateishi, Y. Abe and K. Okumura. Weekly paclitaxel and nedaplatin with concurrent radiotherapy for locally advanced non-small-cell lung cancer: a phase I/II study. Jpn J Clin Oncol 2004 34(11): 647-53. NRP

Hata, K. Tokuuye, K. Kagei, S. Sugahara, H. Nakayama, N. Fukumitsu, T. Hashimoto, M. Mizumoto, K. Ohara and Y. Akine. Hypofractionated high-dose proton beam therapy for stage I non-small-cell lung cancer: preliminary results of a phase I/II clinical study. Int J Radiat Oncol Biol Phys 2007 68(3): 786-93. NRP

Hatton, M. Nankivell, E. Lyn, S. Falk, C. Pugh, N. Navani, R. Stephens and M. Parmar. Induction chemotherapy and continuous hyperfractionated accelerated radiotherapy (chart) for patients with locally advanced inoperable non-small-cell lung cancer: the MRC INCH randomized trial. Int J Radiat Oncol Biol Phys 2011 81(3): 712-8. NRP

Havemann, M. Wolf, C. Goerg, C. Faoro, R. Pfab and K. Diergarten. Paclitaxel and simultaneous radiation in the treatment of stage III A/B non-small cell lung cancer. Semin Oncol 1995 22(6 Suppl 14): 19-22. NRP

Hayakawa, N. Mitsuhashi, M. Furuta, Y. Saito, Y. Nakayama, S. Katano, M. Yamakawa, I. Hashida and Niibe. High-dose radiation therapy for inoperable non-small cell lung cancer without mediastinal involvement (clinical stage N0, N1). Strahlenther Onkol 1996 172(9): 489-95. NRI

Hayakawa, N. Mitsuhashi, S. Katano, Y. Saito, Y. Nakayama, H. Sakurai, T. Akimoto, M. Hasegawa, M. Yamakawa and H. Niibe. High-dose radiation therapy for elderly patients with inoperable or unresectable non-small cell lung cancer. Lung Cancer 2001 32(1): 81-8. NRP

Hayakawa, N. Mitsuhashi, Y. Saito, M. Furuta, Y. Nakayama, S. Katano, H. Sakurai, T. Takahashi, O. Mitomo and H. Niibe. Impact of tumor extent and location on treatment outcome in patients with stage III non-small cell lung cancer treated with radiation therapy. Jpn J Clin Oncol 1996 26(4): 221-8. NRP

Hayakawa, N. Mitsuhashi, Y. Saito, Y. Nakayama, M. Furuta, H. Sakurai, M. Kawashima, T. Ohno, S. Nasu and H. Niibe. Limited field irradiation for medically inoperable patients with peripheral stage I non-small cell lung cancer. Lung Cancer 1999 26(3): 137-42. NRI

Hayakawa, N. Mitsuhashi, Y. Saito, Y. Nakayama, M. Furuta, S. Nakamoto, M. Kawashima and H. Niibe. Effect of Krestin as adjuvant treatment following radical radiotherapy in non-small cell lung cancer patients. Cancer Detect Prev 1997 21(1): 71-7. NRP

Hayakawa, N. Mitsuhashi, Y. Saito, Y. Nakayama, S. Katano, M. Furuta, H. Sakurai, T. Takahashi and H. Niibe. Definitive radiation therapy for medically inoperable patients with stage I and II non-small cell lung cancer. Radiation Oncology Investigations 1996 4(4): 165-170. NRI

Hayman, M. K. Martel, R. K. Ten Haken, D. P. Normolle, R. F. Todd, 3rd, J. F. Littles, M. A. Sullivan, P. W. Possert, A. T. Turrisi and A. S. Lichter. Dose escalation in non-small-cell lung cancer using three-dimensional conformal radiation therapy: update of a phase I trial. J Clin Oncol 2001 19(1): 127-36. NRP

Hayman, P. H. Abrahamse, I. Lakhani, C. C. Earle and S. J. Katz. Use of palliative radiotherapy among patients with metastatic non-small-cell lung cancer. Int J Radiat Oncol Biol Phys 2007 69(4): 1001-7. NRP

Hehr, G. Friedel, V. Steger, W. Spengler, S. M. Eschmann, M. Bamberg and W. Budach. Neoadjuvant chemoradiation with paclitaxel/carboplatin for selected Stage III non-small-cell lung cancer: long-term results of a trimodality Phase II protocol. Int J Radiat Oncol Biol Phys 2010 76(5): 1376-81. NRP

Heinzerling, H. Choy, R. S. Hughes, R. Govindan, J. D. Bradley, L. S. Schwartzberg, G. Peng, J. Treat, T. Tran and C. Obasaju. Toxicity and response of pemetrexed plus carboplatin or cisplatin with concurrent chest radiation therapy for patients with locally advanced non-small cell lung cancer: A phase i trial. Journal of Thoracic Oncology 2010 5(9): 1391-1396. NRP

Henderson, D. J. Hoopes, J. W. Fletcher, P. F. Lin, M. Tann, C. T. Yiannoutsos, M. D. Williams, A. J. Fakiris, R. C. McGarry and R. D. Timmerman. A pilot trial of serial 18F-fluorodeoxyglucose positron emission tomography in patients with medically inoperable stage I non-small-cell lung cancer treated with hypofractionated stereotactic body radiotherapy. Int J Radiat Oncol Biol Phys 2010 76(3): 789-95. OPP

Henderson, R. McGarry, C. Yiannoutsos, A. Fakiris, D. Hoopes, M. Williams and R. Timmerman. Baseline pulmonary function as a predictor for survival and decline in pulmonary function over time in patients undergoing stereotactic body radiotherapy for the treatment of stage I non-small-cell lung cancer. Int J Radiat Oncol Biol Phys 2008 72(2): 404-9. OPP

Hennequin, J. Trédaniel, C. Durdux, A. Salemkour, G. Zalcman, A. Hirsch, M. Housset and C. Maylin. Concomitant radiochemotherapy in inoperable non-small cell lung cancer. 1997 1(): 143-7. FLA

Hepp, C. Pottgen, T. Gauler, P. Erichsen, C. Le Pechoux, D. Grunenwald, S. Welter, G. Stamatis, M. Stuschke and W. E. E. Eberhardt. Long-term survival results and prognostic factor analysis of two consecutive trimodality Phase-II trials in stage IIIA(N2) and selected stage IIIB non-small-cell lung cancer (NSCLC). Strahlentherapie und Onkologie 2011 187(): 68-69. NRD

Herse, H. Dalichau, B. Wormann, B. Hemmerlein, H. Schmidberger, C. F. Hess, P. Hannemann, C. P. Criee, W. Hiddemann and F. Griesinger. Induction combination chemotherapy with docetaxel and carboplatin in advanced non-small-cell lung cancer. Thorac Cardiovasc Surg 1998 46(5): 298-302. NRP

Herskovic, C. Scott, W. Demas, L. Gaspar and A. Trotti. Accelerated hyperfractionation for bronchogenic cancer: Radiation Therapy Oncology Group 9205. Am J Clin Oncol 2000 23(2): 207-12. NRP

Herth, S. Peter, F. Baty, R. Eberhardt, J. D. Leuppi and P. N. Chhajed. Combined airway and oesophageal stenting in malignant airway-oesophageal fistulas: A prospective study. European Respiratory Journal 2010 36(6): 1370-1374. NRP

Hicks, M. P. Mac Manus, J. P. Matthews, A. Hogg, D. Binns, D. Rischin, D. L. Ball and L. J. Peters. Early FDG-PET imaging after radical radiotherapy for non-small-cell lung cancer: inflammatory changes in normal tissues correlate with tumor response and do not confound therapeutic response evaluation. Int J Radiat Oncol Biol Phys 2004 60(2): 412-8. NRP

Higgins, J. P. Chino, L. B. Marks, N. Ready, T. A. D'Amico, R. W. Clough and C. R. Kelsey. Preoperative chemotherapy versus preoperative chemoradiotherapy for stage III (N2) non-small-cell lung cancer. Int J Radiat Oncol Biol Phys 2009 75(5): 1462-7. NRP

Hill, C. E. Nwogu, G. Loewen, J. Pelow, T. J. Dougherty and T. M. Anderson. Off-Label Management of Primary and Metastatic Endobronchial Tumors with Photodynamic Therapy. Clinical Pulmonary Medicine 2004 11(2): 107-111. NRP

Hillas, P. Bakakos, M. Trichas and F. Vlastos. The disparity of health facilities in an urban area discourages proposed treatment application in inoperable lung cancer patients. Cancer Manag Res 2010 2(): 287-91. NRP

Hiraki, H. Gobara, H. Mimura, S. Toyooka, H. Fujiwara, K. Yasui, Y. Sano, T. Iguchi, J. Sakurai, N. Tajiri, T. Mukai, Y. Matsui and S. Kanazawa. Radiofrequency ablation of lung cancer at Okayama University Hospital: a review of 10 years of experience. Acta Med Okayama 2011 65(5): 287-97. NRD

Hiraki, H. Gobara, H. Mimura, Y. Matsui, S. Toyooka and S. Kanazawa. Percutaneous radiofrequency ablation of clinical stage I non-small cell lung cancer. J Thorac Cardiovasc Surg 2011 142(1): 24-30. USD

Hiraki, H. Gobara, T. Iishi, Y. Sano, T. Iguchi, H. Fujiwara, N. Tajiri, J. Sakurai, H. Date, H. Mimura and S. Kanazawa. Percutaneous radiofrequency ablation for clinical stage I non-small cell lung cancer: results in 20 nonsurgical candidates. J Thorac Cardiovasc Surg 2007 134(5): 1306-12. NRP

Hiraoka and S. Ishikura. A Japan clinical oncology group trial for stereotactic body radiation therapy of non-small cell lung cancer. Journal of Thoracic Oncology 2007 2(7 SUPPL.3): S115-S117. NRD

Hiraoka and Y. Nagata. Stereotactic body radiation therapy for early-stage non-small-cell lung cancer: the Japanese experience. Int J Clin Oncol 2004 9(5): 352-5. NRD

Hiraoka, Y. Matsuo and Y. Nagata. Stereotactic body radiation therapy (SBRT) for early-stage lung cancer. Cancer Radiother 2007 11(1-2): 32-5. NRD

Hirose, Y. Mizutani, T. Ohmori, H. Ishida, T. Hosaka, K. Ando, T. Shirai, K. Okuda, T. Ohnishi, N. Horichi, H. Kubota and M. Adachi. The combination of cisplatin and vinorelbine with concurrent thoracic radiation therapy for locally advanced stage IIIA or IIIB non-small-cell lung cancer. Cancer Chemother Pharmacol 2006 58(3): 361-7. NRP

Hirsh, D. Soulieres, M. Duclos, S. Faria, P. Del Vecchio, L. Ofiara, J. P. Ayoub, D. Charpentier, J. Gruber, L. Portelance and L. Souhami. Phase II multicenter trial with carboplatin and gemcitabine induction chemotherapy followed by radiotherapy concomitantly with low-dose paclitaxel and gemcitabine for stage IIIA and IIIB non-small cell lung cancer. J Thorac Oncol 2007 2(10): 927-32. NRP

Hodge, W. A. Tome, H. A. Jaradat, N. P. Orton, D. Khuntia, A. Traynor, T. Weigel and M. P. Mehta. Feasibility report of image guided stereotactic body radiotherapy (IG-SBRT) with tomotherapy for early stage medically inoperable lung cancer using extreme hypofractionation. Acta Oncol 2006 45(7): 890-6. NRO

Hoekstra, S. C. Stroobants, E. F. Smit, J. Vansteenkiste, H. Van Tinteren, P. E. Postmus, R. P. Golding, B. Biesma, F. J. H. M. Schramel, N. Van Zandwijk, A. A. Lammertsma and O. S. Hoekstra. Prognostic relevance of response evaluation using [18F]-2- fluoro-2-deoxy-D-glucose positron emission tomography in patients with locally advanced non-small-cell lung cancer. Journal of Clinical Oncology 2005 23(33): 8362-8370. NRP

Hof, K. K. Herfarth, M. Munter, A. Hoess, J. Motsch, M. Wannenmacher and J. J. Debus. Stereotactic single-dose radiotherapy of stage I non-small-cell lung cancer (NSCLC). Int J Radiat Oncol Biol Phys 2003 56(2): 335-41. USD

Hof, M. Muenter, D. Oetzel, A. Hoess, J. Debus and K. Herfarth. Stereotactic single-dose radiotherapy (radiosurgery) of early stage nonsmall-cell lung cancer (NSCLC). Cancer 2007 110(1): 148-55. NRP

Hoffman, E. E. Cohen, G. A. Masters, D. J. Haraf, A. M. Mauer, C. M. Rudin, S. A. Krauss, D. Huo and E. E. Vokes. Carboplatin plus vinorelbine with concomitant radiation therapy in advanced non-small cell lung cancer: a phase I study. Lung Cancer 2002 38(1): 65-71. NRP

Hongwu, Z. Yunzhi, L. Dongmei, Z. Hang and L. Lingfei. Place of cryotherapy, argon plasma coagulation? Photodynamic therapy and stents in therapeutic bronchoscopy of lung cancers. Photodiagnosis and Photodynamic Therapy 2011 8(2): 176. NRD

Hoopes, M. Tann, J. W. Fletcher, J. A. Forquer, P. F. Lin, S. S. Lo, R. D. Timmerman and R. C. McGarry. FDG-PET and stereotactic body radiotherapy (SBRT) for stage I non-small-cell lung cancer. Lung Cancer 2007 56(2): 229-34. NRI, USD

Hoppe, B. Laser, A. V. Kowalski, S. C. Fontenla, E. Pena-Greenberg, E. D. Yorke, D. M. Lovelock, M. A. Hunt and K. E. Rosenzweig. Acute skin toxicity following stereotactic body radiation therapy for stage I non-small-cell lung cancer: who's at risk?. Int J Radiat Oncol Biol Phys 2008 72(5): 1283-6. NRP

Hoyer, H. Roed, A. T. Hansen, L. Ohlhuis, J. Petersen, H. Nellemann, A. K. Berthelsen, C. Grau, S. A. Engelholm and H. von der Maase. Prospective study on stereotactic radiotherapy of limited-stage non-small-cell lung cancer. International Journal of Radiation Oncology Biology Physics 2006 66(4 SUPPL.): S128-S135. NRP

Hsie, S. Morbidini-Gaffney, L. J. Kohman, E. Dexter, E. M. Scalzetti and J. A. Bogart. Definitive treatment of poor-risk patients with stage I lung cancer: a single institution experience. J Thorac Oncol 2009 4(1): 69-73. USD

Hu, E. L. Chang, S. J. Hassenbusch, 3rd, P. K. Allen, S. Y. Woo, A. Mahajan, R. Komaki and Z. Liao. Nonsmall cell lung cancer presenting with synchronous solitary brain metastasis. Cancer 2006 106(9): 1998-2004. NRP

Huang, Z. Liao, J. D. Cox, T. M. Guerrero, J. Y. Chang, M. Jeter, Y. Borghero, X. Wei, F. Fossella, R. S. Herbst, G. R. Blumenschein, Jr., C. Moran, P. K. Allen and R. Komaki. Comparison of outcomes for patients with unresectable, locally advanced non-small-cell lung cancer treated with induction chemotherapy followed by concurrent chemoradiation vs. concurrent chemoradiation alone. Int J Radiat Oncol Biol Phys 2007 68(3): 779-85. NRP

Huber, A. Borgmeier, M. Flentje, J. Willner, M. Schmidt, C. Manegold, P. Bramlage and J. Debus. Concurrent chemoradiation therapy with docetaxel/cisplatin followed by docetaxel consolidation therapy in inoperable stage IIIA/B non-small-cell lung cancer: results of a phase I study. Clin Lung Cancer 2010 11(1): 45-50. NRP

Huber, M. Flentje, M. Schmidt, B. Pollinger, H. Gosse, J. Willner and K. Ulm. Simultaneous chemoradiotherapy compared with radiotherapy alone after induction chemotherapy in inoperable stage IIIA or IIIB non-small-cell lung cancer: study CTRT99/97 by the Bronchial Carcinoma Therapy Group. J Clin Oncol 2006 24(27): 4397-404. NRP

Huber, R. Fischer, H. Hautmann, B. Pollinger, K. Haussinger and T. Wendt. Does additional brachytherapy improve the effect of external irradiation? A prospective, randomized study in central lung tumors. Int J Radiat Oncol Biol Phys 1997 38(3): 533-40. NRD

Hughes, J. Liong, A. Miah, S. Ahmad, M. Leslie, P. Harper, J. Prendiville, J. Shamash, R. Subramaniam, A. Gaya, J. Spicer and D. Landau. A brief report on the safety study of induction chemotherapy followed by synchronous radiotherapy and cetuximab in stage III non-small cell lung cancer (NSCLC): SCRATCH study. J Thorac Oncol 2008 3(6): 648-51. NRP

Huisman, G. Giaccone, C. J. van Groeningen, G. Sutedja, P. E. Postmus and E. F. Smit. Combination of gemcitabine and cisplatin for advanced non-small cell lung cancer: a phase II study with emphasis on scheduling. Lung Cancer 2001 33(2-3): 267-75. NRP

Iaffaioli, F. Caponigro, A. Tortoriello, G. Facchini, V. Ravo, M. Maccauro, P. Dimitri, F. Crovella and P. Muto. Accelerated split-course (type B) thoracic radiation therapy plus vinorelbine/carboplatin combination chemotherapy in stage III inoperable non-small cell lung cancer. Eur J Cancer 1996 32A(11): 1901-4. NRP

Ichinose, T. Seto, T. Sasaki, T. Yamanaka, I. Okamoto, K. Takeda, M. Tanaka, N. Katakami, T. Sawa, S. Kudoh, H. Saka, Y. Nishimura, K. Nakagawa and M. Fukuoka. S-1 Plus Cisplatin with Concurrent Radiotherapy for Locally Advanced Non-small Cell Lung Cancer: A Multi-Institutional Phase II Trial (West Japan Thoracic Oncology Group 3706). J Thorac Oncol 2011 6(12): 2069-2075. NRP

Ichinose, T. Yano, H. Asoh, H. Yokoyama, R. Maruyama, C. Ushijima, T. Uehara, T. Kanematsu, T. Yohena and S. Wada. UFT plus cisplatin with concurrent radiotherapy for locally advanced non-small-cell lung cancer. Oncology (Williston Park) 1999 13(7 Suppl 3): 98-101. NRP

Ichinose, Y. Fukuyama, H. Asoh, C. Ushijima, T. Okamoto, J. Ikeda, J. Okamoto and M. Sakai. Induction chemoradiotherapy and surgical resection for selected stage IIIB non-small-cell lung cancer. Ann Thorac Surg 2003 76(6): 1810-4; discussion 1815. NRP

Ichinose, Y. Nakai, S. Kudoh, H. Semba, S. Yoshida, T. Nukiwa, H. Yamamoto, Y. Yamane and H. Niitani. Uracil/tegafur plus cisplatin with concurrent radiotherapy for locally advanced non-small-cell lung cancer: a multi-institutional phase II trial. Clin Cancer Res 2004 10(13): 4369-73. NRP

Iranzo, R. M. Bremnes, P. Almendros, J. Gavila, A. Blasco, R. Sirera and C. Camps. Induction chemotherapy followed by concurrent chemoradiation for patients with non-operable stage III non-small-cell lung cancer. Lung Cancer 2009 63(1): 63-7. NRP

Isakovic-Vidovic, L. Radosevic-Jelic and N. Borojevic. Combined chemoradiotherapy in the treatment of locally advanced non-small cell lung cancer. J BUON 2002 7(1): 47-51. NRP

Ishikawa, Y. Nakayama, Y. Kitamoto, T. Nonaka, H. Kawamura, K. Shirai, H. Sakurai, K. Hayakawa, H. Niibe and T. Nakano. Effect of histologic type on recurrence pattern in radiation therapy for medically inoperable patients with stage I non-small-cell lung cancer. Lung 2006 184(6): 347-53. NRI

Ishikura, Y. Ohe, K. Nihei, K. Kubota, R. Kakinuma, H. Ohmatsu, K. Goto, S. Niho, Y. Nishiwaki and T. Ogino. A phase II study of hyperfractionated accelerated radiotherapy (HART) after induction cisplatin (CDDP) and vinorelbine (VNR) for stage III non-small-cell lung cancer (NSCLC). Int J Radiat Oncol Biol Phys 2005 61(4): 1117-22. NRP

Isokangas, H. Joensuu, M. Halme, A. Jekunen and K. Mattson. Paclitaxel (Taxol) and carboplatin followed by concomitant paclitaxel, cisplatin and radiotherapy for inoperable stage III NSCLC. Lung Cancer 1998 20(2): 127-33. NRP

Itoh, N. Fuwa, A. Matumoto, A. Asano and K. Morita. Continuous infusion low-dose CDDP/5-FU plus radiation in inoperable or recurrent non-small-cell lung cancer: preliminary experience. Am J Clin Oncol 2002 25(3): 230-4. NRP

Iwasaki, S. Ohsugi, A. Natsuhara, T. Tsubokura, H. Harada, M. Ueda, T. Arimoto, H. Hara, T. Yamada, T. Takesako, K. Kohno, S. Hosogi, M. Nakanishi, Y. Marunaka and T. Nishimura. Phase I/II trial of biweekly docetaxel and cisplatin with concurrent thoracic radiation for stage III non-small-cell lung cancer. Cancer Chemother Pharmacol 2006 58(6): 735-41. NRP

Iwata, Y. Shibamoto, F. Baba, C. Sugie, H. Ogino, R. Murata, T. Yanagi, S. Otsuka, K. Kosaki, T. Murai and A. Miyakawa. Correlation between the serum KL-6 level and the grade of radiation pneumonitis after stereotactic body radiotherapy for stage i lung cancer or small lung metastasis. Radiotherapy and Oncology 2011 101(2): 267-270. NRO

Izmirli, F. Yaman, M. Y. Buyukpolat, A. Yoney and M. Unsal. An accelerated radiotherapy scheme using a concomitant boost technique for the treatment of unresectable stage III non-small cell lung cancer. Jpn J Clin Oncol 2005 35(5): 239-44. NRP

Jager, H. J. Groen, A. van der Leest, J. W. van Putten, R. M. Pieterman, E. G. de Vries and D. A. Piers. L-3-[123I]iodo-alpha-methyl-tyrosine SPECT in non-small cell lung cancer: preliminary observations. J Nucl Med 2001 42(4): 579-85. NRP

Jain, R. S. Hughes, A. B. Sandler, A. Dowlati, L. S. Schwartzberg, T. Dobbs, L. Schlabach, J. Wu, N. J. Muldowney and H. Choy. A phase II study of concurrent chemoradiation with weekly docetaxel, carboplatin, and radiation therapy followed by consolidation chemotherapy with docetaxel and carboplatin for locally advanced inoperable non-small cell lung cancer (NSCLC). J Thorac Oncol 2009 4(6): 722-7. NRP

Jakse, K. S. Kapp, E. Geyer, A. Oechs, A. Maier, S. Gabor and F. M. Juttner. IORT and external beam irradiation (EBI) in clinical stage I-II NSCLC patients with severely compromised pulmonary function: an 52-patient single-institutional experience. Strahlenther Onkol 2007 183 Spec No 2(): 24-5. NRI

Jatoi, S. E. Schild, N. Foster, G. T. Henning, K. J. Dornfeld, P. J. Flynn, T. R. Fitch, S. R. Dakhil, K. M. Rowland, P. J. Stella, G. S. Soori and A. A. Adjei. A phase II study of cetuximab and radiation in elderly and/or poor performance status patients with locally advanced non-small-cell lung cancer (N0422). Ann Oncol 2010 21(10): 2040-4. NRP

Jazieh, A. Younas, M. Safa, K. Redmond, R. Buncher and J. Howington. Phase I clinical trial of concurrent paclitaxel, carboplatin, and external beam chest irradiation with glutamine in patients with locally advanced non-small cell lung cancer. Cancer Invest 2007 25(5): 294-8. NRP

Jenkins, S. Anderson, S. Wronski and A. Ashton. A phase II trial of induction chemotherapy followed by continuous hyperfractionated accelerated radiotherapy in locally advanced non-small-cell lung cancer. Radiother Oncol 2009 93(3): 396-401. NRP

Jensen, M. W. Munter, H. G. Bischoff, R. Haselmann, U. Haberkorn, P. E. Huber, M. Thomas, J. Debus and K. K. Herfarth. Combined treatment of nonsmall cell lung cancer NSCLC stage III with intensity-modulated RT radiotherapy and cetuximab: the NEAR trial. Cancer 2011 117(13): 2986-94. NRP

Jeong, J. H. Jung, J. H. Han, J. H. Kim, Y. W. Choi, H. W. Lee, S. Y. Kang, Y. H. Hwang, M. S. Ahn, J. H. Choi, Y. T. Oh, M. Chun, S. Kang, K. J. Park, S. C. Hwang and S. S. Sheen. Expression of Bcl-2 predicts outcome in locally advanced non-small cell lung cancer patients treated with cisplatin-based concurrent chemoradiotherapy. Lung Cancer 2010 68(2): 288-94. NRP

Jeremic and B. Milicic. From conventionally fractionated radiation therapy to hyperfractionated radiation therapy alone and with concurrent chemotherapy in patients with early-stage nonsmall cell lung cancer. Cancer 2008 112(4): 876-84. NRI

Jeremic and Y. Shibamoto. Effect of interfraction interval in hyperfractionated radiotherapy with or without concurrent chemotherapy for stage III nonsmall cell lung cancer. Int J Radiat Oncol Biol Phys 1996 34(2): 303-8. NRP

Jeremic and Y. Shibamoto. Pre-treatment prognostic factors in patients with stage III non-small cell lung cancer treated with hyperfractionated radiation therapy with or without concurrent chemotherapy. Lung Cancer 1995 13(1): 21-30. NRP

Jeremic, B. Milicic and S. Milisavljevic. Clinical prognostic factors in patients with locally advanced (stage III) nonsmall cell lung cancer treated with hyperfractionated radiation therapy with and without concurrent chemotherapy: single-Institution Experience in 600 Patients. Cancer 2011 117(13): 2995-3003. NRP

Jeremic, B. Milicic and S. Milisavljevic. Concurrent Hyperfractionated Radiation Therapy and Chemotherapy in Locally Advanced (Stage III) non-Small-cell lung Cancer: Single Institution Experience with 600 Patients. Int J Radiat Oncol Biol Phys 2011 (): . NRP

Jeremic, B. Milicic, A. Dagovic, J. Aleksandrovic and S. Milisavljevic. Interfraction interval in patients with stage III non-small-cell lung cancer treated with hyperfractionated radiation therapy with or without concurrent chemotherapy: final results in 536 patients. Am J Clin Oncol 2004 27(6): 616-25. NRP

Jeremic, B. Milicic, A. Dagovic, J. Aleksandrovic and S. Milisavljevic. Stage III non-small-cell lung cancer treated with high-dose hyperfractionated radiation therapy and concurrent low-dose daily chemotherapy with or without weekend chemotherapy: retrospective analysis of 301 patients. Am J Clin Oncol 2004 27(4): 350-60. NRP

Jeremic, B. Milicic, A. Dagovic, L. Acimovic and S. Milisavljevic. Pretreatment prognostic factors in patients with early-stage (I/II) non-small-cell lung cancer treated with hyperfractionated radiation therapy alone. Int J Radiat Oncol Biol Phys 2006 65(4): 1112-9. NRI

Jeremic, B. Milicic, L. Acimovic and S. Milisavljevic. Concurrent hyperfractionated radiotherapy and low-dose daily carboplatin and paclitaxel in patients with stage III non-small-cell lung cancer: long-term results of a phase II study. J Clin Oncol 2005 23(6): 1144-51. NRP

Jeremic, F. B. Zimmermann, C. Nieder and M. M. Molls. Radiation therapy alone as an alternative to surgery in patients with early stage non-small-cell lung cancer having cardiovascular (and other) comorbidity. Eur J Cardiothorac Surg 2004 25(2): 297. NRD

Jeremic, Y. Shibamoto, B. Milicic, A. Dagovic, J. Aleksandrovic, N. Nikolic and I. Igrutinovic. No thoracic radiation myelitis after spinal cord dose > or = 50.4 Gy using 1.2. Gy b.i.d. fractionation in patients with Stage III non-small cell lung cancer treated with hyperfractionated radiation therapy with and without concurrent chemotherapy. Lung Cancer 2002 35(3): 287-92. NRP

Jeremic, Y. Shibamoto, B. Milicic, A. Dagovic, N. Nikolic, J. Aleksandrovic, L. Acimovic and S. Milisavljevic. Impact of treatment interruptions due to toxicity on outcome of patients with early stage (I/II) non-small-cell lung cancer (NSCLC) treated with hyperfractionated radiation therapy alone. Lung Cancer 2003 40(3): 317-23. NRI

Jeremic, Y. Shibamoto, B. Milicic, L. Acimovic and S. Milisavljevic. Absence of thoracic radiation myelitis after hyperfractionated radiation therapy with and without concurrent chemotherapy for Stage III nonsmall-cell lung cancer. Int J Radiat Oncol Biol Phys 1998 40(2): 343-6. NRP

Jeremic, Y. Shibamoto, B. Milicic, N. Nikolic, A. Dagovic and S. Milisavljevic. Concurrent radiochemotherapy for patients with stage III non-small-cell lung cancer (NSCLC): long-term results of a phase II study. Int J Radiat Oncol Biol Phys 1998 42(5): 1091-6. NRP

Jeremic, Y. Shibamoto, B. Milicic, S. Milisavljevic, N. Nikolic, A. Dagovic and G. Radosavljevic-Asic. Short-term chemotherapy and palliative radiotherapy for elderly patients with stage IV non-small cell lung cancer: a phase II study. Lung Cancer 1999 24(1): 1-9. NRP

Jeremic, Y. Shibamoto, B. Milicic, S. Milisavljevic, N. Nikolic, A. Dagovic, J. Aleksandrovic and G. Radosavljevic-Asic. A phase II study of concurrent accelerated hyperfractionated radiotherapy and carboplatin/oral etoposide for elderly patients with stage III non-small-cell lung cancer. Int J Radiat Oncol Biol Phys 1999 44(2): 343-8. NRP

Jeremic, Y. Shibamoto, L. Acimovic and L. Djuric. Randomized trial of hyperfractionated radiation therapy with or without concurrent chemotherapy for stage III non-small-cell lung cancer. J Clin Oncol 1995 13(2): 452-8. NRP

Jeremic, Y. Shibamoto, L. Acimovic and S. Milisavljevic. Hyperfractionated radiation therapy with or without concurrent low-dose daily carboplatin/etoposide for stage III non-small-cell lung cancer: a randomized study. J Clin Oncol 1996 14(4): 1065-70. NRP

Jeremic, Y. Shibamoto, L. Acimovic and S. Milisavljevic. Hyperfractionated radiotherapy alone for clinical stage I nonsmall cell lung cancer. Int J Radiat Oncol Biol Phys 1997 38(3): 521-5. NRI

Jeremic, Y. Shibamoto, L. Acimovic, B. Milicic, S. Milisavljevic, N. Nikolic, A. Dagovic, J. Aleksandrovic and G. Radosavljevic-Asic. Hyperfractionated radiation therapy and concurrent low-dose, daily carboplatin/etoposide with or without weekend carboplatin/etoposide chemotherapy in stage III non-small-cell lung cancer: a randomized trial. Int J Radiat Oncol Biol Phys 2001 50(1): 19-25. NRP

Jiang, K. Yang, R. Komaki, X. Wei, S. L. Tucker, Y. Zhuang, M. K. Martel, S. Vedam, P. Balter, G. Zhu, D. Gomez, C. Lu, R. Mohan, J. D. Cox and Z. Liao. Long-Term Clinical Outcome of Intensity-Modulated Radiotherapy for Inoperable Non-Small-Cell Lung Cancer: The MD Anderson Experience. Int J Radiat Oncol Biol Phys 2011 (): . NRP

Jiang, W. Yan, J. Ming and Y. Yu. Docetaxel weekly regimen in conjunction with RF hyperthermia for pretreated locally advanced non-small cell lung cancer: a preliminary study. BMC Cancer 2007 7(): 189. NRP

Jin, H. S. Ji, H. Y. Song, J. Y. Ohm, M. L. Jae, H. L. Dae and S. W. Kim. Palliative treatment of inoperable malignant tracheobronchial obstruction: Temporary stenting combined with radiation therapy and/or chemotherapy. American Journal of Roentgenology 2009 193(1): W38-W42. USD

Jin, S. L. Tucker, H. H. Liu, X. Wei, S. S. Yom, S. Wang, R. Komaki, Y. Chen, M. K. Martel, R. Mohan, J. D. Cox and Z. Liao. Dose-volume thresholds and smoking status for the risk of treatment-related pneumonitis in inoperable non-small cell lung cancer treated with definitive radiotherapy. Radiother Oncol 2009 91(3): 427-32. NRO

Jin, Y. M. Han, Y. S. Lee and Y. C. Lee. Radiofrequency ablation using a monopolar wet electrode for the treatment of inoperable non-small cell lung cancer: a preliminary report. Korean J Radiol 2008 9(2): 140-7. NRO

Jiwnani, G. Karimundackal and C. S. Pramesh. Stereotactic radiotherapy versus sublobar lung resection in medically unfit patients with early-stage non-small-cell lung cancer. J Clin Oncol 2010 28(29): e569-70; author reply e571-2. NRD

Johnstone, R. W. Byhardt, D. Ettinger and C. B. Scott. Phase III study comparing chemotherapy and radiotherapy with preoperative chemotherapy and surgical resection in patients with non-small-cell lung cancer with spread to mediastinal lymph nodes (N2); final report of RTOG 89-01. Radiation Therapy Oncology Group. Int J Radiat Oncol Biol Phys 2002 54(2): 365-9. NRP

Kadono, T. Homma, K. Kamahara, M. Nakayama, H. Satoh, K. Sekizawa and T. Miyamoto. Effect of heavy-ion radiotherapy on pulmonary function in stage I non-small cell lung cancer patients. Chest 2002 122(6): 1925-32. NRI

Kaira, N. Sunaga, N. Yanagitani, T. Kawata, M. Utsugi, K. Shimizu, T. Ebara, H. Kawamura, T. Nonaka, H. Ishikawa, H. Sakurai, T. Suga, K. Hara, T. Hisada, T. Ishizuka, T. Nakano and M. Mori. Phase I study of oral S-1 plus Cisplatin with concurrent radiotherapy for locally advanced non-small-cell lung cancer. Int J Radiat Oncol Biol Phys 2009 75(1): 109-14. NRP

Kalemkerian, K. Belzer, A. J. Wozniak, L. E. Gaspar, M. Valdivieso and M. J. Kraut. Phase I trial of concurrent thoracic radiation and continuous infusion cisplatin and etoposide in stage III non-small cell lung cancer. Lung Cancer 1999 25(3): 175-82. NRP

Kang, Y. C. Ahn, D. H. Lim, K. Park, J. O. Park, Y. M. Shim, J. Kim and K. Kim. Preoperative concurrent radiochemotherapy and surgery for stage IIIA non-small cell lung cancer. J Korean Med Sci 2006 21(2): 229-35. NRP

Kaplan, M. Altynbas, C. Eroglu, E. Karahacioglu, O. Er, M. Ozkan, M. Bilgin, O. Canoz, I. Gulmez and M. Gulec. Preliminary results of a phase II study of weekly paclitaxel (PTX) and carboplatin (CBDCA) administered concurrently with thoracic radiation therapy (TRT) followed by consolidation chemotherapy with PTX/CBDCA for stage III unresectable non-small-cell lung cancer (NSCLC). Am J Clin Oncol 2004 27(6): 603-10. NRP

Kappers, J. S. Belderbos, J. A. Burgers, N. van Zandwijk, H. J. Groen and H. M. Klomp. Non-small cell lung carcinoma of the superior sulcus: favourable outcomes of combined modality treatment in carefully selected patients. Lung Cancer 2008 59(3): 385-90. NRP

Kappers, J. W. van Sandick, J. A. Burgers, J. S. Belderbos, M. W. Wouters, N. van Zandwijk and H. M. Klomp. Results of combined modality treatment in patients with non-small-cell lung cancer of the superior sulcus and the rationale for surgical resection. Eur J Cardiothorac Surg 2009 36(4): 741-6. NRP

Kappers, J. W. van Sandick, S. A. Burgers, J. S. Belderbos, N. van Zandwijk and H. M. Klomp. Surgery after induction chemotherapy in stage IIIA-N2 non-small cell lung cancer: why pneumonectomy should be avoided. Lung Cancer 2010 68(2): 222-7. NRP

Karasawa, N. Okano, Y. Machitori, T. C. Chang, G. Kuga, N. Mitsui, N. Hanyu and N. Kunishima. 3-D non-coplanar conformal radiotherapy for the treatment of stage I NSCLC - Its usefulness for central tumors. Radiotherapy and Oncology 2011 99(): S340-S341. NRD

Katakami, M. Okazaki, S. Nishiuchi, H. Fukuda, T. Horikawa, H. Nishiyama, H. Inui and K. Bando. Induction chemoradiotherapy for advanced stage III non-small cell lung cancer: long-term follow-up in 42 patients. Lung Cancer 1998 22(2): 127-37. NRP

Katayama, H. Ueoka, K. Kiura, M. Tabata, T. Kozuki, M. Tanimoto, T. Fujiwara, N. Tanaka, H. Date, M. Aoe, N. Shimizu, M. Takemoto and Y. Hiraki. Preoperative concurrent chemoradiotherapy with cisplatin and docetaxel in patients with locally advanced non-small-cell lung cancer. Br J Cancer 2004 90(5): 979-84. NRP

Kato, A. Nambu, H. Onishi, A. Saito, K. Kuriyama, T. Komiyama, K. Marino and T. Araki. Computed tomography appearances of local recurrence after stereotactic body radiation therapy for stage I non-small-cell lung carcinoma. Jpn J Radiol 2010 28(4): 259-65. NRO

Kawaguchi, M. Takada, M. Ando, K. Okishio, S. Atagi, Y. Fujita, Y. Tomizawa, K. Hayashihara, Y. Okano, F. Takahashi, R. Saito, A. Matsumura and A. Tamura. A multi-institutional phase II trial of consolidation S-1 after concurrent chemoradiotherapy with cisplatin and vinorelbine for locally advanced non-small cell lung cancer. European Journal of Cancer 2011 (): . NRP

Kaya, S. Buyukberber, M. Benekli, U. Coskun, A. Sevinc, M. Akmansu, R. Yildiz, B. Ozturk, E. Yaman, M. E. Kalender, O. Orhan, D. Yamac and A. Uner. Concomitant chemoradiotherapy with cisplatin and docetaxel followed by surgery and consolidation chemotherapy in patients with unresectable locally advanced non-small cell lung cancer. Med Oncol 2010 27(1): 152-7. NRP

Ke, G. Fu, Y. Bian, D. Jiang and J. Yang. Concurrent gemcitabine and cisplatin combined with 3D conformal radiotherapy for stage III non-small cell lung cancer. Chinese-German Journal of Clinical Oncology 2009 8(3): 156-159. NRP

Keene, E. M. Harman, D. G. Knauf, D. McCarley and R. A. Zlotecki. Five-year results of a phase II trial of hyperfractionated radiotherapy and concurrent daily cisplatin chemotherapy for stage III non-small-cell lung cancer. Am J Clin Oncol 2005 28(3): 217-22. NRP

Kelly, K. Chansky, L. E. Gaspar, K. S. Albain, J. Jett, Y. C. Ung, D. H. Lau, J. J. Crowley and D. R. Gandara. Phase III trial of maintenance gefitinib or placebo after concurrent chemoradiotherapy and docetaxel consolidation in inoperable stage III non-small-cell lung cancer: SWOG S0023. J Clin Oncol 2008 26(15): 2450-6. NRP

Kelly, M. Hazuka, Z. Pan, J. Murphy, J. Caskey, C. Leonard and P. A. Bunn, Jr.. A phase I study of daily carboplatin and simultaneous accelerated, hyperfractionated chest irradiation in patients with regionally inoperable non-small cell lung cancer. Int J Radiat Oncol Biol Phys 1998 40(3): 559-67. NRP

Kelly, P. A. Balter, N. Rebueno, H. J. Sharp, Z. Liao, R. Komaki and J. Y. Chang. Stereotactic body radiation therapy for patients with lung cancer previously treated with thoracic radiation. Int J Radiat Oncol Biol Phys 2010 78(5): 1387-93. NRP

Kepka, D. Tyc-Szczepaniak and K. Bujko. Dose-per-fraction escalation of accelerated hypofractionated three-dimensional conformal radiotherapy in locally advanced non-small cell lung cancer. J Thorac Oncol 2009 4(7): 853-61. NRP

Kepka, K. Bujko and A. Zolciak-Siwinska. Risk of isolated nodal failure for non-small cell lung cancer (NSCLC) treated with the elective nodal irradiation (ENI) using 3D-conformal radiotherapy (3D-CRT) techniques--a retrospective analysis. Acta Oncol 2008 47(1): 95-103. NRP

Kerner, L. F. A. Van Dullemen, E. M. Wiegman, A. H. D. Van Der Leest, J. Widder, J. F. Ubbels, T. J. N. Hiltermann and H. J. M. Groen. Gemcitabine and cisplatin followed by concurrent gemcitabine and radiotherapy or sequential radiotherapy alone in unresectable stage III non-small cell lung cancer (NSCLC). European Journal of Cancer 2011 47(): S600. NRD

Kim, H. J. Han, S. J. Park, K. H. Min, M. H. Lee, C. R. Chung, M. H. Kim, G. Y. Jin and Y. C. Lee. Comparison between surgery and radiofrequency ablation for stage I non-small cell lung cancer. Eur J Radiol 2011 (): . USD

Kim, S. H. Yang, S. H. Lee, Y. S. Park, Y. H. Im, W. K. Kang, S. H. Ha, C. I. Park, D. S. Heo, Y. J. Bang and N. K. Kim. A phase III randomized trial of combined chemoradiotherapy versus radiotherapy alone in locally advanced non-small-cell lung cancer. Am J Clin Oncol 2002 25(3): 238-43. NRP

Kim, S. M. Yoon, E. K. Choi, B. Y. Yi, J. H. Kim, S. D. Ahn, S. W. Lee, S. S. Shin, J. S. Lee, C. Suh, S. W. Kim, D. S. Kim, W. S. Kim, H. J. Park and C. I. Park. Phase II study of radiotherapy with three-dimensional conformal boost concurrent with paclitaxel and cisplatin for Stage IIIB non-small-cell lung cancer. Int J Radiat Oncol Biol Phys 2005 62(1): 76-81. NRP

Kim, Y. C. Ahn, H. C. Park, H. Lim do and H. Nam. Results and prognostic factors of hypofractionated stereotactic radiation therapy for primary or metastatic lung cancer. J Thorac Oncol 2010 5(4): 526-32. USD

Kim, Y. C. Ahn, H. Lim do and H. R. Nam. High-dose thoracic radiation therapy at 3.0 Gy/fraction in inoperable stage I/II non-small cell lung cancer. Jpn J Clin Oncol 2008 38(2): 92-8. NRI

Kim, Y. C. Ahn, H. Lim do, J. Han, K. Park, J. O. Park, K. Kim, J. Kim and Y. M. Shim. Analyses on prognostic factors following tri-modality therapy for stage IIIa non-small cell lung cancer. Lung Cancer 2007 55(3): 329-36. NRP

Kim, Y. J. Kim, M. D. Seo, H. G. Yi, S. H. Lee, S. M. Lee, D. W. Kim, S. C. Yang, C. T. Lee, J. S. Lee, Y. W. Kim and D. S. Heo. Patterns of palliative procedures and clinical outcomes in patients with advanced non-small cell lung cancer. Lung Cancer 2009 65(2): 242-6. NRP

Kim, Y. Shyr, B. Shaktour, W. Akerley, D. H. Johnson and H. Choy. Long term follow up and analysis of long term survivors in patients treated with paclitaxel-based concurrent chemo/radiation therapy for locally advanced non-small cell lung cancer. Lung Cancer 2005 50(2): 235-45. NRP

Kim, Y. Shyr, H. Chen, W. Akerley, D. H. Johnson and H. Choy. Response to combined modality therapy correlates with survival in locally advanced non-small-cell lung cancer. Int J Radiat Oncol Biol Phys 2005 63(4): 1029-36. NRP

King, J. C. Acker, P. S. Kussin, L. B. Marks, K. J. Weeks and K. A. Leopold. High-dose, hyperfractionated, accelerated radiotherapy using a concurrent boost for the treatment of nonsmall cell lung cancer: unusual toxicity and promising early results. Int J Radiat Oncol Biol Phys 1996 36(3): 593-9. NRI

Kirkbride, K. Gelmon and E. Eisenhauer. Paclitaxel and concurrent radiotherapy in locally advanced non-small cell lung cancer: the Canadian experience. Semin Radiat Oncol 1999 9(2 Suppl 1): 102-7. NRP

Kirkbride, K. Gelmon, E. Eisenhauer, B. Fisher and H. Dulude. A phase I/II study of paclitaxel (TAXOL) and concurrent radiotherapy in advanced nonsmall cell lung cancer. Int J Radiat Oncol Biol Phys 1997 39(5): 1107-11. NRP

Kishida, T. Hirose, T. Shirai, T. Sugiyama, S. Kusumoto, T. Yamaoka, K. Okuda, M. Adachi and A. Nakamura. Myelosuppression induced by concurrent hemoradiotherapy as a prognostic factor for patients with locally advanced non-small cell lung cancer. Oncology Letters 2011 2(5): 949-955. NRP

Kiura, H. Ueoka, Y. Segawa, M. Tabata, H. Kamei, N. Takigawa, S. Hiraki, Y. Watanabe, A. Bessho, K. Eguchi, N. Okimoto, S. Harita, M. Takemoto, Y. Hiraki, M. Harada and M. Tanimoto. Phase I/II study of docetaxel and cisplatin with concurrent thoracic radiation therapy for locally advanced non-small-cell lung cancer. Br J Cancer 2003 89(5): 795-802. NRP

Kobayashi, K. Matsui, T. Hirashima, T. Nitta, S. Sasada, T. Tada, K. Minakuchi, M. Furukawa, Y. Ogata and I. Kawase. Phase I study of weekly cisplatin, vinorelbine, and concurrent thoracic radiation therapy in patients with locally advanced non-small-cell lung cancer. Int J Clin Oncol 2006 11(4): 314-9. NRP

Kobayashi, T. Uno, K. Isobe, N. Ueno, M. Watanabe, R. Harada, Y. Takiguchi, K. Tatsumi and H. Ito. Radiation pneumonitis following twice-daily radiotherapy with concurrent carboplatin and paclitaxel in patients with stage III non-small-cell lung cancer. Jpn J Clin Oncol 2010 40(5): 464-9. NRP

Koc, M. D. Onuk, M. Koruk and F. Memik. Therapeutic effect of oral recombinant human granulocyte macrophage-colony stimulating factor in radiotherapy-induced esophagitis. Hepatogastroenterology 2003 50(53): 1297-300. NRP

Kocak, A. Ozkan, A. Mayadagli, C. Parlak, A. Bilici, M. Seker, B. B. Oven Ustaalioglu, M. Gumus, M. Eren, S. G. Karabulut and F. Oruc. Induction chemotherapy and chemoradiation therapy for inoperable locally advanced non-small-cell lung cancer: a single-institution review of two different regimens. Clin Lung Cancer 2009 10(2): 124-9. NRP

Koeppler, J. Heymanns, J. Thomalla, K. Kleboth, U. Mergenthaler and R. Weide. Treatment of advanced non small cell lung cancer in routine care: a retrospective analysis of 212 consecutive patients treated in a community based oncology group practice. Clin Med Oncol 2009 3(): 63-70. NRP

Komaki, C. B. Scott, W. T. Sause, D. H. Johnson, S. G. t. Taylor, J. S. Lee, B. Emami, R. W. Byhardt, W. J. Curran, Jr., A. R. Dar and J. D. Cox. Induction cisplatin/vinblastine and irradiation vs. irradiation in unresectable squamous cell lung cancer: failure patterns by cell type in RTOG 88-08/ECOG 4588. Radiation Therapy Oncology Group. Eastern Cooperative Oncology Group. Int J Radiat Oncol Biol Phys 1997 39(3): 537-44. NRP

Komaki, C. Scott, D. Ettinger, J. S. Lee, F. V. Fossella, W. Curran, R. F. Evans, P. Rubin and R. W. Byhardt. Randomized study of chemotherapy/radiation therapy combinations for favorable patients with locally advanced inoperable nonsmall cell lung cancer: Radiation Therapy Oncology Group (RTOG) 92-04. Int J Radiat Oncol Biol Phys 1997 38(1): 149-55. NRP

Komaki, C. Scott, J. S. Lee, R. C. Urtasun, R. W. Byhardt, B. Emami, E. J. Andras, S. O. Asbell, M. Rotman and J. D. Cox. Impact of adding concurrent chemotherapy to hyperfractionated radiotherapy for locally advanced non-small cell lung cancer (NSCLC): comparison of RTOG 83-11 and RTOG 91-06. Am J Clin Oncol 1997 20(5): 435-40. NRI

Komaki, J. A. Roth, G. L. Walsh, J. B. Putnam, A. Vaporciyan, J. S. Lee, F. V. Fossella, M. Chasen, M. E. Delclos and J. D. Cox. Outcome predictors for 143 patients with superior sulcus tumors treated by multidisciplinary approach at the University of Texas M. D. Anderson Cancer Center. Int J Radiat Oncol Biol Phys 2000 48(2): 347-54. NRP

Komaki, J. S. Lee, B. Kaplan, P. Allen, J. F. Kelly, Z. Liao, C. W. Stevens, F. V. Fossella, R. Zinner, V. Papadimitrakopoulou, F. Khuri, B. Glisson, K. Pisters, J. Kurie, R. Herbst, L. Milas, J. Ro, H. D. Thames, W. K. Hong and J. D. Cox. Randomized phase III study of chemoradiation with or without amifostine for patients with favorable performance status inoperable stage II-III non-small cell lung cancer: preliminary results. Semin Radiat Oncol 2002 12(1 Suppl 1): 46-9. NRP

Komaki, J. S. Lee, L. Milas, H. K. Lee, F. V. Fossella, R. S. Herbst, P. K. Allen, Z. Liao, C. W. Stevens, C. Lu, R. G. Zinner, V. A. Papadimitrakopoulou, M. S. Kies, G. R. Blumenschein, Jr., K. M. Pisters, B. S. Glisson, J. Kurie, B. Kaplan, V. P. Garza, D. Mooring, S. L. Tucker and J. D. Cox. Effects of amifostine on acute toxicity from concurrent chemotherapy and radiotherapy for inoperable non-small-cell lung cancer: report of a randomized comparative trial. Int J Radiat Oncol Biol Phys 2004 58(5): 1369-77. NRP

Komaki, J. Y. Chang, X. Wu, P. K. Allen, L. Milas, Z. Liao, F. V. Fossella, E. Travis and M. R. Spitz. Mutagen sensitivity may predict lung protection by amifostine for patients with locally advanced non-small cell lung cancer treated by chemoradiotherapy. Semin Oncol 2005 32(2 Suppl 3): S92-8. NRP

Komaki, W. Seiferheld, D. Ettinger, J. S. Lee, B. Movsas and W. Sause. Randomized phase II chemotherapy and radiotherapy trial for patients with locally advanced inoperable non-small-cell lung cancer: long-term follow-up of RTOG 92-04. Int J Radiat Oncol Biol Phys 2002 53(3): 548-57. NRP

Komaki, X. Wei, P. K. Allen, R. Amos, R. Mohan, J. Y. Chang, Z. Liao, L. Dong and J. D. Cox. Protons compared to X-IMRT compared to 3D in locally advanced NSCLC. Radiotherapy and Oncology 2011 99(): S89-S90. NRD

Kong, J. A. Hayman, K. A. Griffith, G. P. Kalemkerian, D. Arenberg, S. Lyons, A. Turrisi, A. Lichter, B. Fraass, A. Eisbruch, T. S. Lawrence and R. K. Ten Haken. Final toxicity results of a radiation-dose escalation study in patients with non-small-cell lung cancer (NSCLC): predictors for radiation pneumonitis and fibrosis. Int J Radiat Oncol Biol Phys 2006 65(4): 1075-86. NRO

Kong, R. K. Ten Haken, M. J. Schipper, M. A. Sullivan, M. Chen, C. Lopez, G. P. Kalemkerian and J. A. Hayman. High-dose radiation improved local tumor control and overall survival in patients with inoperable/unresectable non-small-cell lung cancer: long-term results of a radiation dose escalation study. Int J Radiat Oncol Biol Phys 2005 63(2): 324-33. NRP

Koshy, O. Goloubeva and M. Suntharalingam. Impact of neoadjuvant radiation on survival in stage III non-small-cell lung cancer. Int J Radiat Oncol Biol Phys 2011 79(5): 1388-94. NRP

Kosmidis, G. Fountzilas, S. Baka, E. Samantas, A. M. Dimopoulos, H. Gogas, D. Skarlos, P. Papacostas, J. Boukovinas, C. Bakogiannis, P. Pantelakos, H. Athanasiou, D. Misailidou, P. Tsekeris and N. Pavlidis. Combination chemotherapy with paclitaxel and gemcitabine followed by concurrent chemoradiotherapy in non-operable localized non-small cell lung cancer. A hellenic cooperative oncology group (HeCOG) phase II study. Anticancer Res 2007 27(6C): 4391-5. NRP

Koto, Y. Takai, Y. Ogawa, H. Matsushita, K. Takeda, C. Takahashi, K. R. Britton, K. Jingu, K. Takai, M. Mitsuya, K. Nemoto and S. Yamada. A phase II study on stereotactic body radiotherapy for stage I non-small cell lung cancer. Radiother Oncol 2007 85(3): 429-34. USD

Koukourakis, C. Kourousis, M. Kamilaki, S. Koukouraki, A. Giatromanolaki, S. Kakolyris, A. Kotsakis, N. Androulakis, N. Bahlitzanakis and V. Georgoulias. Weekly docetaxel and concomitant boost radiotherapy for non-small cell lung cancer. A phase I/II dose escalation trial. Eur J Cancer 1998 34(6): 838-44. NRP

Koukourakis, G. Patlakas, M. E. Froudarakis, G. Kyrgias, J. Skarlatos, I. Abatzoglou, G. Bougioukas and D. Bouros. Hypofractionated accelerated radiochemotherapy with cytoprotection (Chemo-HypoARC) for inoperable non-small cell lung carcinoma. Anticancer Res 2007 27(5B): 3625-31. NRP

Koukourakis, J. Skarlatos, L. Kosma, A. Giatromanolaki and D. Yannakakis. Radiotherapy alone for non-small cell lung carcinoma. Five-year disease-free survival and patterns of failure. Acta Oncol 1995 34(4): 525-30. NRI

Koukourakis, N. Bahlitzanakis, M. Froudarakis, A. Giatromanolaki, V. Georgoulias, S. Koumiotaki, M. Christodoulou, G. Kyrias, J. Skarlatos, J. Kostantelos and K. Beroukas. Concurrent conventionally factionated radiotherapy and weekly docetaxel in the treatment of stage IIIb non-small-cell lung carcinoma. Br J Cancer 1999 80(11): 1792-6. NRP

Koukourakis, P. G. Tsoutsou and I. Abatzoglou. Computed tomography assessment of lung density in patients with lung cancer treated with accelerated hypofractionated radio-chemotherapy supported with amifostine. Am J Clin Oncol 2009 32(3): 258-61. NRP

Koukourakis, S. Koukouraki, A. Giatromanolaki, S. C. Archimandritis, J. Skarlatos, K. Beroukas, J. G. Bizakis, G. Retalis, N. Karkavitsas and E. S. Helidonis. Liposomal doxorubicin and conventionally fractionated radiotherapy in the treatment of locally advanced non-small-cell lung cancer and head and neck cancer. J Clin Oncol 1999 17(11): 3512-21. NRP

Koutaissoff, D. Wellmann, P. Coucke, M. Ozsahin, S. Pampallona and R. O. Mirimanoff. Hyperfractionated accelerated radiotherapy (HART) for inoperable, nonmetastatic non-small cell lung carcinoma of the lung (NSCLC): results of a phase II study for patients ineligible for combination radiochemotherapy. Int J Radiat Oncol Biol Phys 1999 45(5): 1151-6. NRI

Kozak, J. D. Murphy, M. L. Schipper, J. S. Donington, L. Zhou, R. I. Whyte, J. B. Shrager, C. D. Hoang, J. Bazan, P. G. Maxim, E. E. Graves, M. Diehn, W. Y. Hara, A. Quon, Q. T. Le, H. A. Wakelee and B. W. Loo, Jr.. Tumor volume as a potential imaging-based risk-stratification factor in trimodality therapy for locally advanced non-small cell lung cancer. J Thorac Oncol 2011 6(5): 920-6. NRP

Kramer, S. L. Wanders, E. M. Noordijk, E. J. Vonk, H. C. van Houwelingen, W. B. van den Hout, R. B. Geskus, M. Scholten and J. W. Leer. Results of the Dutch National study of the palliative effect of irradiation using two different treatment schemes for non-small-cell lung cancer. J Clin Oncol 2005 23(13): 2962-70. NRP

Krol, P. Aussems, E. M. Noordijk, J. Hermans and J. W. Leer. Local irradiation alone for peripheral stage I lung cancer: could we omit the elective regional nodal irradiation?. Int J Radiat Oncol Biol Phys 1996 34(2): 297-302. NRI

Krzakowski, M. Provencio, B. Utracka-Hutka, E. Villa, M. Codes, A. Kuten, M. Henke, M. Lopez, D. Bell, G. Biti, O. Merimsky, A. Beorchia, M. Riggi, N. R. Caux, J. C. Pouget, B. Dubray and P. David. Oral vinorelbine and cisplatin as induction chemotherapy and concomitant chemo-radiotherapy in stage III non-small cell lung cancer: final results of an international phase II trial. J Thorac Oncol 2008 3(9): 994-1002. NRP

Kubota, T. Tamura, M. Fukuoka, K. Furuse, H. Ikegami, Y. Ariyoshi, Y. Kurita and N. Saijo. Phase II study of concurrent chemotherapy and radiotherapy for unresectable stage III non-small-cell lung cancer: long-term follow-up results. Japan Clinical Oncology Group Protocol 8902. Ann Oncol 2000 11(4): 445-50. NRP

Kumar, J. Herndon, 2nd, M. Langer, L. J. Kohman, A. D. Elias, F. C. Kass, W. L. Eaton, S. L. Seagren, M. R. Green and D. J. Sugarbaker. Patterns of disease failure after trimodality therapy of nonsmall cell lung carcinoma pathologic stage IIIA (N2). Analysis of Cancer and Leukemia Group B Protocol 8935. Cancer 1996 77(11): 2393-9. NRP

Kunitoh, K. Watanabe, A. Nagatomo, H. Okamoto and K. Kimbara. Concurrent daily carboplatin and accelerated hyperfractionated thoracic radiotherapy in locally advanced nonsmall cell lung cancer. Int J Radiat Oncol Biol Phys 1997 37(1): 103-9. NRP

Kupelian, R. Komaki and P. Allen. Prognostic factors in the treatment of node-negative nonsmall cell lung carcinoma with radiotherapy alone. Int J Radiat Oncol Biol Phys 1996 36(3): 607-13. NRI

Kusumoto, T. Hirose, M. Fukayama, D. Kataoka, K. Hamada, T. Sugiyama, T. Shirai, T. Yamaoka, K. Okuda, T. Ohnishi, T. Ohmori, M. Kadokura and M. Adachi. Induction chemoradiotherapy followed by surgery for locally advanced non-small cell lung cancer. Oncol Rep 2009 22(5): 1157-62. NRP

Kuten, Y. Anacak, R. Abdah-Bortnyak, L. Chetver, I. Zen Al Deen, K. Daoud, R. Nijem, S. Billan and L. Best. Neoadjuvant radiotherapy concurrent with weekly paclitaxel and carboplatin and followed by surgery in locally advanced non-small-cell lung cancer. Am J Clin Oncol 2003 26(2): 184-7. NRP

Kwak, W. C. Kim and H. J. Kim. Treatment results of cyberknife radiosurgery for patients with primary or recurrent non-small cell lung cancer. Respirology 2011 16(): 163-164. NRD

Kwon, S. K. Kim, W. K. Chung, M. J. Cho, J. S. Kim, S. R. Moon, W. Y. Park, S. J. Ahn, Y. K. Oh, H. G. Yun and B. S. Na. Effect of pentoxifylline on radiation response of non-small cell lung cancer: a phase III randomized multicenter trial. Radiother Oncol 2000 56(2): 175-9. NRP

Kyasa and A. R. Jazieh. Characteristics and outcomes of patients with unresected early-stage non-small cell lung cancer. South Med J 2002 95(10): 1149-52. NRI

Lafitte, M. E. Ribet, B. M. Prevost, B. H. Gosselin, M. C. Copin and A. H. Brichet. Postresection irradiation for T2 N0 M0 non-small cell carcinoma: a prospective, randomized study. Ann Thorac Surg 1996 62(3): 830-4. NRI

Lagerwaard, C. J. Haasbeek, E. F. Smit, B. J. Slotman and S. Senan. Outcomes of risk-adapted fractionated stereotactic radiotherapy for stage I non-small-cell lung cancer. Int J Radiat Oncol Biol Phys 2008 70(3): 685-92. USD

Lagerwaard, S. Senan, J. P. van Meerbeeck and W. J. Graveland. Has 3-D conformal radiotherapy (3D CRT) improved the local tumour control for stage I non-small cell lung cancer?. Radiother Oncol 2002 63(2): 151-7. NRP

Lam, S. Berman, R. Thurer, S. Ashiku, M. DeCamp, M. Goldstein, S. Schumer, B. Halmos, D. Karp, D. Coute, M. Bergman, C. Boyd-Sirard, S. H. Ou, A. Muzikansky, C. Woodard and M. Huberman. Phase II trial of sequential chemotherapy followed by chemoradiation, surgery, and postoperative chemotherapy for the treatment of stage IIIA/IIIB non-small-cell lung cancer. Clin Lung Cancer 2006 8(2): 122-9. NRP

Lan and Y. Jiang. The therapeutic effects of the radiotherapy plus TCM treatment observed in senile non-parvicellular lung cancer patients at the late stage. J Tradit Chin Med 2003 23(1): 32-4. NRP

Langendijk, F. B. Thunnissen, R. J. Lamers, J. M. de Jong, G. P. ten Velde and E. F. Wouters. The prognostic significance of accumulation of p53 protein in stage III non-small cell lung cancer treated by radiotherapy. Radiother Oncol 1995 36(3): 218-24. NRP

Langendijk, G. P. ten Velde, N. K. Aaronson, J. M. de Jong, M. J. Muller and E. F. Wouters. Quality of life after palliative radiotherapy in non-small cell lung cancer: a prospective study. Int J Radiat Oncol Biol Phys 2000 47(1): 149-55. NRI

Langendijk, J. de Jong, R. Wanders, P. Lambin and B. Slotman. The importance of pre-treatment haemoglobin level in inoperable non-small cell lung carcinoma treated with radical radiotherapy. Radiother Oncol 2003 67(3): 321-5. NRI

Langendijk, M. K. Tjwa, J. M. de Jong, G. P. ten Velde and E. F. Wouters. Massive haemoptysis after radiotherapy in inoperable non-small cell lung carcinoma: is endobronchial brachytherapy really a risk factor?. Radiother Oncol 1998 49(2): 175-83. NRP

Langendijk, N. K. Aaronson, G. P. ten Velde, J. M. de Jong, M. J. Muller and E. F. Wouters. Pretreatment quality of life of inoperable non-small cell lung cancer patients referred for primary radiotherapy. Acta Oncol 2000 39(8): 949-58. NRI

Langendijk, N. K. Aaronson, J. M. de Jong, G. P. ten Velde, M. J. Muller and M. Wouters. The prognostic impact of quality of life assessed with the EORTC QLQ-C30 in inoperable non-small cell lung carcinoma treated with radiotherapy. Radiother Oncol 2000 55(1): 19-25. NRI

Langendijk, N. K. Aaronson, J. M. de Jong, G. P. ten Velde, M. J. Muller, B. J. Slotman and E. F. Wouters. Quality of life after curative radiotherapy in Stage I non-small-cell lung cancer. Int J Radiat Oncol Biol Phys 2002 53(4): 847-53. NRI

Langer, B. Movsas, R. Hudes, J. Schol, E. Keenan, D. Kilpatrick, C. Yeung and W. Curran. Induction paclitaxel and carboplatin followed by concurrent chemoradiotherapy in patients with unresectable, locally advanced non-small cell lung carcinoma: report of Fox Chase Cancer Center study 94-001. Semin Oncol 1997 24(4 Suppl 12): S12-89-S12-95. NRP

Langer, R. Somer, S. Litwin, S. Feigenberg, B. Movsas, C. Maiale, E. Sherman, M. Millenson, N. Nicoloau, C. Huang and J. Treat. Phase I study of radical thoracic radiation, weekly irinotecan, and cisplatin in locally advanced non-small cell lung carcinoma. J Thorac Oncol 2007 2(3): 203-9. NRP

Langer, W. J. Curran, S. M. Keller, R. B. Catalano, S. Litwin, K. B. Blankstein, N. Haas, S. N. Campli and R. L. Comis. Long-term survival results for patients with locally advanced, initially unresectable non-small cell lung cancer treated with aggressive concurrent chemoradiation. Cancer J Sci Am 1996 2(2): 99-105. NRP

Langer. Concurrent chemoradiation using paclitaxel and carboplatin in locally advanced non-small cell lung cancer. Semin Radiat Oncol 1999 9(2 Suppl 1): 108-16. NRP

Langer. The emerging role of gemcitabine in combination with radiation in locally advanced, unresectable non-small-cell lung cancer. Clin Lung Cancer 2003 4 Suppl 2(): S45-9. NRD

Lanni, Jr., I. S. Grills, L. L. Kestin and J. M. Robertson. Stereotactic radiotherapy reduces treatment cost while improving overall survival and local control over standard fractionated radiation therapy for medically inoperable non-small-cell lung cancer. Am J Clin Oncol 2011 34(5): 494-8. USD

Lanuti, A. Sharma, S. R. Digumarthy, C. D. Wright, D. M. Donahue, J. C. Wain, D. J. Mathisen and J. A. Shepard. Radiofrequency ablation for treatment of medically inoperable stage I non-small cell lung cancer. J Thorac Cardiovasc Surg 2009 137(1): 160-6. USD

Lau, B. Leigh, D. Gandara, M. Edelman, R. Morgan, V. Israel, P. Lara, R. Wilder, J. Ryu and J. Doroshow. Twice-weekly paclitaxel and weekly carboplatin with concurrent thoracic radiation followed by carboplatin/paclitaxel consolidation for stage III non-small-cell lung cancer: a California Cancer Consortium phase II trial. J Clin Oncol 2001 19(2): 442-7. NRP

Lau, J. J. Crowley, D. R. Gandara, M. B. Hazuka, K. S. Albain, B. Leigh, W. S. Fletcher, K. S. Lanier, W. L. Keiser and R. B. Livingston. Southwest Oncology Group phase II trial of concurrent carboplatin, etoposide, and radiation for poor-risk stage III non-small-cell lung cancer. J Clin Oncol 1998 16(9): 3078-81. NRP

Lau, J. K. Ryu and D. R. Gandara. Chemoradiotherapy for poor-risk stage III non-small cell lung cancer. Semin Oncol 1997 24(4 Suppl 12): S12-110-S12-112. NRP

Lau, J. K. Ryu, D. R. Gandara and S. A. Rosenthal. Concurrent carboplatin, etoposide and thoracic radiation for poor-risk stage III non-small-cell lung carcinoma: a pilot study. Int J Radiat Oncol Biol Phys 1997 38(1): 157-61. NRP

Lau, J. K. Ryu, D. R. Gandara, R. Morgan, J. Doroshow, R. Wilder and B. Leigh. Twice-weekly paclitaxel and radiation for stage III non-small cell lung cancer. Semin Oncol 1997 24(4 Suppl 12): S12-106-S12-109. NRP

Lau, J. Ryu, D. Gandara, R. Morgan, J. Doroshow, R. Wilder and B. Leigh. Concurrent twice-weekly paclitaxel and thoracic irradiation for stage III non-small cell lung cancer. Semin Radiat Oncol 1999 9(2 Suppl 1): 117-20. NRP

Law, D. D. Karp, T. Dipetrillo and B. T. Daly. Emergence of increased cerebral metastasis after high-dose preoperative radiotherapy with chemotherapy in patients with locally advanced nonsmall cell lung carcinoma. Cancer 2001 92(1): 160-4. NRP

Lazarov, I. Mihaylova, N. Gesheva-Atanasova and S. Bakardjiev. Comparative analysis of two radiotherapy regimens for the treatment of patients with non-small cell lung cancer. Radiotherapy and Oncology 2011 99(): S341. NRD

Le Pechoux, R. Arriagada, T. Le Chevalier, J. J. Bretel, B. P. Cosset, P. Ruffie, P. Baldeyrou and D. Grunenwald. Concurrent cisplatin-vindesine and hyperfractionated thoracic radiotherapy in locally advanced nonsmall cell lung cancer. Int J Radiat Oncol Biol Phys 1996 35(3): 519-25. NRP

Le, B. W. Loo, A. Ho, C. Cotrutz, A. C. Koong, H. Wakelee, S. T. Kee, D. Constantinescu, R. I. Whyte and J. Donington. Results of a phase I dose-escalation study using single-fraction stereotactic radiotherapy for lung tumors. J Thorac Oncol 2006 1(8): 802-9. USD

Lee, C. Scott, R. Komaki, F. V. Fossella, G. S. Dundas, S. McDonald, R. W. Byhardt and W. J. Curran, Jr.. Concurrent chemoradiation therapy with oral etoposide and cisplatin for locally advanced inoperable non-small-cell lung cancer: radiation therapy oncology group protocol 91-06. J Clin Oncol 1996 14(4): 1055-64. NRP

Lee, E. K. Choi, J. S. Lee, S. D. Lee, C. Suh, S. W. Kim, W. S. Kim, S. D. Ahn, B. Y. Yi, J. H. Kim, Y. J. Noh, S. S. Kim, Y. Koh, D. S. Kim and W. D. Kim. Phase II study of three-dimensional conformal radiotherapy and concurrent mitomycin-C, vinblastine, and cisplatin chemotherapy for Stage III locally advanced, unresectable, non-small-cell lung cancer. Int J Radiat Oncol Biol Phys 2003 56(4): 996-1004. NRP

Lee, G. Y. Jin, S. N. Goldberg, Y. C. Lee, G. H. Chung, Y. M. Han, S. Y. Lee and C. S. Kim. Percutaneous radiofrequency ablation for inoperable non-small cell lung cancer and metastases: preliminary report. Radiology 2004 230(1): 125-34. USD

Lee, G. Y. Jin, Y. M. Han, G. H. Chung, Y. C. Lee, K. S. Kwon and D. Lynch. Comparison of Survival Rate in Primary Non-Small-Cell Lung Cancer Among Elderly Patients Treated With Radiofrequency Ablation, Surgery, or Chemotherapy. Cardiovasc Intervent Radiol 2011 (): . NRP

Lee, J. H. Choi, H. Y. Lim, J. S. Park, H. C. Kim, S. Kang, Y. T. Oh, M. Chun, S. S. Sheen, Y. J. Oh, K. J. Park and S. C. Hwang. The addition of induction chemotherapy with etoposide, ifosfamide, and cisplatin failed to improve therapeutic outcome of concurrent chemoradiotherapy in patients with locally advanced non-small cell lung cancer - - single institution retrospective analysis. Neoplasma 2006 53(1): 30-6. NRP

Lee, J. Y. Han, K. H. Cho, H. R. Pyo, H. Y. Kim, S. J. Yoon and J. S. Lee. Phase II study of induction chemotherapy with gemcitabine and vinorelbine followed by concurrent chemoradiotherapy with oral etoposide and cisplatin in patients with inoperable stage III non-small-cell lung cancer. Int J Radiat Oncol Biol Phys 2005 63(4): 1037-44. NRP

Lee, R. Komaki, F. V. Fossella, B. S. Glisson, W. K. Hong and J. D. Cox. A pilot trial of hyperfractionated thoracic radiation therapy with concurrent cisplatin and oral etoposide for locally advanced inoperable non-small-cell lung cancer: a 5-year follow-up report. Int J Radiat Oncol Biol Phys 1998 42(3): 479-86. NRP

Lee, T. E. Stinchcombe, D. T. Moore, D. E. Morris, D. N. Hayes, J. Halle, J. G. Rosenman, M. P. Rivera and M. A. Socinski. Late complications of high-dose (>/=66 Gy) thoracic conformal radiation therapy in combined modality trials in unresectable stage III non-small cell lung cancer. J Thorac Oncol 2009 4(1): 74-9. NRP

Lee, Y. S. Kim, J. H. Kang, S. N. Lee, Y. K. Kim, M. I. Ahn, D. H. Han, R. Yoo Ie, Y. P. Wang, J. G. Park, S. C. Yoon, H. S. Jang and B. O. Choi. Clinical Responses and Prognostic Indicators of Concurrent Chemoradiation for Non-small Cell Lung Cancer. Cancer Res Treat 2011 43(1): 32-41. NRP

Leon, J. F. Cueva-Banuelos, G. Huidobro, J. L. Firvida, M. Amenedo, M. Lazaro, C. Romero, S. V. Estevez, F. J. Baron, C. Grande, J. Garcia Mata, A. Gonzalez, J. Castellanos, A. Gomez, M. Caeiro, M. R. Rodriguez and J. Casal. Gemcitabine, cisplatin and vinorelbine as induction chemotherapy followed by radical therapy in stage III non-small-cell lung cancer: a multicentre study of galician-lung-cancer-group. Lung Cancer 2003 40(2): 215-20. NRP

Leong, E. H. Tan, K. W. Fong, E. Wilder-Smith, Y. K. Ong, B. C. Tai, L. Chew, S. H. Lim, J. Wee, K. M. Lee, K. F. Foo, P. Ang and P. T. Ang. Randomized double-blind trial of combined modality treatment with or without amifostine in unresectable stage III non-small-cell lung cancer. J Clin Oncol 2003 21(9): 1767-74. NRP

Leong, K. W. Fong, W. T. Lim, C. K. Toh, S. P. Yap, S. W. Hee and E. H. Tan. A phase II trial of induction gemcitabine and vinorelbine followed by concurrent vinorelbine and radiotherapy in locally advanced non-small cell lung cancer. Lung Cancer 2010 67(3): 325-9. NRP

Leong, K. W. Fong, Y. K. Ong, K. F. Foo, P. Ang, J. Wee, K. M. Lee and E. H. Tan. Chemo-radiotherapy for stage III unresectable non-small cell lung cancer long-term results of a prospective study. Respir Med 2004 98(11): 1080-6. NRP

Lester, F. R. Macbeth, A. E. Brewster, J. B. Court and N. Iqbal. CT-planned accelerated hypofractionated radiotherapy in the radical treatment of non-small cell lung cancer. Lung Cancer 2004 45(2): 237-42. USD

Li, A. H. Shi, F. H. Li, R. Yu and G. Y. Zhu. Phase i study to determine MTD of docetaxel and cisplatin with concurrent radiation therapy for stage III non-small cell lung cancer. Chinese Journal of Cancer Research 2011 23(2): 129-133. NRP

Li, C. H. Dai, L. C. Yu, P. Chen, X. Q. Li, S. B. Shi and J. R. Wu. Results of trimodality therapy in patients with stage IIIA (N2-bulky) and stage IIIB non-small-cell lung cancer. Clin Lung Cancer 2009 10(5): 353-9. NRP

Li, C. H. Dai, S. B. Shi, P. Chen, L. C. Yu and J. R. Wu. Prognostic factors and long term results of neo adjuvant therapy followed by surgery in stage IIIA N2 non-small cell lung cancer patients. Annals of Thoracic Medicine 2009 4(4): 201-207. NRP

Li, H. Bai, X. Li, M. Wu, R. Yu, A. Shi, L. Yin, J. Wang and G. Zhu. Role of EGFR mutation status in patients with stage III non-squamous non-small cell lung cancer treated with chemoradiotherapy. Chinese Journal of Lung Cancer 2011 14(9): 715-718. FLA

Li, H. Y. Gong, W. Huang, Y. Yi, J. M. Yu, Z. T. Wang, Z. C. Zhang, H. F. Sun, H. S. Li and L. Y. Wang. Phase I Study of Pemetrexed, Cisplatin, and Concurrent Radiotherapy in Patients With Locally Advanced Non-small Cell Lung Cancer. Am J Clin Oncol 2011 (): . NRP

Li, J. M. Yu, L. G. Xing, G. R. Yang, X. D. Sun, J. Xu, H. Zhu and J. B. Yue. Hypoxic imaging with 99mTc-HL91 single photon emission computed tomography in advanced nonsmall cell lung cancer. Chin Med J (Engl) 2006 119(17): 1477-80. NRO

Li, M. Hu, H. Zhu, W. Zhao, G. Yang and J. Yu. Comparison of 18F-Fluoroerythronitroimidazole and 18F-fluorodeoxyglucose positron emission tomography and prognostic value in locally advanced non-small-cell lung cancer. Clin Lung Cancer 2010 11(5): 335-40. NRP

Li, S. H. Zhang, Z. Zhang and R. L. Wang. Efficacy of gemcitabine with concurrent radiotherapy on stage III,inoperable non-small cell lung cancer. 2007 26(): 1377-80. FLA

Liao, J. Zhao and Y. Zhou. Multimodality therapy of late stage lung cancer. 1995 17(): 384-6. FLA

Liao, R. Komaki, C. Stevens, J. Kelly, F. Fossella, J. S. Lee, P. Allen and J. D. Cox. Twice daily irradiation increases locoregional control in patients with medically inoperable or surgically unresectable stage II-IIIB non-small-cell lung cancer. Int J Radiat Oncol Biol Phys 2002 53(3): 558-65. NRP

Liao, R. Komaki, L. Milas, C. Yuan, M. Kies, J. Y. Chang, M. Jeter, T. Guerrero, G. Blumenschien, C. M. Smith, F. Fossella, B. Brown and J. D. Cox. A phase I clinical trial of thoracic radiotherapy and concurrent celecoxib for patients with unfavorable performance status inoperable/unresectable non-small cell lung cancer. Clin Cancer Res 2005 11(9): 3342-8. NRI

Liao, R. R. Komaki, H. D. Thames, Jr., H. H. Liu, S. L. Tucker, R. Mohan, M. K. Martel, X. Wei, K. Yang, E. S. Kim, G. Blumenschein, W. K. Hong and J. D. Cox. Influence of technologic advances on outcomes in patients with unresectable, locally advanced non-small-cell lung cancer receiving concomitant chemoradiotherapy. Int J Radiat Oncol Biol Phys 2010 76(3): 775-81. NRP

Lilenbaum, M. Samuels, M. Taffaro-Neskey, M. Cusnir, J. Pizzolato and A. Blaustein. Phase II trial of combined modality therapy with myeloid growth factor support in patients with locally advanced non-small cell lung cancer. J Thorac Oncol 2010 5(6): 837-40. NRP

Lin, D. J. Stewart, M. R. Spitz, M. A. Hildebrandt, C. Lu, J. Lin, J. Gu, M. Huang, S. M. Lippman and X. Wu. Genetic variations in the transforming growth factor-beta pathway as predictors of survival in advanced non-small cell lung cancer. Carcinogenesis 2011 32(7): 1050-6. NRP

Lin, J. Wang, L. Yue'E, H. Su, N. Wang, Y. Huang, C. X. Liu, P. Zhang, Y. Zhao and K. Chen. High-dose 3-dimensional conformal radiotherapy with concomitant vinorelbine plus carboplatin in patients with non-small cell lung cancer: A feasibility study. Oncology Letters 2011 2(4): 669-674. NRP

Lind, F. J. Lagerwaard, E. F. Smit, P. E. Postmus, B. J. Slotman and S. Senan. Time for reappraisal of extracranial treatment options? Synchronous brain metastases from nonsmall cell lung cancer. Cancer 2011 117(3): 597-605. NRP

Liu, H. L. Li and T. R. Zheng. Long term results of bronchial arterial infusion with chemotherapeutic agents plus radiation therapy in the teratment of locally advanced non small cell lung cancer. Chinese Journal of Cancer Research 1999 11(1): 66-69. NRP

Livartowski, B. Dubray, A. Dierick, P. Beuzeboc, P. Pouillart and J. M. Cosset. A combined radiochemotherapy trial for non-small cell lung cancers: initial results. 1997 1(): 170-3. FLA

Lochrin, G. Goss, D. J. Stewart, P. Cross, O. Agboola, S. Dahrouge, E. Tomiak and W. K. Evans. Concurrent chemotherapy with hyperfractionated accelerated thoracic irradiation in stage III non-small cell lung cancer. Lung Cancer 1999 23(1): 19-30. NRP

Lokich, M. Auerbach, L. Essig, J. Fryer and D. Fryer. Etoposide plus cisplatin followed by thoracic radiation for stage IIIB non-small cell lung cancer: MAOP study 2188. J Infus Chemother 1995 5(2): 70-2. NRP

Lonardi, M. Coeli, G. Pavanato, F. Adami, G. Gioga and F. Campostrini. Radiotherapy for non-small cell lung cancer in patients aged 75 and over: safety, effectiveness and possible impact on survival. Lung Cancer 2000 28(1): 43-50. NRP

Lopez-Picazo, I. Azinovic, J. J. Aristu, R. Martinez Monge, M. Moreno Jimenez, E. Calvo Aller, C. Beltran, J. M. Aramendia, J. Rebollo and A. Brugarolas. Induction platinum-based chemotherapy followed by radical hyperfractionated radiotherapy with concurrent chemotherapy in the treatment of locally advanced non-small-cell carcinoma of the lung. Am J Clin Oncol 1999 22(2): 203-8. NRP

Louie, G. Rodrigues, M. Hannouf, F. Lagerwaard, D. Palma, G. S. Zaric, C. Haasbeek and S. Senan. Withholding stereotactic radiotherapy in elderly patients with stage I non-small cell lung cancer and co-existing COPD is not justified: outcomes of a Markov model analysis. Radiother Oncol 2011 99(2): 161-5. NRD

Louie, G. Rodrigues, M. Hannouf, G. S. Zaric, D. A. Palma, J. Q. Cao, B. P. Yaremko, R. Malthaner and J. D. Mocanu. Stereotactic body radiotherapy versus surgery for medically operable Stage I non-small-cell lung cancer: a Markov model-based decision analysis. Int J Radiat Oncol Biol Phys 2011 81(4): 964-73. NRD

Low, W. Y. Koh, S. P. Yap and K. W. Fong. Radical radiotherapy in stage I non-small cell lung cancer (NSCLC)--Singapore National Cancer Centre experience. Ann Acad Med Singapore 2007 36(9): 778-83. NRI

Lu, J. J. Lee, R. Komaki, R. S. Herbst, L. Feng, W. K. Evans, H. Choy, P. Desjardins, B. T. Esparaz, M. T. Truong, S. Saxman, J. Kelaghan, A. Bleyer and M. J. Fisch. Chemoradiotherapy with or without AE-941 in stage III non-small cell lung cancer: a randomized phase III trial. J Natl Cancer Inst 2010 102(12): 859-65. NRP

Lunn, J. Stroud, L. Tripcony, M. Dauth and M. Lehman. Factors influencing survival in patients with synchronous solitary cerebral metastatic from non-small cell cancer of the lung. Journal of Thoracic Oncology 2011 6(3): S9. NRD

Lupattelli, E. Maranzano, R. Bellavita, F. Chionne, S. Darwish, F. Piro and P. Latini. Short-course palliative radiotherapy in non-small-cell lung cancer: results of a prospective study. Am J Clin Oncol 2000 23(1): 89-93. NRP

Lupattelli, M. Massetti, R. Bellavita, L. Falcinelli, G. Capezzali, M. P. Leogrande, P. Salustri, S. Saccia and C. Aristei. High dose-rate (HDR) brachitherapy in non-small cell lung cancer: A monoistitutional experience. Radiotherapy and Oncology 2011 99(): S342. NRD

Lutz, D. T. Huang, C. L. Ferguson, B. D. Kavanagh, O. F. Tercilla and J. Lu. A retrospective quality of life analysis using the Lung Cancer Symptom Scale in patients treated with palliative radiotherapy for advanced nonsmall cell lung cancer. Int J Radiat Oncol Biol Phys 1997 37(1): 117-22. NRP

Maas, I. van der Lee, K. Bolt, P. Zanen, J. W. Lammers and F. M. Schramel. Lung function changes and pulmonary complications in patients with stage III non-small cell lung cancer treated with gemcitabine/cisplatin as part of combined modality treatment. Lung Cancer 2003 41(3): 345-51. NRP

Maas, S. Y. El Sharouni, E. C. Phernambucq, J. A. Stigt, H. J. Groen, G. J. Herder, B. E. Van Den Borne, S. Senan, M. A. Paul, E. F. Smit and F. M. Schramel. Weekly chemoradiation (docetaxel/cisplatin) followed by surgery in stage III NSCLC; a multicentre phase II study. Anticancer Res 2010 30(10): 4237-43. NRP

Mac Manus, K. Wong, R. J. Hicks, J. P. Matthews, A. Wirth and D. L. Ball. Early mortality after radical radiotherapy for non-small-cell lung cancer: comparison of PET-staged and conventionally staged cohorts treated at a large tertiary referral center. Int J Radiat Oncol Biol Phys 2002 52(2): 351-61. NRP

Mac Manus, R. J. Hicks, J. P. Matthews, A. McKenzie, D. Rischin, E. K. Salminen and D. L. Ball. Positron emission tomography is superior to computed tomography scanning for response-assessment after radical radiotherapy or chemoradiotherapy in patients with non-small-cell lung cancer. J Clin Oncol 2003 21(7): 1285-92. NRI

Macbeth, J. J. Bolger, P. Hopwood, N. M. Bleehen, J. Cartmell, D. J. Girling, D. Machin, R. J. Stephens and A. J. Bailey. Randomized trial of palliative two-fraction versus more intensive 13-fraction radiotherapy for patients with inoperable non-small cell lung cancer and good performance status. Medical Research Council Lung Cancer Working Party. Clin Oncol (R Coll Radiol) 1996 8(3): 167-75. NRP

Macbeth, T. E. Wheldon, D. J. Girling, R. J. Stephens, D. Machin, N. M. Bleehen, A. Lamont, D. J. Radstone and N. S. Reed. Radiation myelopathy: estimates of risk in 1048 patients in three randomized trials of palliative radiotherapy for non-small cell lung cancer. The Medical Research Council Lung Cancer Working Party. Clin Oncol (R Coll Radiol) 1996 8(3): 176-81. NRD

Macha, B. Wahlers, C. Reichle and D. von Zwehl. Endobronchial radiation therapy for obstructing malignancies: ten years' experience with iridium-192 high-dose radiation brachytherapy afterloading technique in 365 patients. Lung 1995 173(5): 271-80. USD

Machtay, C. Hsu, R. Komaki, W. T. Sause, R. S. Swann, C. J. Langer, R. W. Byhardt and W. J. Curran. Effect of overall treatment time on outcomes after concurrent chemoradiation for locally advanced non-small-cell lung carcinoma: analysis of the Radiation Therapy Oncology Group (RTOG) experience. Int J Radiat Oncol Biol Phys 2005 63(3): 667-71. NRP

Machtay, C. Washam and P. Devine. Pilot study of accelerated radiotherapy with concurrent chemotherapy for stage III non-small cell lung cancer. Semin Oncol 2005 32(2 Suppl 3): S9-12. NRP

Machtay, J. H. Lee, J. P. Stevenson, J. B. Shrager, K. M. Algazy, J. Treat and L. R. Kaiser. Two commonly used neoadjuvant chemoradiotherapy regimens for locally advanced stage III non-small cell lung carcinoma: long-term results and associations with pathologic response. J Thorac Cardiovasc Surg 2004 127(1): 108-13. NRP

Machtay, W. Seiferheld, R. Komaki, J. D. Cox, W. T. Sause and R. W. Byhardt. Is prolonged survival possible for patients with supraclavicular node metastases in non-small cell lung cancer treated with chemoradiotherapy?: Analysis of the Radiation Therapy Oncology Group experience. Int J Radiat Oncol Biol Phys 1999 44(4): 847-53. NRP

MacRae, Y. Shyr, D. Johnson and H. Choy. Declining hemoglobin during chemoradiotherapy for locally advanced non-small cell lung cancer is significant. Radiother Oncol 2002 64(1): 37-40. NRP

Maguire, G. S. Sibley, S. M. Zhou, T. A. Jamieson, K. L. Light, P. A. Antoine, J. E. Herndon, 2nd, M. S. Anscher and L. B. Marks. Clinical and dosimetric predictors of radiation-induced esophageal toxicity. Int J Radiat Oncol Biol Phys 1999 45(1): 97-103. NRP

Maiwand. The role of cryosurgery in palliation of tracheo-bronchial carcinoma. Eur J Cardiothorac Surg 1999 15(6): 764-8. NRP

Mak, E. Doran, A. Muzikansky, J. Kang, J. W. Neal, E. H. Baldini, N. C. Choi, H. Willers, D. M. Jackman and L. V. Sequist. Outcomes after combined modality therapy for EGFR-mutant and wild-type locally advanced NSCLC. Oncologist 2011 16(6): 886-95. NRP

Mallick, S. C. Sharma and D. Behera. Endobronchial brachytherapy for symptom palliation in non-small cell lung cancer--analysis of symptom response, endoscopic improvement and quality of life. Lung Cancer 2007 55(3): 313-8. USD

Manegold and D. Latz. Concurrent radiochemotherapy with ifosfamide in locally advanced unresectable non-small-cell lung cancer. Onkologie 1998 21(SUPPL. 2): 15-18. NRP

Mantz, D. E. Dosoretz, J. H. Rubenstein, P. H. Blitzer, M. J. Katin, G. R. Garton, B. M. Nakfoor, A. D. Siegel, K. A. Tolep, S. E. Hannan, R. Dosani, A. Feroz, C. Maas, S. Bhat, G. Panjikaran, S. Lalla, K. Belani and R. H. Ross. Endobronchial brachytherapy and optimization of local disease control in medically inoperable non-small cell lung carcinoma: a matched-pair analysis. Brachytherapy 2004 3(4): 183-90. NRP

Mao, Z. Kocak, S. Zhou, J. Garst, E. S. Evans, J. Zhang, N. A. Larrier, D. R. Hollis, R. J. Folz and L. B. Marks. The Impact of Induction Chemotherapy and the Associated Tumor Response on Subsequent Radiation-Related Changes in Lung Function and Tumor Response. International Journal of Radiation Oncology Biology Physics 2007 67(5): 1360-1369. NRP

Marangolo, E. Emiliani, G. Rosti, M. Giannini, B. Vertogen and F. Zumaglini. Paclitaxel and radiotherapy in the treatment of advanced non-small cell lung cancer. Semin Oncol 1996 23(6 Suppl 15): 31-4. NRP

Marasso, V. Bernardi, R. Gai, E. Gallo, G. M. Massaglia, M. Onoscuri and S. B. Cardaci. Radiofrequency resection of bronchial tumours in combination with cryotherapy: evaluation of a new technique. Thorax 1998 53(2): 106-9. NRP

Mariotta, B. Sposato, E. Li Bianchi, F. Fiorucci, A. Ricci, F. Carbone, M. Crescenzi and G. Schmid. Combined treatment in advanced stages (IIIb-IV) of non-small cell lung cancer. Eur Rev Med Pharmacol Sci 2002 6(2-3): 49-54. NRP

Marks, J. Garst, M. A. Socinski, G. Sibley, A. W. Blackstock, J. E. Herndon, S. Zhou, T. Shafman, A. Tisch, R. Clough, X. Yu, A. Turrisi, M. Anscher, J. Crawford and J. Rosenman. Carboplatin/paclitaxel or carboplatin/vinorelbine followed by accelerated hyperfractionated conformal radiation therapy: report of a prospective phase I dose escalation trial from the Carolina Conformal Therapy Consortium. J Clin Oncol 2004 22(21): 4329-40. NRP

Martel, M. Strawderman, M. B. Hazuka, A. T. Turrisi, B. A. Fraass and A. S. Lichter. Volume and dose parameters for survival of non-small cell lung cancer patients. Radiother Oncol 1997 44(1): 23-9. NRP

Martin, R. J. Ginsberg, E. S. Venkatraman, M. S. Bains, R. J. Downey, R. J. Korst, M. G. Kris and V. W. Rusch. Long-term results of combined-modality therapy in resectable non-small-cell lung cancer. J Clin Oncol 2002 20(8): 1989-95. NRP

Martins, R. Dienstmann, P. de Biasi, K. Dantas, V. Santos, E. Toscano, W. Roriz, M. Zamboni, A. Sousa, I. A. Small, D. Moreira, C. G. Ferreira and M. Zukin. Phase II trial of neoadjuvant chemotherapy using alternating doublets in non-small-cell lung cancer. Clin Lung Cancer 2007 8(4): 257-63. NRP

Maruyama, F. Hirai, K. Ondo, T. Kometani, M. Hamatake, T. Seto, K. Sugio and Y. Ichinose. Concurrent chemoradiotherapy using cisplatin plus S-1, an oral fluoropyrimidine, followed by surgery for selected patients with stage III non-small cell lung cancer: a single-center feasibility study. Surg Today 2011 41(11): 1492-7. NRP

Masciullo, F. Casamassima, C. Menichelli, I. Bonucci, L. Masi and R. Doro. Stereotactic body radiation therapy for inoperable NSCLC with stage I-II: A mono-institutional retrospective study. Radiotherapy and Oncology 2011 99(): S346. NRD

Massabeau, T. Filleron, G. Wakil, I. Rouquette, J. M. Bachaud, S. Leguellec, M. B. Delisle, C. Toulas, J. Mazieres and E. C. Moyal. The Prognostic Significance of Lymphovascular Invasion on Biopsy Specimens in Lung Cancer Treated With Definitive Chemoradiotherapy. Clin Lung Cancer 2011 (): . NRI

Masters, X. Wang, L. Hodgson, T. Shea, E. Vokes and M. Green. A phase II trial of high dose carboplatin and paclitaxel with G-CSF and peripheral blood stem cell support followed by surgery and/or chest radiation in patients with stage III non-small cell lung cancer: CALGB 9531. Lung Cancer 2011 74(2): 258-63. NRP

Mathisen, J. C. Wain, C. Wright, N. Choi, R. Carey, A. Hilgenberg, M. Grossbard, T. Lynch and H. Grillo. Assessment of preoperative accelerated radiotherapy and chemotherapy in stage IIIA (N2) non-small-cell lung cancer. J Thorac Cardiovasc Surg 1996 111(1): 123-31; discussion 131-3. NRP

Matsuo, K. Shibuya, Y. Nagata, K. Takayama, Y. Norihisa, T. Mizowaki, M. Narabayashi, K. Sakanaka and M. Hiraoka. Prognostic factors in stereotactic body radiotherapy for non-small-cell lung cancer. Int J Radiat Oncol Biol Phys 2011 79(4): 1104-11. USD

Matsuura, T. Kimura, K. Kashiwado, K. Fujita, Y. Akagi, S. Yuki, Y. Murakami, K. Wadasaki, Y. Monzen, A. Ito, M. Kagemoto, M. Mori, K. Ito and Y. Nagata. Results of a preliminary study using hypofractionated involved-field radiation therapy and concurrent carboplatin/paclitaxel in the treatment of locally advanced non-small-cell lung cancer. Int J Clin Oncol 2009 14(5): 408-15. NRP

Mattson, R. P. Abratt, G. ten Velde and K. Krofta. Docetaxel as neoadjuvant therapy for radically treatable stage III non-small-cell lung cancer: a multinational randomised phase III study. Ann Oncol 2003 14(1): 116-22. NRP

Mattson. Docetaxel (Taxotere) in the neo-adjuvant setting in non-small-cell lung cancer. Ann Oncol 1999 10 Suppl 5(): S69-72. NRP

Mattson. Neoadjuvant chemotherapy with docetaxel in non--small cell lung cancer. Semin Oncol 2001 28(3 Suppl 9): 33-6. NRP

Mauer, G. A. Masters, D. J. Haraf, P. C. Hoffman, S. M. Watson, H. M. Golomb and E. E. Vokes. Phase I study of docetaxel with concomitant thoracic radiation therapy. J Clin Oncol 1998 16(1): 159-64. NRP

Maurel, J. Martinez-Trufero, A. Artal, C. Martin, T. Puertolas, M. Zorrrilla, A. Herrero, A. Anton and R. Rosell. Prognostic impact of bulky mediastinal lymph nodes (N2>2.5 cm) in patients with locally advanced non-small-cell lung cancer (LA-NSCLC) treated with platinum-based induction chemotherapy. Lung Cancer 2000 30(2): 107-16. NRP

McAleer, J. Moughan, R. W. Byhardt, J. D. Cox, W. T. Sause and R. Komaki. Does response to induction chemotherapy predict survival for locally advanced non-small-cell lung cancer? Secondary analysis of RTOG 8804/8808. Int J Radiat Oncol Biol Phys 2010 76(3): 802-8. NRP

McGarry, G. Song, P. des Rosiers and R. Timmerman. Observation-only management of early stage, medically inoperable lung cancer: poor outcome. Chest 2002 121(4): 1155-8. NRI

McGarry, L. Papiez, M. Williams, T. Whitford and R. D. Timmerman. Stereotactic body radiation therapy of early-stage non-small-cell lung carcinoma: phase I study. Int J Radiat Oncol Biol Phys 2005 63(4): 1010-5. NRI, USD

McGovern, Z. Liao, M. K. Bucci, M. F. McAleer, M. D. Jeter, J. Y. Chang, M. S. O'Reilly, J. D. Cox, P. K. Allen and R. Komaki. Is sex associated with the outcome of patients treated with radiation for nonsmall cell lung cancer?. Cancer 2009 115(14): 3233-42. NRI

McGrath, D. Warriner and P. Anderson. The Insertion of Self Expanding Metal Stents With Flexible Bronchoscopy Under Sedation for Malignant Tracheobronchial Stenosis: A Single-Center Retrospective Analysis. Arch Bronconeumol 2011 (): . FLA

Mehi, B., Zuti, H., Dizdarevi, Z., Lomigori and J.. Effectiveness of gemcitabine in combination with cisplatin in a randomized study of untreated patients with advanced non-small-cell lung carcinoma. 2004 58(): 11-3. FLA

Mehta, S. P. Tannehill, S. Adak, L. Martin, D. G. Petereit, H. Wagner, J. F. Fowler and D. Johnson. Phase II trial of hyperfractionated accelerated radiation therapy for nonresectable non-small-cell lung cancer: results of Eastern Cooperative Oncology Group 4593. J Clin Oncol 1998 16(11): 3518-23. NRP

Melotti, M. Guaraldi, F. Sperandi, C. Zamagni, S. Giaquinta, G. Oliverio and A. A. Martoni. Long-term results of a pilot study on an intensive induction regimen for unresectable stage III non-small-cell lung cancer. Tumori 2010 96(1): 42-7. NRP

Merchant, K. Kim, M. P. Mehta, G. H. Ripple, M. L. Larson, D. J. Brophy, L. C. Hammes and J. H. Schiller. Pilot and safety trial of carboplatin, paclitaxel, and thalidomide in advanced non-small-cell lung cancer. Clinical Lung Cancer 2000 2(1): 48-52. NRP

Metcalfe, M. T. Milano, K. Bylund, T. Smudzin, P. Rubin and Y. Chen. Split-course palliative radiotherapy for advanced non-small cell lung cancer. J Thorac Oncol 2010 5(2): 185-90. NRI

Meydan, S. Cakir, N. Ozbek, B. Gursel and O. Karaoglanoglu. Neoadjuvant chemotherapy and concomitant boost radiotherapy in locally advanced non-small cell lung cancer. Turkish Journal of Cancer 2006 36(4): 162-168. NRP

Michael, A. Wirth, D. L. Ball, M. MacManus, D. Rischin, L. Mileshkin, B. Solomon, J. McKendrick and A. D. Milner. A phase I trial of high-dose palliative radiotherapy plus concurrent weekly Vinorelbine and Cisplatin in patients with locally advanced and metastatic NSCLC. Br J Cancer 2005 93(6): 652-61. NRD

Migliorino, F. De Marinis, F. Nelli, F. Facciolo, M. V. Ammaturo, A. Cipri, R. Belli, O. Ariganello, F. Diana, M. Di Molfetta and O. Martelli. A 3-week schedule of gemcitabine plus cisplatin as induction chemotherapy for Stage III non-small cell lung cancer. Lung Cancer 2002 35(3): 319-27. NRP

Milano, Y. Chen, A. W. Katz, A. Philip, M. C. Schell and P. Okunieff. Central thoracic lesions treated with hypofractionated stereotactic body radiotherapy. Radiotherapy and Oncology 2009 91(3): 301-306. NRP

Milker-Zabel, A. Zabel, C. Manegold, I. Zuna, M. Wannenmacher and J. Debus. Calcification in coronary arteries as quantified by CT scans correlated with tobacco consumption in patients with inoperable non-small cell lung cancer treated with three-dimensional radiotherapy. Br J Radiol 2003 76(912): 891-6. USD

Milstein, A. Kuten, M. Saute, L. A. Best, K. Daoud, I. Zen-Al-Deen, J. Dale and E. Robinson. Preoperative concurrent chemoradiotherapy for unresectable Stage III nonsmall cell lung cancer. Int J Radiat Oncol Biol Phys 1996 34(5): 1125-32. NRP

Minnich, A. S. Bryant, A. Dooley and R. J. Cerfolio. Photodynamic laser therapy for lesions in the airway. Ann Thorac Surg 2010 89(6): 1744-8; discussion 1748-9. NRP

Mirimanoff, D. Moro, M. Bolla, G. Michel, C. Brambilla, B. Mermillod, R. Miralbell and P. Alberto. Alternating radiotherapy and chemotherapy for inoperable Stage III non-small-cell lung cancer: long-term results of two Phase II GOTHA trials. Groupe d'Oncologie Thoracique Alpine. Int J Radiat Oncol Biol Phys 1998 42(3): 487-94. NRP

Misirlioglu, H. Erkal, Y. Elgin, I. Ugur and K. Altundag. Effect of concomitant use of pentoxifylline and alpha-tocopherol with radiotherapy on the clinical outcome of patients with stage IIIB non-small cell lung cancer: a randomized prospective clinical trial. Med Oncol 2006 23(2): 185-9. NRP

Misirlioglu, T. Demirkasimoglu, B. Kucukplakci, E. Sanri and K. Altundag. Pentoxifylline and alpha-tocopherol in prevention of radiation-induced lung toxicity in patients with lung cancer. 2007 24(): 308-11. NRP

Mitchell, V. Thursfield, G. Wright, D. Ball, G. Richardson, L. Irving and G. Giles. Management of lung cancer in Victoria: Have we made progress?. Journal of Thoracic Oncology 2011 6(3): S8. NRD

Mitsumori, Z. F. Zeng, P. Oliynychenko, J. H. Park, I. B. Choi, H. Tatsuzaki, Y. Tanaka and M. Hiraoka. Regional hyperthermia combined with radiotherapy for locally advanced non-small cell lung cancers: a multi-institutional prospective randomized trial of the International Atomic Energy Agency. Int J Clin Oncol 2007 12(3): 192-8. NRP

Miyaji. Radiotherapy following bronchial artery infusion (BAI) chemotherapy for lung cancer - Analysis of long-term treatment results of 168 patients. Journal of JASTRO 1995 7(4): 331-340. NRI

Miyamoto, M. Baba, N. Yamamoto, M. Koto, T. Sugawara, T. Yashiro, K. Kadono, H. Ezawa, H. Tsujii, J. E. Mizoe, K. Yoshikawa, S. Kandatsu and T. Fujisawa. Curative treatment of Stage I non-small-cell lung cancer with carbon ion beams using a hypofractionated regimen. Int J Radiat Oncol Biol Phys 2007 67(3): 750-8. NRI

Miyamoto, M. Baba, T. Sugane, M. Nakajima, T. Yashiro, K. Kagei, N. Hirasawa, T. Sugawara, N. Yamamoto, M. Koto, H. Ezawa, K. Kadono, H. Tsujii, J. E. Mizoe, K. Yoshikawa, S. Kandatsu and T. Fujisawa. Carbon ion radiotherapy for stage I non-small cell lung cancer using a regimen of four fractions during 1 week. J Thorac Oncol 2007 2(10): 916-26. NRI

Miyamoto, N. Yamamoto, H. Nishimura, M. Koto, H. Tsujii, J. E. Mizoe, T. Kamada, H. Kato, S. Yamada, S. Morita, K. Yoshikawa, S. Kandatsu and T. Fujisawa. Carbon ion radiotherapy for stage I non-small cell lung cancer. Radiother Oncol 2003 66(2): 127-40. NRI

Moghissi, K. Dixon, M. Stringer, T. Freeman, A. Thorpe and S. Brown. The place of bronchoscopic photodynamic therapy in advanced unresectable lung cancer: experience of 100 cases. Eur J Cardiothorac Surg 1999 15(1): 1-6. USD

Moghissi, M. G. Bond, R. J. Sambrook, R. J. Stephens, P. Hopwood and D. J. Girling. Treatment of endotracheal or endobronchial obstruction by non-small cell lung cancer: lack of patients in an MRC randomized trial leaves key questions unanswered. Medical Research Council Lung Cancer Working Party. 1999 11(): 179-83. USD

Mohammed, I. S. Grills, C. Y. O. Wong, A. P. Galerani, K. Chao, R. Welsh, G. Chmielewski, D. Yan and L. L. Kestin. Radiographic and metabolic response rates following image-guided stereotactic radiotherapy for lung tumors. Radiotherapy and Oncology 2011 99(1): 18-22. NRO

Momm, M. Kaden, I. Tannock, M. Schumacher, J. Hasse and M. Henke. Dose escalation of gemcitabine concomitant with radiation and cisplatin for nonsmall cell lung cancer: a phase 1-2 study. Cancer 2010 116(20): 4833-9. NRP

Moreno, J. Aristu, L. I. Ramos, L. Arbea, J. M. Lopez-Picazo, M. Cambeiro and R. Martinez-Monge. Predictive factors for radiation-induced pulmonary toxicity after three-dimensional conformal chemoradiation in locally advanced non-small-cell lung cancer. Clin Transl Oncol 2007 9(9): 596-602. NRP

Moreno-Jimenez, J. Aristu, J. M. Lopez-Picazo, L. I. Ramos, A. Gurpide, A. Gomez-Iturriaga, J. Valero and R. Martinez-Monge. Dosimetric analysis of the patterns of local failure observed in patients with locally advanced non-small cell lung cancer treated with neoadjuvant chemotherapy and concurrent conformal (3D-CRT) chemoradiation. Radiother Oncol 2008 88(3): 342-50. NRP

Morita, N. Fuwa, Y. Suzuki, M. Nishio, K. Sakai, Y. Tamaki, H. Niibe, M. Chujo, S. Wada, T. Sugawara and M. Kita. Radical radiotherapy for medically inoperable non-small cell lung cancer in clinical stage I: a retrospective analysis of 149 patients. Radiother Oncol 1997 42(1): 31-6. NRI

Morris, J. M. Budde, K. D. Godette, T. L. Kerwin, J. I. Miller Jr, C. E. Reed and R. J. Cerfolio. Palliative management of malignant airway obstruction. Annals of Thoracic Surgery 2002 74(6): 1928-1933. USD

Moscetti, F. Nelli, A. Felici, M. Rinaldi, S. De Santis, G. D'Auria, G. Mansueto, G. Tonini, I. Sperduti and F. C. Pollera. Up-front chemotherapy and radiation treatment in newly diagnosed nonsmall cell lung cancer with brain metastases: survey by Outcome Research Network for Evaluation of Treatment Results in Oncology. Cancer 2007 109(2): 274-81. NRP

Mostafa, A. Khatab, E. R. Al-Adwy and G. M. Al-Assal. Limited Field Radiotherapy Concomitant with Cisplatin/Etoposide Followed by Consolidation Docetaxel for the Treatment of Inoperable Stage III Non-Small Cell Lung Cancer. J Egypt Natl Canc Inst 2007 19(1): 28-38. NRP

Movsas, C. J. Langer, H. J. Ross, L. Wang, R. M. Jotte, S. Feigenberg, F. Xu, C. H. Huang, M. J. Monberg and C. K. Obasaju. Randomized phase II trial of cisplatin, etoposide, and radiation followed by gemcitabine alone or by combined gemcitabine and docetaxel in stage III A/B unresectable non-small cell lung cancer. J Thorac Oncol 2010 5(5): 673-9. NRP

Movsas, C. Scott, C. Langer, M. Werner-Wasik, N. Nicolaou, R. Komaki, M. Machtay, C. Smith, R. Axelrod, L. Sarna, T. Wasserman and R. Byhardt. Randomized trial of amifostine in locally advanced non-small-cell lung cancer patients receiving chemotherapy and hyperfractionated radiation: radiation therapy oncology group trial 98-01. J Clin Oncol 2005 23(10): 2145-54. NRP

Movsas, C. Scott, W. Sause, R. Byhardt, R. Komaki, J. Cox, D. Johnson, C. Lawton, A. R. Dar, T. Wasserman, M. Roach, J. S. Lee and E. Andras. The benefit of treatment intensification is age and histology-dependent in patients with locally advanced non-small cell lung cancer (NSCLC): a quality-adjusted survival analysis of radiation therapy oncology group (RTOG) chemoradiation studies. Int J Radiat Oncol Biol Phys 1999 45(5): 1143-9. NRP

Movsas, J. Moughan, L. Sarna, C. Langer, M. Werner-Wasik, N. Nicolaou, R. Komaki, M. Machtay, T. Wasserman and D. W. Bruner. Quality of life supersedes the classic prognosticators for long-term survival in locally advanced non-small-cell lung cancer: an analysis of RTOG 9801. J Clin Oncol 2009 27(34): 5816-22. NRP

Movsas, R. S. Hudes, J. Schol, M. Mellenson, E. Rosvold, N. Nicolaou, S. Litwin, H. Wang, E. Keenan, W. J. Curran, Jr. and C. J. Langer. Induction and concurrent paclitaxel/carboplatin every 3 weeks with thoracic radiotherapy in locally advanced non-small-cell lung cancer: an interim report. Clin Lung Cancer 2001 3(2): 125-32; discussion 133. NRP

Mudad, M. Ramsey, K. Kovitz, T. J. Curiel, R. Hartz, L. L. Nedzi, R. S. Weiner and E. L. Zakris. Concomitant weekly docetaxel, cisplatin and radiation therapy in locally advanced non-small cell lung cancer: a dose finding study. Lung Cancer 2003 39(2): 173-7. NRP

Murai, Y. Shibamoto, F. Baba, C. Hashizume, Y. Mori, S. Ayakawa, T. Kawai, S. Takemoto, C. Sugie and H. Ogino. Progression of Non-Small-Cell Lung Cancer During the Interval Before Stereotactic Body Radiotherapy. Int J Radiat Oncol Biol Phys 2010 (): . NRO

Murakami, Y. Kuroda, A. Sano, S. Noma, N. Kanaoka, S. Ishikura, K. Yamada, M. Takamori, T. Mori and T. Okada. Therapeutic results of non-small cell lung cancer in stage III: combined synchronous irradiation with bronchial artery infusion of CDDP. 1995 55(): 44-9. FLA

Mutter, B. Lu, D. P. Carbone, I. Csiki, L. Moretti, D. H. Johnson, J. D. Morrow, A. B. Sandler, Y. Shyr, F. Ye and H. Choy. A phase II study of celecoxib in combination with paclitaxel, carboplatin, and radiotherapy for patients with inoperable stage IIIA/B non-small cell lung cancer. Clin Cancer Res 2009 15(6): 2158-65. NRP

Naito, K. Kubota, K. Nihei, T. Fujii, K. Yoh, S. Niho, K. Goto, H. Ohmatsu, N. Saijo and Y. Nishiwaki. Concurrent chemoradiotherapy with cisplatin and vinorelbine for stage III non-small cell lung cancer. J Thorac Oncol 2008 3(6): 617-22. NRP

Nakamura, N. Fuwa, T. Kodaira, H. Tachibana, T. Tomoda, R. Nakahara and H. Inokuchi. Clinical outcome of stage III non-small-cell lung cancer patients after definitive radiotherapy. Lung 2008 186(2): 91-6. NRP

Nakamura, N. Kawasaki, M. Hagiwara, A. Ogata, M. Saito, C. Konaka and H. Kato. Early hilar lung cancer--risk for multiple lung cancers and clinical outcome. Lung Cancer 2001 33(1): 51-7. USD

Nakamura, T. Koizumi, M. Hayasaka, M. Yasuo, K. Tsushima, K. Kubo, K. Gomi and N. Shikama. Cisplatin and weekly docetaxel with concurrent thoracic radiotherapy for locally advanced stage III non-small-cell lung cancer. Cancer Chemother Pharmacol 2009 63(6): 1091-6. NRP

Nakano, T. Hiramoto, M. Kanehara, M. Doi, Y. Hada and K. Nakamura. Concurrent high-dose thoracic irradiation plus daily low-dose cisplatin and vindesine in locally advanced unresectable stage III non-small cell lung cancer. Japanese Journal of Lung Cancer 2000 40(2): 111-115. FLA

Nakayama, H. Satoh, K. Kurishima, H. Ishikawa and K. Tokuuye. High-dose conformal radiotherapy for patients with stage III non-small-cell lung carcinoma. Int J Radiat Oncol Biol Phys 2010 78(3): 645-50. NRP

Nakayama, H. Satoh, S. Sugahara, K. Kurishima, K. Tsuboi, H. Sakurai, S. Ishikawa and K. Tokuuye. Proton beam therapy of Stage II and III non-small-cell lung cancer. Int J Radiat Oncol Biol Phys 2011 81(4): 979-84. NRP

Nakayama, K. Hayakawa, N. Mitsuhashi, Y. Saito and H. Niibe. Long-term survivors of non-small cell lung cancer after radiation therapy: the significance of histological type. Anticancer Res 1997 17(4A): 2769-73. NRP

Nath, A. P. Sandhu, D. Kim, A. Bharne, P. D. Nobiensky, J. D. Lawson, M. Fuster, L. Bazhenova, W. Y. Song and A. J. Mundt. Locoregional and distant failure following image-guided stereotactic body radiation for early-stage primary lung cancer. Radiotherapy and Oncology 2011 99(1): 12-17. USD

Nawrocki, M. Krzakowski, E. Wasilewska-Tesluk, D. Kowalski, M. Rucinska, R. Dziadziuszko and A. Sowa. Concurrent chemotherapy and short course radiotherapy in patients with stage IIIA to IIIB non-small cell lung cancer not eligible for radical treatment: results of a randomized phase II study. J Thorac Oncol 2010 5(8): 1255-62. NRP

Nestle, C. Nieder, K. Walter, M. Niewald, B. Motaref, A. Braun-Fischer, D. Ukena, G. W. Sybrecht and K. Schnabel. Palliative accelerated irradiation for advanced non-small-cell lung bronchial carcinoma: results of a pilot study. 1999 53(): 385-92. FLA

Nestle, C. Nieder, K. Walter, U. Abel, D. Ukena, G. W. Sybrecht and K. Schnabel. A palliative accelerated irradiation regimen for advanced non-small-cell lung cancer vs. conventionally fractionated 60 GY: results of a randomized equivalence study. Int J Radiat Oncol Biol Phys 2000 48(1): 95-103. NRP

Nestle, C. Nieder, U. Abel, M. Niewald, D. Ukena, W. Berberich and K. Schnabel. A palliative accelerated irradiation regimen (PAIR) for advanced non-small-cell lung cancer (NSCLC). Radiother Oncol 1996 38(3): 195-203. NRP

Nestle, D. Hellwig, J. Fleckenstein, K. Walter, D. Ukena, C. Rube, C. M. Kirsch and M. Baumann. Comparison of early pulmonary changes in 18FDG-PET and CT after combined radiochemotherapy for advanced non-small-cell lung cancer: a study in 15 patients. Front Radiat Ther Oncol 2002 37(): 26-33. NRP

Ng, S. Y. Tung and V. Y. Wong. Hypofractionated stereotactic radiotherapy for medically inoperable stage I non-small cell lung cancer--report on clinical outcome and dose to critical organs. Radiother Oncol 2008 87(1): 24-8. USD

Nguyen, J. M. Leonardo, U. Karlsson, P. Vos, L. Bullock, P. Thomas, P. Lepera, A. Ludin, C. Chu, M. Salehpour, G. Jendrasiak and S. Sallah. Efficacy of combined radiation, paclitaxel and carboplatin for locally advanced non-small cell lung carcinoma. Anticancer Res 2002 22(6B): 3429-35. NRP

Nguyen, R. Komaki, P. Allen, R. A. Schea and L. Milas. Effectiveness of accelerated radiotherapy for patients with inoperable non-small cell lung cancer (NSCLC) and borderline prognostic factors without distant metastasis: a retrospective review. Int J Radiat Oncol Biol Phys 1999 44(5): 1053-6. NRP

Nieder, U. Nestle, K. Walter, M. Niewald and K. Schnabel. Dose-response relationships for radiotherapy of brain metastases: role of intermediate-dose stereotactic radiosurgery plus whole-brain radiotherapy. Am J Clin Oncol 2000 23(6): 584-8. NRP

Nihei, S. Ishikura, M. Kawashima, T. Ogino, Y. Ito and H. Ikeda. Short-course palliative radiotherapy for airway stenosis in non-small cell lung cancer. Int J Clin Oncol 2002 7(5): 284-8. NRP

Nihei, T. Ogino, S. Ishikura and H. Nishimura. High-dose proton beam therapy for Stage I non-small-cell lung cancer. Int J Radiat Oncol Biol Phys 2006 65(1): 107-11. USD

Nishimura, K. Nakagawa, K. Takeda, M. Tanaka, Y. Segawa, K. Tsujino, S. Negoro, N. Fuwa, T. Hida, M. Kawahara, N. Katakami, K. Hirokawa, N. Yamamoto, M. Fukuoka and Y. Ariyoshi. Phase I/II trial of sequential chemoradiotherapy using a novel hypoxic cell radiosensitizer, doranidazole (PR-350), in patients with locally advanced non-small-cell lung Cancer (WJTOG-0002). Int J Radiat Oncol Biol Phys 2007 69(3): 786-92. NRP

Nuyttens, J. B. Prevost, J. Praag, M. Hoogeman, R. J. Van Klaveren, P. C. Levendag and P. M. Pattynama. Lung tumor tracking during stereotactic radiotherapy treatment with the CyberKnife: Marker placement and early results. Acta Oncol 2006 45(7): 961-5. NRO

Nyman, B. Bergman and C. Mercke. Accelerated hyperfractionated radiotherapy combined with induction and concomitant chemotherapy for inoperable non-small-cell lung cancer--impact of total treatment time. Acta Oncol 1998 37(6): 539-45. NRI

Nyman, S. Friesland, A. Hallqvist, M. Seke, S. Bergstrom, L. Thaning, B. Loden, C. Sederholm and G. Wagenius. How to improve loco-regional control in stages IIIa-b NSCLC? Results of a three-armed randomized trial from the Swedish Lung Cancer Study Group. Lung Cancer 2009 65(1): 62-7. NRP

Ohashi, K. Takahashi, K. Miura, T. Ishiwata, S. Sakuraba and Y. Fukuchi. Prognostic factors in patients with inoperable non-small cell lung cancer--an analysis of long-term survival patients. Gan To Kagaku Ryoho 2006 33(11): 1595-602. NRP

Ohe, N. Ishizuka, T. Tamura, I. Sekine, Y. Nishiwaki and N. Saijo. Long-term follow-up of patients with unresectable locally advanced non-small cell lung cancer treated with chemoradiotherapy: a retrospective analysis of the data from the Japan Clinical Oncology Group trials (JCOG0003A). Cancer Sci 2003 94(8): 729-34. NRD

Ohguri, H. Imada, K. Yahara, T. Morioka, K. Nakano, H. Terashima and Y. Korogi. Radiotherapy with 8-MHz radiofrequency-capacitive regional hyperthermia for stage III non-small-cell lung cancer: the radiofrequency-output power correlates with the intraesophageal temperature and clinical outcomes. Int J Radiat Oncol Biol Phys 2009 73(1): 128-35. NRP

Ohnishi, J. Okada, M. Yamaguchi, H. Ogata, K. Hatano, Y. Takizawa, Y. Imai, R. Hara and T. Araki. Effect of daily administration of oral etoposide for non-small cell lung cancer treated with concurrent radiation therapy. 1997 57(): 510-4. FLA

Ohyanagi, N. Yamamoto, A. Horiike, H. Harada, T. Kozuka, H. Murakami, K. Gomi, T. Takahashi, M. Morota, T. Nishimura, M. Endo, Y. Nakamura, A. Tsuya, T. Horai and M. Nishio. Phase II trial of S-1 and cisplatin with concurrent radiotherapy for locally advanced non-small-cell lung cancer. Br J Cancer 2009 101(2): 225-31. NRP

Oka, M. Fukuda, A. Kinoshita, M. Kuba, M. Ichiki, T. Rikimaru, H. Soda, H. Takatani, F. Narasaki, S. Nagashima, Y. Nakamura, N. Hayashi and S. Kohno. Phase I study of irinotecan and cisplatin with concurrent split-course radiotherapy in unresectable and locally advanced non-small cell lung cancer. Eur J Cancer 2001 37(11): 1359-65. NRP

Okamoto, M. Murakami, T. Mizowaki, T. Nakajima and Y. Kuroda. Radiotherapy for stage I-II non-small cell lung cancer. International Journal of Clinical Oncology 1999 4(6): 372-377. NRI

Okamoto, R. Maruyama, F. Shoji, H. Asoh, J. Ikeda, T. Miyamoto, T. Nakamura, T. Miyake and Y. Ichinose. Long-term survivors in stage IV non-small cell lung cancer. Lung Cancer 2005 47(1): 85-91. NRP

Okamoto, T. Takahashi, H. Okamoto, K. Nakagawa, K. Watanabe, K. Nakamatsu, Y. Nishimura, M. Fukuoka and N. Yamamoto. Single-agent gefitinib with concurrent radiotherapy for locally advanced non-small cell lung cancer harboring mutations of the epidermal growth factor receptor. Lung Cancer 2011 72(2): 199-204. NRP

Ong, D. Palma, W. F. Verbakel, B. J. Slotman and S. Senan. Treatment of large stage I-II lung tumors using stereotactic body radiotherapy (SBRT): planning considerations and early toxicity. Radiother Oncol 2010 97(3): 431-6. NRP

Onimaru, M. Fujino, K. Yamazaki, Y. Onodera, H. Taguchi, N. Katoh, F. Hommura, S. Oizumi, M. Nishimura and H. Shirato. Steep dose-response relationship for stage I non-small-cell lung cancer using hypofractionated high-dose irradiation by real-time tumor-tracking radiotherapy. Int J Radiat Oncol Biol Phys 2008 70(2): 374-81. USD

Onishi, H. Shirato, Y. Nagata, M. Hiraoka, M. Fujino, K. Gomi, Y. Niibe, K. Karasawa, K. Hayakawa, Y. Takai, T. Kimura, A. Takeda, A. Ouchi, M. Hareyama, M. Kokubo, R. Hara, J. Itami, K. Yamada and T. Araki. Hypofractionated stereotactic radiotherapy (HypoFXSRT) for stage I non-small cell lung cancer: updated results of 257 patients in a Japanese multi-institutional study. J Thorac Oncol 2007 2(7 Suppl 3): S94-100. USD

Onishi, K. Kuriyama, M. Yamaguchi, T. Komiyama, S. Tanaka, T. Araki, K. Nishikawa and H. Ishihara. Concurrent two-dimensional radiotherapy and weekly docetaxel in the treatment of stage III non-small cell lung cancer: a good local response but no good survival due to radiation pneumonitis. Lung Cancer 2003 40(1): 79-84. NRP

Onishi, K. Kuriyama, T. Komiyama, S. Tanaka, N. Sano, K. Marino, S. Ikenaga, T. Araki and M. Uematsu. Clinical outcomes of stereotactic radiotherapy for stage I non-small cell lung cancer using a novel irradiation technique: patient self-controlled breath-hold and beam switching using a combination of linear accelerator and CT scanner. Lung Cancer 2004 45(1): 45-55. OPP

Onishi, T. Araki, H. Shirato, Y. Nagata, M. Hiraoka, K. Gomi, T. Yamashita, Y. Niibe, K. Karasawa, K. Hayakawa, Y. Takai, T. Kimura, Y. Hirokawa, A. Takeda, A. Ouchi, M. Hareyama, M. Kokubo, R. Hara, J. Itami and K. Yamada. Stereotactic hypofractionated high-dose irradiation for stage I nonsmall cell lung carcinoma: clinical outcomes in 245 subjects in a Japanese multiinstitutional study. Cancer 2004 101(7): 1623-31. OPP

Oral, A. Aydiner, Y. Eralp and E. Topuz. Induction and concurrent chemotherapy with concomitant boost radiotherapy in non-small cell lung cancer. Med Oncol 2005 22(4): 367-74. NRP

Oral, S. Bavbek, A. Kizir, N. Tenececi, A. Yoney, E. Kaytan and E. Topuz. Preliminary analysis of a phase II study of Paclitaxel and CHART in locally advanced non-small cell lung cancer. Lung Cancer 1999 25(3): 191-8. NRP

Oral. Long term results of CHART and weekly Paclitaxel in locally advanced non-small cell lung cancer. Lung Cancer 2005 49(3): 421-2. NRD

Oshita, M. Ohe, T. Honda, S. Murakami, T. Kondo, H. Saito, K. Noda, K. Yamashita, Y. Nakayama and K. Yamada. Phase II study of nedaplatin and irinotecan with concurrent thoracic radiotherapy in patients with locally advanced non-small-cell lung cancer. Br J Cancer 2010 103(9): 1325-30. NRP

Oshita, Y. Kato, K. Yamada, I. Nomura, M. Sugiyama, K. Yamashita, T. Kitamura and K. Noda. A feasibility study of continuous etoposide infusion combined with thoracic radiation for non-small cell lung cancer. Oncol Rep 1999 6(2): 263-8. NRP

Ozkaya, S. Findik, A. G. Atici and A. Dirica. Cisplatin-based chemotherapy in elderly patients with advanced stage (IIIB and IV) non-small cell lung cancer patients. Neoplasma 2011 58(4): 348-51. NRP

Ozkok, A. B. Aras, M. A. Esassolak, A. H. Arican, D. Yalman and A. Haydaroglu. Hyperfractionated radiotherapy combined with simultaneous chemotherapy in inoperable non-small cell lung cancer: a pilot study. Monaldi Arch Chest Dis 1995 50(6): 443-7. NRP

Ozkok, O. Karakoyun-Celik, T. Goksel, N. Mogulkoc, D. Yalman, G. Gok and Y. Bolukbasi. High dose rate endobronchial brachytherapy in the management of lung cancer: response and toxicity evaluation in 158 patients. Lung Cancer 2008 62(3): 326-33. NRP

Palazzi, B. Morrica, P. Montanaro, L. Cerizza and M. Leoni. Hyperfractionated radiotherapy and concomitant cisplatin in stage III non-small cell lung cancer: a phase II study by the AIRO-Lombardia Cooperative Group. Lung Cancer 1996 15(1): 85-91. NRP

Pallares, J. Capdevila, A. Paredes, N. Farre, J. P. Ciria, I. Membrive, L. Basterrechea, G. Gomez-Segura and A. Barnadas. Induction chemotherapy with paclitaxel plus carboplatin followed by paclitaxel with concurrent radiotherapy in stage IIIB non-small-cell lung cancer (NSCLC) patients: a phase II trial. Lung Cancer 2007 58(2): 238-45. NRP

Palma, O. Visser, F. J. Lagerwaard, J. Belderbos, B. J. Slotman and S. Senan. Impact of introducing stereotactic lung radiotherapy for elderly patients with stage I non-small-cell lung cancer: a population-based time-trend analysis. J Clin Oncol 2010 28(35): 5153-9. NRP

Palma, O. Visser, F. J. Lagerwaard, J. Belderbos, B. Slotman and S. Senan. Treatment of stage i NSCLC in elderly patients: A population-based matched-pair comparison of stereotactic radiotherapy versus surgery. Radiotherapy and Oncology 2011 101(2): 240-244. USD

Palma, S. Tyldesley, F. Sheehan, I. G. Mohamed, S. Smith, E. Wai, N. Murray and S. Senan. Stage I non-small cell lung cancer (NSCLC) in patients aged 75 years and older: does age determine survival after radical treatment?. J Thorac Oncol 2010 5(6): 818-24. NRI

Paludan, A. Traberg Hansen, J. Petersen, C. Grau and M. Hoyer. Aggravation of dyspnea in stage I non-small cell lung cancer patients following stereotactic body radiotherapy: Is there a dose-volume dependency?. Acta Oncol 2006 45(7): 818-22. NRO

Paprota, B. Karczmarek-Borowska, B. Budny and F. Furmanik. Efficacy of combined treatment (chemotherapy + radiotherapy) of non-small cell lung cancer in stage IIIA. Onkologia Polska 2001 4(2): 69-74. FLA

Parashar, A. Edwards, R. Mehta, M. Pasmantier, A. G. Wernicke, A. Sabbas, R. S. Kerestez, D. Nori and K. S. Chao. Chemotherapy significantly increases the risk of radiation pneumonitis in radiation therapy of advanced lung cancer. Am J Clin Oncol 2011 34(2): 160-4. NRP

Parisi, A. Romeo, G. Ghigi, S. Bellia, M. Giannini, S. Micheletti, E. Neri, A. D'Angelo, C. Fabbri, E. Menghi, A. Sarnelli and R. Polico. Accelerated hypofractionated radiotherapy in inoperable locally advanced lung cancer using tomotherapy: Our experience. Strahlentherapie und Onkologie 2011 187(10): 680. NRD

Park, J. O. Park, H. Kim, Y. C. Ahn, Y. S. Choi, K. Kim, J. Kim, Y. M. Shim, J. S. Ahn and K. Park. Is trimodality approach better then bimodality in stage IIIA, N2 positive non-small cell lung cancer?. Lung Cancer 2006 53(3): 323-30. NRP

Park, M. K. Kim, S. Y. Kyung, Y. H. Lim, C. H. An, J. W. Park, S. H. Jeong, J. W. Lee, K. C. Lee, E. K. Cho, S. M. Bang, D. B. Shin and J. H. Lee. A phase II study of weekly paclitaxel, cisplatin and concurrent radiation therapy for locally-advanced unresectable non-small cell lung cancer: early closure due to lack of efficacy. Cancer Res Treat 2004 36(5): 293-7. NRP

Park, Y. C. Ahn, H. Kim, S. H. Lee, S. H. Park, K. E. Lee, D. H. Lim, K. Kim, C. W. Jung, Y. H. Im, W. K. Kang, M. H. Lee and K. Park. A phase II trial of concurrent chemoradiation therapy followed by consolidation chemotherapy with oral etoposide and cisplatin for locally advanced inoperable non-small cell lung cancers. Lung Cancer 2003 42(2): 227-35. NRP

Patel, J. Jenkins, N. Papadopolous, M. Andrew Burgess, C. Plager, J. Gutterman and R. S. Benjamin. Dose-escalating conformal thoracic radiation therapy with induction and concurrent carboplatin/paclitaxel in unresectable stage IIIA/B nonsmall cell lung carcinoma: A modified phase I/II trial. Cancer 2001 92(5): 1213-1223. NRP

Patel, M. Ajlouni, R. Chapman, M. Lu, B. Movsas and J. H. Kim. A prospective phase II study of induction carboplatin and vinorelbine followed by concomitant topotecan and accelerated radiotherapy (ART) in locally advanced non-small cell lung cancer (NSCLC). J Thorac Oncol 2007 2(9): 831-7. NRP

Patel, M. J. Edelman, Y. Kwok, M. J. Krasna and M. Suntharalingam. Predictors of acute esophagitis in patients with non-small-cell lung carcinoma treated with concurrent chemotherapy and hyperfractionated radiotherapy followed by surgery. Int J Radiat Oncol Biol Phys 2004 60(4): 1106-12. NRP

Pennathur, G. Abbas, W. E. Gooding, M. J. Schuchert, S. Gilbert, N. A. Christie, R. J. Landreneau and J. D. Luketich. Image-guided radiofrequency ablation of lung neoplasm in 100 consecutive patients by a thoracic surgical service. Ann Thorac Surg 2009 88(5): 1601-6; discussion 1607-8. NRP

Pennathur, J. D. Luketich, D. E. Heron, M. J. Schuchert, S. Burton, G. Abbas, W. E. Gooding, P. F. Ferson, C. Ozhasoglu, S. Gilbert, R. J. Landreneau and N. A. Christie. Stereotactic radiosurgery for the treatment of lung neoplasm: experience in 100 consecutive patients. Ann Thorac Surg 2009 88(5): 1594-600; discussion 1600. USD

Pennathur, J. D. Luketich, S. Burton, G. Abbas, D. E. Heron, H. C. Fernando, W. E. Gooding, C. Ozhasoglu, J. Ireland, R. J. Landreneau and N. A. Christie. Stereotactic radiosurgery for the treatment of lung neoplasm: initial experience. Ann Thorac Surg 2007 83(5): 1820-4; discussion 1824-5. USD

Pergolizzi, A. Santacaterina, C. D. Renzis, N. Settineri, M. Gaeta, P. Frosina, E. G. Russi and G. Altavilla. Older people with non small cell lung cancer in clinical stage IIIA and co-morbid conditions. Is curative irradiation feasible? Final results of a prospective study. Lung Cancer 2002 37(2): 201-6. NRP

Pergolizzi, N. Settineri, R. Maisano, A. Santacaterina, C. Faranda, E. Russi, L. Raffaele and V. Adamo. Curative radiotherapy (RT) using limited RT treatment fields in elderly patients with non-small cell lung cancer in clinical stage IIIA. Oncol Rep 1997 4(5): 961-5. NRP

Pettersson, J. Nyman and K. A. Johansson. Radiation-induced rib fractures after hypofractionated stereotactic body radiation therapy of non-small cell lung cancer: a dose- and volume-response analysis. Radiother Oncol 2009 91(3): 360-8. OPP

Phernambucq, B. Biesma, E. F. Smit, M. A. Paul, A. vd Tol, F. M. Schramel, R. J. Bolhuis and P. E. Postmus. Multicenter phase II trial of accelerated cisplatin and high-dose epirubicin followed by surgery or radiotherapy in patients with stage IIIa non-small-cell lung cancer with mediastinal lymph node involvement (N2-disease). Br J Cancer 2006 95(4): 470-4. NRP

Phernambucq, F. O. Spoelstra, M. A. Paul, S. Senan, C. F. Melissant, P. E. Postmus and E. F. Smit. Evaluation of a treatment strategy for optimising preoperative chemoradiotherapy in stage III non-small-cell lung cancer. Eur J Cardiothorac Surg 2009 36(6): 1052-7. NRP

Phernambucq, F. O. Spoelstra, W. F. Verbakel, P. E. Postmus, C. F. Melissant, K. I. Maassen van den Brink, V. Frings, P. M. van de Ven, E. F. Smit and S. Senan. Outcomes of concurrent chemoradiotherapy in patients with stage III non-small-cell lung cancer and significant comorbidity. Ann Oncol 2011 22(1): 132-8. NRP

Photodynamic therapy for palliation of locally advanced lung cancer. Oncology 1999 13(5): 608+613. NRD

Pignon, S. Ruggieri, C. Boutin, J. Gouvernet, M. Irisson, P. Juin and P. Astoul. Alternating chemotherapy and accelerated split-course irradiation in locally advanced nonsmall cell lung carcinoma. Cancer 1999 85(10): 2144-50. NRP

Pijls-Johannesma, R. Houben, L. Boersma, J. Grutters, K. Seghers, P. Lambin, R. Wanders and D. De Ruysscher. High-dose radiotherapy or concurrent chemo-radiation in lung cancer patients only induces a temporary, reversible decline in QoL. Radiother Oncol 2009 91(3): 443-8. NRP

Pisch, A. M. Berson, S. Malamud, E. J. Beattie, J. Harvey and B. Vikram. Chemoradiation in advanced nonsmall cell lung cancer. Int J Radiat Oncol Biol Phys 1995 33(1): 183-8. NRP

Pisch, J. C. Harvey, N. Panigrahi and Beattie E.J, Jr.. Iodine-125 volume implant in patients with medically unresectable stage I lung cancer. Endocurietherapy/Hyperthermia Oncology 1996 12(3): 165-170. NRI

Pisch, T. Moskovitz, O. Esik, P. Homel and S. Keller. Concurrent paclitaxel-cisplatin and twice-a-day irradiation in stage IIIA and IIIB NSCLC shows improvement in local control and survival with acceptable hematologic toxicity. Pathol Oncol Res 2002 8(3): 163-9. NRP

Pitz, K. W. Maas, H. A. Van Swieten, A. B. de la Riviere, P. Hofman and F. M. Schramel. Surgery as part of combined modality treatment in stage IIIB non-small cell lung cancer. Ann Thorac Surg 2002 74(1): 164-9. NRP

Planting, P. Helle, P. Drings, O. Dalesio, A. Kirkpatrick, G. McVie and G. Giaccone. A randomized study of high-dose split course radiotherapy preceded by high-dose chemotherapy versus high-dose radiotherapy only in locally advanced non-small-cell lung cancer. An EORTC Lung Cancer Cooperative Group trial. Ann Oncol 1996 7(2): 139-44. NRP

Plataniotis, J. R. Kouvaris, C. Dardoufas, V. Kouloulias, M. A. Theofanopoulou and L. Vlahos. A short radiotherapy course for locally advanced non-small cell lung cancer (NSCLC): effective palliation and patients' convenience. Lung Cancer 2002 35(2): 203-7. NRP

Plumridge, M. J. Millward, D. Rischin, M. P. Macmanus, A. Wirth, M. Michael, K. Yuen and D. L. Ball. Long-term survival following chemoradiation for inoperable non-small cell lung cancer. Med J Aust 2008 189(10): 557-9. NRP

Pohl, G. Krajnik, R. Malayeri, R. M. Muller, W. Klepetko, F. Eckersberger, C. Schafer-Prokop, B. Pokrajac, S. Schmeikal, A. Maier, G. Ambrosch, M. Woltsche, W. Minar and R. Pirker. Induction chemotherapy with the TIP regimen (paclitaxel/ifosfamide/cisplatin) in stage III non-small cell lung cancer. Lung Cancer 2006 54(1): 63-7. NRP

Pottgen, W. E. Eberhardt, T. Gauler, T. Krbek, K. Berkovic, J. A. Jawad, S. Korfee, H. Teschler, G. Stamatis and M. Stuschke. Intensified high-dose chemoradiotherapy with induction chemotherapy in patients with locally advanced non-small-cell lung cancer-safety and toxicity results within a prospective trial. Int J Radiat Oncol Biol Phys 2010 76(3): 809-15. NRP

Pottgen, W. Eberhardt, S. Bildat, G. Stuben, G. Stamatis, L. Hillejan, S. Sohrab, H. Teschler, S. Seeber, H. Sack and M. Stuschke. Induction chemotherapy followed by concurrent chemotherapy and definitive high-dose radiotherapy for patients with locally advanced non-small-cell lung cancer (stages IIIa/IIIb): a pilot phase I/II trial. Ann Oncol 2002 13(3): 403-11. NRP

Pourel, N. Santelmo, N. Naafa, A. Serre, W. Hilgers, L. Mineur, N. Molinari and F. Reboul. Concurrent cisplatin/etoposide plus 3D-conformal radiotherapy followed by surgery for stage IIB (superior sulcus T3N0)/III non-small cell lung cancer yields a high rate of pathological complete response. Eur J Cardiothorac Surg 2008 33(5): 829-36. NRP

Pradier, K. Lederer, A. Hille, E. Weiss, H. Christiansen, H. Schmidberger and C. F. Hess. Concurrent low-dose cisplatin and thoracic radiotherapy in patients with inoperable stage III non-small cell lung cancer: a phase II trial with special reference to the hemoglobin level as prognostic parameter. J Cancer Res Clin Oncol 2005 131(4): 261-9. NRP

Pujol, T. Lafontaine, X. Quantin, M. Reme-Saumon, D. Cupissol, F. Khial and F. B. Michel. Neoadjuvant etoposide, ifosfamide, and cisplatin followed by concomitant thoracic radiotherapy and continuous cisplatin infusion in stage IIIb non-small cell lung cancer. Chest 1999 115(1): 144-50. NRP

Qiao, L. Xin and H. Liu. The combined therapy of carboplatin, fluorouracil and radiotherapy for moderate and advanced non-small cell lung cancer. 1999 22(): 536-7. FLA

Qiao, Y. H. Zhao, Y. B. Zhao and R. Z. Wang. Clinical and dosimetric factors of radiation-induced esophageal injury: Radiation-induced esophageal toxicity. World Journal of Gastroenterology 2005 11(17): 2626-2629. NRP

Quddus, G. R. Kerr, A. Price and A. Gregor. Long-term survival in patients with non-small cell lung cancer treated with palliative radiotherapy. Clin Oncol (R Coll Radiol) 2001 13(2): 95-8. NRP

Ranson, N. Davidson, M. Nicolson, S. Falk, J. Carmichael, P. Lopez, H. Anderson, N. Gustafson, A. Jeynes, G. Gallant, T. Washington and N. Thatcher. Randomized trial of paclitaxel plus supportive care versus supportive care for patients with advanced non-small-cell lung cancer. J Natl Cancer Inst 2000 92(13): 1074-80. NRI

Ratanatharathorn, V. Lorvidhaya, P. Kraipiboon, E. Sirachainan, S. Maoleekoonpairoj, P. Phromratanapongse, A. Cheirsilpa, S. Tangkaratt, V. Srimuninnimit, P. Pattaranutaporn and P. Lertsanguansinchai. Phase II study of concurrent chemoradiotherapy for inoperable (bulky) stage III (A/B) non-small cell lung cancer (NSCLC): a preliminary report. J Med Assoc Thai 2000 83(1): 85-92. NRP

Ratanatharathorn, V. Lorvidhaya, S. Maoleekoonpairoj, P. Phromratanapongse, S. Sirilerttrakul, P. Kraipiboon, A. Cheirsilpa, S. Tangkaratt, V. Srimuninnimit and P. Pattaranutaporn. Phase II trial of paclitaxel, carboplatin, and concurrent radiation therapy for locally advanced non-small-cell lung cancer. Lung Cancer 2001 31(2-3): 257-65. NRP

Rathmann, K. A. Leopold and J. R. Rigas. Daily paclitaxel and thoracic radiation therapy for non-small cell lung cancer: preliminary results. Semin Radiat Oncol 1999 9(2 Suppl 1): 130-5. NRP

Razi, R. S. Lebovics, G. Schwartz, M. Sancheti, S. Belsley, C. P. Connery and F. Y. Bhora. Timely airway stenting improves survival in patients with malignant central airway obstruction. Annals of Thoracic Surgery 2010 90(4): 1088-1093. USD

Ready, P. A. Janne, J. Bogart, T. Dipetrillo, J. Garst, S. Graziano, L. Gu, X. Wang, M. R. Green and E. E. Vokes. Chemoradiotherapy and gefitinib in stage III non-small cell lung cancer with epidermal growth factor receptor and KRAS mutation analysis: cancer and leukemia group B (CALEB) 30106, a CALGB-stratified phase II trial. J Thorac Oncol 2010 5(9): 1382-90. NRP

Reboul, Y. Brewer, P. Vincent, B. Chauvet, C. F. Faure and M. Taulelle. Concurrent cisplatin, etoposide, and radiotherapy for unresectable stage III nonsmall cell lung cancer: a phase II study. Int J Radiat Oncol Biol Phys 1996 35(2): 343-50. NRP

Reckzeh, H. Merte, K. H. Pfluger, R. Pfab, M. Wolf and K. Havemann. Severe lymphocytopenia and interstitial pneumonia in patients treated with paclitaxel and simultaneous radiotherapy for non-small-cell lung cancer. J Clin Oncol 1996 14(4): 1071-6. NRP

Reguart, N. Vinolas, F. Casas, J. M. Gimferrer, C. Agusti, R. Molina, M. Martin-Richard, A. Sanchez-Reyes and P. Gascon. Integrating concurrent navelbine and cisplatin to hyperfractionated radiotherapy in locally advanced non-small cell lung cancer patients treated with induction and consolidation chemotherapy: feasibility and activity results. Lung Cancer 2004 45(1): 67-75. NRP

Reinfuss, A. Mucha-Malecka, T. Walasek, P. Blecharz, J. Jakubowicz, P. Skotnicki and T. Kowalska. Palliative thoracic radiotherapy in non-small cell lung cancer. An analysis of 1250 patients. Palliation of symptoms, tolerance and toxicity. Lung Cancer 2011 71(3): 344-9. NRP

Reinfuss, J. Skolyszewski, T. Kowalska, B. Glinski, P. Dymek, T. Walasek, Z. Kojs, P. Skotnicki and A. Michalak. Evaluation of efficacy of combined chemoradiotherapy in locoregional advanced, inoperable Non-Small Cell Lung Cancer (clinical randomized trial). Nowotwory 2005 55(3): 200-206. NRP

Rengan, K. E. Rosenzweig, E. Venkatraman, L. A. Koutcher, J. L. Fox, R. Nayak, H. Amols, E. Yorke, A. Jackson, C. C. Ling and S. A. Leibel. Improved local control with higher doses of radiation in large-volume stage III non-small-cell lung cancer. Int J Radiat Oncol Biol Phys 2004 60(3): 741-7. NRP

Rice, D. J. Adelstein, A. Koka, M. Tefft, T. J. Kirby, M. A. Van Kirk, M. E. Taylor, T. E. Olencki, D. Peereboom and G. T. Budd. Accelerated induction therapy and resection for poor prognosis stage III non-small cell lung cancer. Ann Thorac Surg 1995 60(3): 586-91; discussion 591-2. NRP

Rice, D. J. Adelstein, J. P. Ciezki, M. E. Becker, L. A. Rybicki, C. F. Farver, M. A. Larto and E. H. Blackstone. Short-course induction chemoradiotherapy with paclitaxel for stage III non-small-cell lung cancer. Ann Thorac Surg 1998 66(6): 1909-14. NRP

Robert, S. A. Spencer, H. A. Childs, 3rd, R. Zhang, R. F. Meredith, R. H. Wheeler, M. H. Hawkins and D. Carey. Concurrent chemoradiation therapy with cisplatin and paclitaxel for locally advanced non-small cell lung cancer: long-term follow-up of a phase I trial. Lung Cancer 2002 37(2): 189-99. NRP

Rojas, B. E. Lyn, E. M. Wilson, F. J. Williams, N. Shah, J. Dickson and M. I. Saunders. Toxicity and outcome of a phase II trial of taxane-based neoadjuvant chemotherapy and 3-dimensional, conformal, accelerated radiotherapy in locally advanced nonsmall cell lung cancer. Cancer 2006 107(6): 1321-30. NRP

Rosenman, J. S. Halle, M. A. Socinski, K. Deschesne, D. T. Moore, H. Johnson, R. Fraser and D. E. Morris. High-dose conformal radiotherapy for treatment of stage IIIA/IIIB non-small-cell lung cancer: technical issues and results of a phase I/II trial. Int J Radiat Oncol Biol Phys 2002 54(2): 348-56. NRP

Rosenthal, C. D. Fuller, M. Machtay, K. M. Algazy, D. M. Meyer, L. R. Kaiser, D. A. Yardley, M. E. Loiacano and D. P. Carbone. Phase I study of Paclitaxel given by seven-week continuous infusion concurrent with radiation therapy for locally advanced non-small cell lung cancer. J Thorac Oncol 2006 1(1): 38-45. NRP

Rosenzweig, B. Mychalczak, Z. Fuks, J. Hanley, C. Burman, C. C. Ling, J. Armstrong, R. Ginsberg, M. G. Kris, A. Raben and S. Leibel. Final report of the 70.2-Gy and 75.6-Gy dose levels of a phase I dose escalation study using three-dimensional conformal radiotherapy in the treatment of inoperable non-small cell lung cancer. Cancer J 2000 6(2): 82-7. NRP

Rosenzweig, J. L. Fox, E. Yorke, H. Amols, A. Jackson, V. Rusch, M. G. Kris, C. C. Ling and S. A. Leibel. Results of a phase I dose-escalation study using three-dimensional conformal radiotherapy in the treatment of inoperable nonsmall cell lung carcinoma. Cancer 2005 103(10): 2118-27. USD

Rosenzweig, N. Dladla, R. Schindelheim, S. E. Sim, L. E. Braban, E. S. Venkataraman and S. A. Leibel. Three-dimensional conformal radiation therapy (3D-CRT) for early-stage non-small-cell lung cancer. Clin Lung Cancer 2001 3(2): 141-4. NRP

Rosenzweig, S. E. Sim, B. Mychalczak, L. E. Braban, R. Schindelheim and S. A. Leibel. Elective nodal irradiation in the treatment of non-small-cell lung cancer with three-dimensional conformal radiation therapy. Int J Radiat Oncol Biol Phys 2001 50(3): 681-5. NRP

Rosenzweig, S. Sura, A. Jackson and E. Yorke. Involved-field radiation therapy for inoperable non small-cell lung cancer. J Clin Oncol 2007 25(35): 5557-61. NRO

Rossi, F. Graziano, M. Ugolini, D. Dennetta, P. Alessandroni, V. Catalano, P. Giordani, S. L. Fedeli, A. Fedeli and G. Catalano. Weekly docetaxel as second-line therapy in non-small cell lung cancer: a phase II study. Tumori 2004 90(1): 50-3. NRP

Rossi, R. Dore, A. Cascina, V. Vespro, F. Garbagnati, L. Rosa, V. Ravetta, A. Azzaretti, P. Di Tolla, G. Orlandoni and E. Pozzi. Percutaneous computed tomography-guide radiofrequency thermal ablation of small unresectable lung tumours. European Respiratory Journal 2006 27(3): 556-563. USD

Roszkowski, A. Pluzanska, M. Krzakowski, A. P. Smith, E. Saigi, U. Aasebo, A. Parisi, N. Pham Tran, R. Olivares and J. Berille. A multicenter, randomized, phase III study of docetaxel plus best supportive care versus best supportive care in chemotherapy-naive patients with metastatic or non-resectable localized non-small cell lung cancer (NSCLC). Lung Cancer 2000 27(3): 145-157. NRI

Rothschild, S. E. Bucher, J. Bernier, D. M. Aebersold, A. Zouhair, G. Ries, N. Lombrieser, T. Lippuner, U. M. Lutolf, C. Glanzmann and I. F. Ciernik. Gefitinib in combination with irradiation with or without cisplatin in patients with inoperable stage III non-small cell lung cancer: a phase I trial. Int J Radiat Oncol Biol Phys 2011 80(1): 126-32. NRP

Rowell and C. J. Williams. Radical radiotherapy for stage I/II non-small cell lung cancer in patients not sufficiently fit for or declining surgery (medically inoperable). Cochrane Database Syst Rev 2001 (2): CD002935. NRD

Rusch, D. J. Giroux, M. J. Kraut, J. Crowley, M. Hazuka, D. Johnson, M. Goldberg, F. Detterbeck, F. Shepherd, R. Burkes, T. Winton, C. Deschamps, R. Livingston and D. Gandara. Induction chemoradiation and surgical resection for non-small cell lung carcinomas of the superior sulcus: Initial results of Southwest Oncology Group Trial 9416 (Intergroup Trial 0160). J Thorac Cardiovasc Surg 2001 121(3): 472-83. NRP

Rusch, D. J. Giroux, M. J. Kraut, J. Crowley, M. Hazuka, T. Winton, D. H. Johnson, L. Shulman, F. Shepherd, C. Deschamps, R. B. Livingston and D. Gandara. Induction chemoradiation and surgical resection for superior sulcus non-small-cell lung carcinomas: long-term results of Southwest Oncology Group Trial 9416 (Intergroup Trial 0160). J Clin Oncol 2007 25(3): 313-8. NRP

Rusthoven, S. F. Hammerman, B. D. Kavanagh, M. J. Birtwhistle, M. Stares and D. R. Camidge. Is there a role for consolidative stereotactic body radiation therapy following first-line systemic therapy for metastatic lung cancer? A patterns-of-failure analysis. Acta Oncol 2009 48(4): 578-83. NRP

Rusu, T. E. Ciuleanu, D. Cernea, D. Pelau, V. Gaal, C. Cebotaru, T. Guttman, N. Todor and N. Ghilezan. Concurrent chemoradiotherapy with vinorelbine and a platinum compound followed by consolidation chemotherapy for unresectable stage III non-small cell lung cancer: preliminary results of a phase II study. J BUON 2007 12(1): 33-9. NRP

Rusu, T. E. Ciuleanu, N. Todor, T. Guttman, V. Bogdan and V. Cernea. Dose escalation using 3DCRT in concurrent setting with vinorelbine and a platinum compound in locally advanced NSCLC. Radiotherapy and Oncology 2011 99(): S109-S110. NRD

Saito, K. Hayakawa, Y. Nakayama, S. Katano, M. Furuta, H. Ishikawa, S. Nasu, N. Mitsuhashi and H. Niibe. Radiation therapy for stage III non-small cell lung cancer invading chest wall. Lung Cancer 1997 18(2): 171-8. NRP

Saito, N. Mitsuhashi, K. Hayakawa, Y. Nakayama, T. Kazumoto, M. Furuta, M. Yamakawa, T. Akimoto, H. Sakurai, T. Takahashi and H. Niibe. Prognostic value of pretreatment serum carcinoembryonic antigen and squamous cell carcinoma antigen levels for patients with stage I-III non- small cell lung cancer treated with radiation therapy alone. International Journal of Clinical Oncology 1998 3(1): 27-30. NRD

Saitoh, Y. Saito, T. Kazumoto, S. Kudo, D. Yoshida, A. Ichikawa, H. Sakai, F. Kurimoto, S. Kato and K. Shibuya. Concurrent Chemoradiotherapy Followed by Consolidation Chemotherapy with Bi-Weekly Docetaxel and Carboplatin for Stage III Unresectable, Non-Small-Cell Lung Cancer: Clinical Application of a Protocol Used in a Previous Phase II Study. Int J Radiat Oncol Biol Phys 2011 (): . NRP

Sakai, S. Yoneda, K. Kobayashi, H. Komagata, S. Kosaihira, T. Kazumoto and Y. Saito. Phase II study of bi-weekly docetaxel and carboplatin with concurrent thoracic radiation therapy followed by consolidation chemotherapy with docetaxel plus carboplatin for stage III unresectable non-small cell lung cancer. Lung Cancer 2004 43(2): 195-201. NRP

Sakai, Y. Matsumoto, M. Nishio, S. Hirota, S. Yamada, Y. Hirokawa and H. Inakoshi. Combined chemoradiotherapy with daily low-dose cisplatin in stage III non-small cell lung cancer - An interim report. Journal of JASTRO 2001 13(2): 103-106. NRP

Sakakibara-Konishi, S. Oizumi, I. Kinoshita, N. Shinagawa, J. Kikuchi, M. Kato, T. Inoue, N. Katoh, R. Onimaru, H. Shirato, H. Dosaka-Akita and M. Nishimura. Phase I study of concurrent real-time tumor-tracking thoracic radiation therapy with paclitaxel and carboplatin in locally advanced non-small cell lung cancer. Lung Cancer 2011 74(2): 248-52. NRP

Salama, T. E. Stinchcombe, L. Gu, X. Wang, K. Morano, J. A. Bogart, J. C. Crawford, M. A. Socinski, A. W. Blackstock and E. E. Vokes. Pulmonary toxicity in Stage III non-small cell lung cancer patients treated with high-dose (74 Gy) 3-dimensional conformal thoracic radiotherapy and concurrent chemotherapy following induction chemotherapy: a secondary analysis of Cancer and Leukemia Group B (CALGB) trial 30105. Int J Radiat Oncol Biol Phys 2011 81(4): e269-74. NRP

Salazar, T. S. Sandhu, P. B. Lattin, J. H. Chang, C. K. Lee, G. A. Groshko and C. J. Lattin. Once-weekly, high-dose stereotactic body radiotherapy for lung cancer: 6-year analysis of 60 early-stage, 42 locally advanced, and 7 metastatic lung cancers. Int J Radiat Oncol Biol Phys 2008 72(3): 707-15. NRP

San Jose, M. D. Arnaiz, A. Lucas, V. Navarro, G. Serrano, M. Zaderazjko, B. Jeremic and F. Guedea. Radiation therapy alone in elderly with early stage non-small cell lung cancer. Lung Cancer 2006 52(2): 149-54. USD

Sandhu, K. Messer, M. M. Fuster, E. Ahmad, M. Pu, L. Bazhenova, M. Rose and S. Seagren. Definitive radiation therapy for stage I non-small-cell lung carcinoma: institutional experience with contemporary conformal planning. Clin Lung Cancer 2009 10(6): 433-7. USD

Sangha, R. Prestwich, J. Lilley, A. Needham, H. Summers, R. Stuart, R. Turner, M. Bond, M. Snee and K. N. Franks. Feasibility and early outcomes of stereotactic radiotherapy in early lung cancer at St James's Institute of Oncology. Clinical Oncology 2011 23(3): S51-S52. NRD

Santo, R. Pedersini, F. Pasini, A. Terzi, F. Pari, G. Cartei, A. Sibau, A. Molino, A. Maiorino, N. Panza, M. V. Oletti, S. Maluta, F. Calabro and G. L. Cetto. A phase II study of induction chemotherapy with gemcitabine (G) and cisplatin (P) in locally advanced non-small cell lung cancer: interim analysis. Lung Cancer 2001 34 Suppl 4(): S15-20. NRP

Sarihan, E. Darendeliler, A. Kizir, N. Tuncel, E. N. Oral, A. Karadeniz and N. Bilge. A phase II trial, feasibility of combination of daily cisplatinum and accelerated radiotherapy via concomitant boost in stage III non-small cell lung cancer. Lung Cancer 1998 20(1): 37-46. NRP

Sarihan, U. Kayisogullari, I. Ercan and K. Engin. Randomized phase 2 study of radiotherapy alone versus radiotherapy with paclitaxel in non-small cell lung cancer. J Int Med Res 2004 32(4): 375-83. NRP

Sasaki, R. Komaki, H. Macapinlac, J. Erasmus, P. Allen, K. Forster, J. B. Putnam, R. S. Herbst, C. A. Moran, D. A. Podoloff, J. A. Roth and J. D. Cox. [18F]fluorodeoxyglucose uptake by positron emission tomography predicts outcome of non-small-cell lung cancer. J Clin Oncol 2005 23(6): 1136-43. NRI

Satoh, K. Ohara, H. Fuji, H. Ishikawa, Y. T. Yamashita, H. Kamma, M. Ohtsuka and S. Hasegawa. Use of daily low-dose carboplatin in radiotherapy for non-small cell lung cancer. Anticancer Res 1998 18(6B): 4625-7. NRP

Saunders, A. Rojas, B. E. Lyn, E. Wilson and H. Phillips. Dose-escalation with CHARTWEL (continuous hyperfractionated accelerated radiotherapy week-end less) combined with neo-adjuvant chemotherapy in the treatment of locally advanced non-small cell lung cancer. Clin Oncol (R Coll Radiol) 2002 14(5): 352-60. NRP

Saunders, A. Rojas, B. E. Lyn, K. Pigott, M. Powell, K. Goodchild, P. J. Hoskin, H. Phillips and N. Verma. Experience with dose escalation using CHARTWEL (continuous hyperfractionated accelerated radiotherapy weekend less) in non-small-cell lung cancer. Br J Cancer 1998 78(10): 1323-8. NRI

Saunders, S. Dische, A. Barrett, A. Harvey, D. Gibson and M. Parmar. Continuous hyperfractionated accelerated radiotherapy (CHART) versus conventional radiotherapy in non-small-cell lung cancer: a randomised multicentre trial. CHART Steering Committee. Lancet 1997 350(9072): 161-5. NRP

Saunders, S. Dische, A. Barrett, A. Harvey, G. Griffiths and M. Palmar. Continuous, hyperfractionated, accelerated radiotherapy (CHART) versus conventional radiotherapy in non-small cell lung cancer: mature data from the randomised multicentre trial. CHART Steering committee. Radiother Oncol 1999 52(2): 137-48. NRI

Sause, C. Scott, S. Taylor, D. Johnson, R. Livingston, R. Komaki, B. Emami, W. J. Curran, R. W. Byhardt, A. T. Turrisi and et al.. Radiation Therapy Oncology Group (RTOG) 88-08 and Eastern Cooperative Oncology Group (ECOG) 4588: preliminary results of a phase III trial in regionally advanced, unresectable non-small-cell lung cancer. J Natl Cancer Inst 1995 87(3): 198-205. NRI

Sause, P. Kolesar, S. I. Taylor, D. Johnson, R. Livingston, R. Komaki, B. Emami, W. Curran, Jr., R. Byhardt, A. R. Dar and A. Turrisi, 3rd. Final results of phase III trial in regionally advanced unresectable non-small cell lung cancer: Radiation Therapy Oncology Group, Eastern Cooperative Oncology Group, and Southwest Oncology Group. Chest 2000 117(2): 358-64. NRP

Saynak, G. Aksu, M. Fayda, E. Kaytan, E. Oral, S. Gurocak, A. Kizir and A. Karadeniz. The results of concomitant and sequential chemoradiotherapy with cisplatin and etoposide in patients with locally advanced non-small cell lung cancer. J BUON 2005 10(2): 213-8. NRP

Scagliotti, A. Szczesna, R. Ramlau, F. Cardenal, K. Mattson, N. Van Zandwijk, A. Price, B. Lebeau, J. Debus and C. Manegold. Docetaxel-based induction therapy prior to radiotherapy with or without docetaxel for non-small-cell lung cancer. Br J Cancer 2006 94(10): 1375-82. NRP

Scagliotti, U. Ricardi, L. Crino, E. Maranzano, F. De Marinis, M. G. Morandi, L. Meacci, M. Marangolo, E. Emiliani, G. Rosti, F. Figoli, G. Bolzicco, P. Masiero, A. Gentile and M. Tonato. Phase II study of intensive chemotherapy with carboplatin, ifosfamide and etoposide plus recombinant human granulocyte colony-stimulating factor and sequential radiotherapy in locally advanced, unresectable non-small-cell lung cancer. Cancer Chemother Pharmacol 1996 38(6): 561-5. NRP

Scarda, M. Confalonieri, C. Baghiris, S. Binato, R. Mazzarotto, A. Palamidese, R. Zuin and U. Fantoni. Out-patient high-dose-rate endobronchial brachytherapy for palliation of lung cancer: an observational study. Monaldi Arch Chest Dis 2007 67(3): 128-34. USD

Schaafsma and P. Coy. Response of global quality of life to high-dose palliative radiotherapy for non-small-cell lung cancer. Int J Radiat Oncol Biol Phys 2000 47(3): 691-701. NRD

Schallier, B. Neyns, C. Fontaine, J. V. Steene, J. De Mey, M. Meysman and J. De Greve. A novel triplet regimen with paclitaxel, carboplatin and gemcitabine (PACCAGE) as induction chemotherapy for locally advanced unresectable non small cell lung cancer (NSCLC). Lung Cancer 2007 56(2): 247-54. NRP

Schallier, S. Bral, B. Ilsen, B. Neyns, C. Fontaine, L. Decoster, J. De Mey, M. Meysman and J. De Greve. Final overall results of a study with a novel triplet induction chemotherapy regimen (PACCAGE) followed by consolidation radiotherapy in locally advanced inoperable non-small cell lung cancer (NSCLC). J Thorac Oncol 2009 4(6): 728-35. NRP

Schild, P. J. Stella, S. M. Geyer, J. A. Bonner, R. S. Marks, W. L. McGinnis, S. P. Goetz, S. A. Kuross, J. A. Mailliard, J. W. Kugler, P. L. Schaefer and J. R. Jett. Phase III trial comparing chemotherapy plus once-daily or twice-daily radiotherapy in Stage III non-small-cell lung cancer. Int J Radiat Oncol Biol Phys 2002 54(2): 370-8. NRP

Schild, P. J. Stella, S. M. Geyer, J. A. Bonner, W. L. McGinnis, J. A. Mailliard, J. Brindle, A. Jatoi and J. R. Jett. The outcome of combined-modality therapy for stage III non-small-cell lung cancer in the elderly. J Clin Oncol 2003 21(17): 3201-6. NRP

Schild, S. J. Mandrekar, A. Jatoi, W. L. McGinnis, P. J. Stella, R. L. Deming, J. R. Jett, Y. I. Garces, K. L. Allen and A. A. Adjei. The value of combined-modality therapy in elderly patients with stage III nonsmall cell lung cancer. Cancer 2007 110(2): 363-8. NRP

Schild, W. W. Wong, S. A. Vora, M. Y. Halyard and R. H. Wheeler. Phase I study of hyperfractionated accelerated radiotherapy and escalating doses of daily cisplatin for patients with locally advanced non-small-cell lung cancer. Int J Radiat Oncol Biol Phys 2002 54(3): 729-34. NRP

Schild, W. W. Wong, S. A. Vora, M. Y. Halyard, D. W. Northfelt, H. L. Kogut and R. H. Wheeler. The long-term results of a pilot study of three times a day radiotherapy and escalating doses of daily cisplatin for locally advanced non-small-cell lung cancer. Int J Radiat Oncol Biol Phys 2005 62(5): 1432-7. NRP

Schilder, M. Goldberg, M. M. Millenson, B. Movsas, A. Rogatko, B. Rogers and C. J. Langer. Phase II trial of induction high-dose chemotherapy followed by surgical resection and radiation therapy for patients with marginally resectable non-small cell carcinoma of the lung. Lung Cancer 2000 27(1): 37-45. NRP

Schuette, M. J. Krzakowski, B. Massuti, G. A. Otterson, R. Lizambri, H. Wei, D. P. Berger and Y. Chen. Randomized Phase II Study of Palifermin for Reducing Dysphagia in Patients Receiving Concurrent Chemoradiotherapy for Locally Advanced Unresectable Non-small Cell Lung Cancer. J Thorac Oncol 2011 (): . NRP

Schuster-Uitterhoeve, P. J. van de Vaart, C. C. Schaake-Koning, J. Benraadt, M. G. Koolen, D. Gonzalez Gonzalez and H. Bartelink. Feasibility of escalating daily doses of cisplatin in combination with accelerated radiotherapy in non-small cell lung cancer. Eur J Cancer 1996 32A(8): 1314-9. NRP

Schwarzenberger, A. Fariss, L. Linares, L. Nedzi and O. M. Salazar. Dose escalation of once weekly oral vinorelbine concurrent with weekly split dose hypofractionated chest radiation for palliation of advanced non-small cell lung cancer: a phase I/II study. Am J Med Sci 2011 341(6): 454-9. NRP

Scinto, V. Ferraresi, M. Milella, E. Tucci, C. Santomaggio, R. Pasquali-Lasagni, M. R. Del Vecchio, N. Campioni, M. Nardi and F. Cognetti. Ifosfamide, cisplatin and etoposide combination in locally advanced inoperable non-small-cell lung cancer: a phase II study. Br J Cancer 1999 81(6): 1031-6. NRP

Scorsetti, P. Navarria, P. Mancosu, F. Alongi, S. Castiglioni, R. Cavina, L. Cozzi, A. Fogliata, S. Pentimalli, A. Tozzi and A. Santoro. Large volume unresectable locally advanced non-small cell lung cancer: acute toxicity and initial outcome results with rapid arc. Radiat Oncol 2010 5(): 94. NRP

Sculier, J. J. Lafitte, T. Berghmans, P. Van Houtte, J. Lecomte, J. Thiriaux, A. Efremidis, G. Koumakis, V. Giner, M. Richez, J. L. Corhay, P. Wackenier, P. Lothaire, M. Paesmans, P. Mommen and V. Ninane. A phase III randomised study comparing two different dose-intensity regimens as induction chemotherapy followed by thoracic irradiation in patients with advanced locoregional non-small-cell lung cancer. Ann Oncol 2004 15(3): 399-409. NRI

Sculier, M. Paesmans, J. J. Lafitte, J. Baumohl, J. Thiriaux, O. van Cutsem, P. Recloux, G. Bureau, M. C. Berchier, C. Zacharias, P. Mommen, T. Bosschaerts, T. Berghmans, P. van Houtte, V. Ninane and J. Klastersky. A randomised phase III trial comparing consolidation treatment with further chemotherapy to chest irradiation in patients with initially unresectable locoregional non-small-cell lung cancer responding to induction chemotherapy. European Lung Cancer Working Party. Ann Oncol 1999 10(3): 295-303. NRD

Segawa, H. Ueoka, K. Kiura, H. Kamei, M. Tabata, K. Sakae, Y. Hiraki, S. Kawahara, K. Eguchi, S. Hiraki and M. Harada. A phase II study of cisplatin and 5-fluorouracil with concurrent hyperfractionated thoracic radiation for locally advanced non-small-cell lung cancer: a preliminary report from the Okayama Lung Cancer Study Group. Br J Cancer 2000 82(1): 104-11. NRP

Segawa, K. Kiura, N. Takigawa, H. Kamei, S. Harita, S. Hiraki, Y. Watanabe, K. Sugimoto, T. Shibayama, T. Yonei, H. Ueoka, M. Takemoto, S. Kanazawa, I. Takata, N. Nogami, K. Hotta, A. Hiraki, M. Tabata, K. Matsuo and M. Tanimoto. Phase III trial comparing docetaxel and cisplatin combination chemotherapy with mitomycin, vindesine, and cisplatin combination chemotherapy with concurrent thoracic radiotherapy in locally advanced non-small-cell lung cancer: OLCSG 0007. J Clin Oncol 2010 28(20): 3299-306. NRP

Seiwert, P. P. Connell, A. M. Mauer, P. C. Hoffman, C. M. George, L. Szeto, R. Salgia, K. E. Posther, B. Nguyen, D. J. Haraf and E. E. Vokes. A phase I study of pemetrexed, carboplatin, and concurrent radiotherapy in patients with locally advanced or metastatic non-small cell lung or esophageal cancer. Clin Cancer Res 2007 13(2 Pt 1): 515-22. NRP

Sejpal, R. Komaki, A. Tsao, J. Y. Chang, Z. Liao, X. Wei, P. K. Allen, C. Lu, M. Gillin and J. D. Cox. Early findings on toxicity of proton beam therapy with concurrent chemotherapy for nonsmall cell lung cancer. Cancer 2011 117(13): 3004-13. NRP

Seki, K. Eguchi, N. Katakami, H. Kunikane, K. Takeda, K. Takayama, T. Sawa, H. Saito, M. Harada and Y. Ohashi. Incidence of bone metastases and skeletal-related events in patients with advanced lung cancer - Results of a multicenter, prospective, cohort study (CSP-HOR13). European Journal of Cancer 2011 47(): S638. NRD

Sekine, H. Nokihara, M. Sumi, N. Saijo, Y. Nishiwaki, S. Ishikura, K. Mori, I. Tsukiyama and T. Tamura. Docetaxel consolidation therapy following cisplatin, vinorelbine, and concurrent thoracic radiotherapy in patients with unresectable stage III non-small cell lung cancer. J Thorac Oncol 2006 1(8): 810-5. NRP

Sekine, K. Kubota, S. Niho, M. Sumi, K. Nihei, R. Sekiguchi, J. Funai, S. Enatsu, Y. Ohe and T. Tamura. Phase I trial of pemetrexed and cisplatin combination chemotherapy with concurrent thoracic radiotherapy in Japanese patients with locally advanced non-small-cell lung cancer. European Journal of Cancer 2011 47(): S610. NRD

Sekine, K. Noda, F. Oshita, K. Yamada, M. Tanaka, K. Yamashita, H. Nokihara, N. Yamamoto, H. Kunitoh, Y. Ohe, T. Tamura, T. Kodama, M. Sumi and N. Saijo. Phase I study of cisplatin, vinorelbine, and concurrent thoracic radiotherapy for unresectable stage III non-small cell lung cancer. Cancer Sci 2004 95(8): 691-5. NRP

Sekine, M. Sumi, Y. Ito, C. Tanai, H. Nokihara, N. Yamamoto, H. Kunitoh, Y. Ohe and T. Tamura. Gender difference in treatment outcomes in patients with stage III non-small cell lung cancer receiving concurrent chemoradiotherapy. Jpn J Clin Oncol 2009 39(11): 707-12. NRP

Sekine, M. Sumi, Y. Ito, H. Horinouchi, H. Nokihara, N. Yamamoto, H. Kunitoh, Y. Ohe, K. Kubota and T. Tamura. Phase I Study of Concurrent High-Dose Three-Dimensional Conformal Radiotherapy with Chemotherapy Using Cisplatin and Vinorelbine for Unresectable Stage III Non-Small-Cell Lung Cancer. Int J Radiat Oncol Biol Phys 2011 (): . NRP

Sekine, M. Sumi, Y. Ito, T. Kato, Y. Fujisaka, H. Nokihara, N. Yamamoto, H. Kunitoh, Y. Ohe and T. Tamura. Phase I study of cisplatin analogue nedaplatin, paclitaxel, and thoracic radiotherapy for unresectable stage III non-small cell lung cancer. Jpn J Clin Oncol 2007 37(3): 175-80. NRP

Sekine, Y. Nishiwaki, T. Ogino, A. Yokoyama, M. Saito, K. Mori, I. Tsukiyama, S. Tsuchiya, K. Hayakawa, K. Yoshimura, N. Ishizuka and N. Saijo. Phase II study of twice-daily high-dose thoracic radiotherapy alternating with cisplatin and vindesine for unresectable stage III non-small-cell lung cancer: Japan Clinical Oncology Group Study 9306. J Clin Oncol 2002 20(3): 797-803. NRP

Semik, D. Riesenbeck, A. Linder, C. Schmid, P. Hoffknecht, A. Heinecke, H. Scheld and M. Thomas. Preoperative chemotherapy with and without additional radiochemotherapy: benefit and risk for surgery of stage III non-small cell lung cancer. Eur J Cardiothorac Surg 2004 26(6): 1205-1210. NRP

Semrau, A. Bier, U. Thierbach, C. Virchow, P. Ketterer and R. Fietkau. Concurrent radiochemotherapy with vinorelbine plus cisplatin or carboplatin in patients with locally advanced non-small-cell lung cancer (NSCLC) and an increased risk of treatment complications. Preliminary results. Strahlenther Onkol 2003 179(12): 823-31. NRP

Semrau, A. Bier, U. Thierbach, C. Virchow, P. Ketterer, G. Klautke and R. Fietkau. 6-year experience of concurrent radiochemotherapy with vinorelbine plus a platinum compound in multimorbid or aged patients with inoperable non-small cell lung cancer. Strahlenther Onkol 2007 183(1): 30-5. NRI

Sen, E. K. Saglam, A. Toker, S. Dilege, A. Kizir, E. N. Oral, P. Saip, B. Sakallioglu, E. Topuz and A. Aydiner. Weekly docetaxel and cisplatin with concomitant radiotherapy in addition to surgery and/or consolidation chemotherapy in stage III non-small cell lung cancer. Cancer Chemother Pharmacol 2011 68(6): 1497-505. NRP

Senan and F. J. Lagerwaard. In regard to Rosenman et al., high-dose conformal radiotherapy for treatment of stage III A/B non-small-cell lung cancer: technical issues and results of a phase I/II trial. IJROBP 2002;54:348-356. Int J Radiat Oncol Biol Phys 2003 55(5): 1458-9; author reply 1459-60. NRD

Senan, F. Cardenal, J. Vansteenkiste, J. Stigt, F. Akyol, W. De Neve, J. Bakker, J. M. Dupont, G. V. Scagliotti, U. Ricardi and J. P. van Meerbeeck. A randomized phase II study comparing induction or consolidation chemotherapy with cisplatin-docetaxel, plus radical concurrent chemoradiotherapy with cisplatin-docetaxel, in patients with unresectable locally advanced non-small-cell lung cancer. Ann Oncol 2011 22(3): 553-8. NRP

Senkus-Konefka, R. Dziadziuszko, E. Bednaruk-Mlynski, A. Pliszka, J. Kubrak, A. Lewandowska, K. Malachowski, M. Wierzchowski, M. Matecka-Nowak and J. Jassem. A prospective, randomised study to compare two palliative radiotherapy schedules for non-small-cell lung cancer (NSCLC). Br J Cancer 2005 92(6): 1038-45. NRP

Senzer. A phase III randomized evaluation of amifostine in stage IIIA/IIIB non-small cell lung cancer patients receiving concurrent carboplatin, paclitaxel, and radiation therapy followed by gemcitabine and cisplatin intensification: preliminary findings. Semin Oncol 2002 29(6 Suppl 19): 38-41. NRP

Seung and H. J. Ross. Phase II trial of combined modality therapy with concurrent topotecan plus radiotherapy followed by consolidation chemotherapy for unresectable stage III and selected stage IV non-small-lung cancer. Int J Radiat Oncol Biol Phys 2009 73(3): 802-9. NRP

Sharma, G. K. Rath, S. Thulkar, A. Bahl, S. Pandit and P. K. Julka. Computerized tomography-guided percutaneous high-dose-rate interstitial brachytherapy for malignant lung lesions. Journal of Cancer Research and Therapeutics 2011 7(2): 174-179. NRI

Sharma, R. Sharma and K. T. Bhowmik. Sequential chemoradiotherapy versus radiotherapy in the management of locally advanced non-small-cell lung cancer. Adv Ther 2003 20(1): 14-9. NRP

Shaw, R. L. Deming, E. T. Creagan, S. Nair, J. Q. Su, R. Levitt, P. D. Steen, M. Wiesenfeld and J. A. Mailliard. Pilot study of human recombinant interferon gamma and accelerated hyperfractionated thoracic radiation therapy in patients with unresectable stage IIIA/B nonsmall cell lung cancer. Int J Radiat Oncol Biol Phys 1995 31(4): 827-31. NRP

Shen, A. Denittis, M. Werner-Wasik, R. Axelrod, P. Gilman, T. Meyer, J. Treat, W. J. Curran and M. Machtay. Phase i study of 'dose-dense' pemetrexed plus carboplatin/radiotherapy for locally advanced non-small cell lung carcinoma. Radiat Oncol 2011 6(): 17. NRP

Shepherd, M. R. Johnston, D. Payne, R. Burkes, J. Deslauriers, Y. Cormier, L. D. de Bedoya, J. Ottaway, K. James and B. Zee. Randomized study of chemotherapy and surgery versus radiotherapy for stage IIIA non-small-cell lung cancer: a National Cancer Institute of Canada Clinical Trials Group Study. Br J Cancer 1998 78(5): 683-5. NRP

Shi, G. Zhu, R. Yu, Y. Wang and T. Xia. A randomized phase I/II trial to compare weekly usage with triple weekly usage of paclitaxel in concurrent radiochemotherapy for patients with locally advanced non-small cell lung cancer. 2011 14(): 227-32. FLA

Shi, T. An, G. Zhu, R. Yu, G. Xu, X. Liu and B. Xu. Phase I study to determine the MTD of paclitaxel given three times per week during concurrent radiation therapy for stage III non-small cell lung cancer. Curr Med Res Opin 2007 23(5): 1161-7. NRP

Shibamoto, B. Jeremic, L. Acimovic, B. Milicic and N. Nikolic. Influence of interfraction interval on the efficacy and toxicity of hyperfractionated radiotherapy in combination with concurrent daily chemotherapy in stage III non-small-cell lung cancer. Int J Radiat Oncol Biol Phys 2001 50(2): 295-300. NRP

Shioyama, K. Tokuuye, T. Okumura, K. Kagei, S. Sugahara, K. Ohara, Y. Akine, S. Ishikawa, H. Satoh and K. Sekizawa. Clinical evaluation of proton radiotherapy for non-small-cell lung cancer. Int J Radiat Oncol Biol Phys 2003 56(1): 7-13. USD

Shrimali, G. J. Webster, L. W. Lee, N. Bayman, H. Sheikh, M. Bewley, P. A. Burt, L. Pemberton, M. A. Harris, A. Chittalia and C. Faivre-Finn. Early report of intensity modulated radiotherapy (IMRT) for locally advanced lung cancer at the Christie. Clinical Oncology 2011 23(3): S21-S22. NRD

Sibley, A. J. Mundt, C. Shapiro, R. Jacobs, G. Chen, R. Weichselbaum and S. Vijayakumar. The treatment of stage III nonsmall cell lung cancer using high dose conformal radiotherapy. Int J Radiat Oncol Biol Phys 1995 33(5): 1001-7. NRP

Sibley, T. A. Jamieson, L. B. Marks, M. S. Anscher and L. R. Prosnitz. Radiotherapy alone for medically inoperable stage I non-small-cell lung cancer: the Duke experience. Int J Radiat Oncol Biol Phys 1998 40(1): 149-54. NRI

Sim, K. E. Rosenzweig, R. Schindelheim, K. K. Ng and S. A. Leibel. Induction chemotherapy plus three-dimensional conformal radiation therapy in the definitive treatment of locally advanced non-small-cell lung cancer. Int J Radiat Oncol Biol Phys 2001 51(3): 660-5. NRP

Simon, D. E. Dupuy, T. A. DiPetrillo, H. P. Safran, C. A. Grieco, T. Ng and W. W. Mayo-Smith. Pulmonary radiofrequency ablation: long-term safety and efficacy in 153 patients. Radiology 2007 243(1): 268-75. USD

Singhal, K. Pittman, C. Karapetis, S. Stephens and M. Borg. Oral vinorelbine and cisplatin with concomitant radiotherapy in stage iii non small cell lung cancer (NSCLC) - Covert study. Asia-Pacific Journal of Clinical Oncology 2011 7(): 153. NRD

Sinha and R. C. McGarry. Stereotactic body radiotherapy for bilateral primary lung cancers: the Indiana University experience. Int J Radiat Oncol Biol Phys 2006 66(4): 1120-4. NRP

Smith, D. Palma, T. Parhar, C. S. Alexander and E. S. Wai. Inoperable early stage non-small cell lung cancer: comorbidity, patterns of care and survival. Lung Cancer 2011 72(1): 39-44. NRP

Socinski, A. W. Blackstock, J. A. Bogart, X. Wang, M. Munley, J. Rosenman, L. Gu, G. A. Masters, P. Ungaro, A. Sleeper, M. Green, A. A. Miller and E. E. Vokes. Randomized phase II trial of induction chemotherapy followed by concurrent chemotherapy and dose-escalated thoracic conformal radiotherapy (74 Gy) in stage III non-small-cell lung cancer: CALGB 30105. J Clin Oncol 2008 26(15): 2457-63. NRP

Socinski, C. Zhang, J. E. Herndon, 2nd, R. O. Dillman, G. Clamon, E. Vokes, W. Akerley, J. Crawford, M. C. Perry, S. L. Seagren and M. R. Green. Combined modality trials of the Cancer and Leukemia Group B in stage III non-small-cell lung cancer: analysis of factors influencing survival and toxicity. Ann Oncol 2004 15(7): 1033-41. NRP

Socinski, D. E. Morris, J. S. Halle, D. T. Moore, T. A. Hensing, S. A. Limentani, R. Fraser, M. Tynan, A. Mears, M. P. Rivera, F. C. Detterbeck and J. G. Rosenman. Induction and concurrent chemotherapy with high-dose thoracic conformal radiation therapy in unresectable stage IIIA and IIIB non-small-cell lung cancer: a dose-escalation phase I trial. J Clin Oncol 2004 22(21): 4341-50. NRP

Socinski, J. A. Clark, J. Halle, A. Steagall, B. Kaluzny and J. G. Rosenman. Induction therapy with carboplatin/paclitaxel followed by concurrent carboplatin/paclitaxel and dose-escalating conformal radiotherapy in the treatment of locally advanced, unresectable non-small cell lung cancer: preliminary report of a phase I trial. Semin Oncol 1997 24(4 Suppl 12): S12-117-S12-122. NRP

Socinski, J. G. Rosenman, J. Halle, M. J. Schell, Y. Lin, S. Russo, M. P. Rivera, J. Clark, S. Limentani, R. Fraser, W. Mitchell and F. C. Detterbeck. Dose-escalating conformal thoracic radiation therapy with induction and concurrent carboplatin/paclitaxel in unresectable stage IIIA/B nonsmall cell lung carcinoma: a modified phase I/II trial. Cancer 2001 92(5): 1213-23. NRP

Socinski, J. G. Rosenman, M. J. Schell, J. Halle, S. Russo, M. P. Rivera, J. Clark, S. Limentani, R. Fraser, W. Mitchell and F. C. Detterbeck. Induction carboplatin/paclitaxel followed by concurrent carboplatin/paclitaxel and dose-escalating conformal thoracic radiation therapy in unresectable stage IIIA/B nonsmall cell lung carcinoma: a modified Phase I trial. Cancer 2000 89(3): 534-42. NRP

Soliman, P. Cheung, L. Yeung, I. Poon, J. Balogh, L. Barbera, J. Spayne, C. Danjoux, M. Dahele and Y. Ung. Accelerated hypofractionated radiotherapy for early-stage non-small-cell lung cancer: long-term results. Int J Radiat Oncol Biol Phys 2011 79(2): 459-65. NRI

Solomon, D. L. Ball, G. Richardson, J. G. Smith, M. Millward, M. MacManus, M. Michael, A. Wirth, C. O'Kane, L. Muceniekas, G. Ryan and D. Rischin. Phase I/II study of concurrent twice-weekly paclitaxel and weekly cisplatin with radiation therapy for stage III non-small cell lung cancer. Lung Cancer 2003 41(3): 353-61. NRP

Song, H. Pyo, S. H. Moon, T. H. Kim, D. W. Kim and K. H. Cho. Treatment-related pneumonitis and acute esophagitis in non-small-cell lung cancer patients treated with chemotherapy and helical tomotherapy. Int J Radiat Oncol Biol Phys 2010 78(3): 651-8. NRP

Song, S. H. Benedict, R. M. Cardinale, T. D. Chung, M. G. Chang and R. K. Schmidt-Ullrich. Stereotactic body radiation therapy of lung tumors: preliminary experience using normal tissue complication probability-based dose limits. Am J Clin Oncol 2005 28(6): 591-6. NRP

Sotnikov, G. Panshin, M. Ilin and A. Ivashin. Radiation therapy of non-small cell lung cancer with dose escalation on cobalt 60 gamma units. Four years results. Radiotherapy and Oncology 2011 99(): S345. NRD

Souquet, P. Fournel, C. H. Bohas, I. C. Fortune and G. Chatte. Cisplatin and ifosfamide with various doses of vinorelbine (navelbine) in advanced non-small lung cancer. Semin Oncol 1996 23(2 Suppl 5): 8-10. NRP

Spiro, R. M. Rudd, R. L. Souhami, J. Brown, D. J. Fairlamb, N. H. Gower, L. Maslove, R. Milroy, V. Napp, M. K. Parmar, M. D. Peake, R. J. Stephens, H. Thorpe, D. A. Waller and P. West. Chemotherapy versus supportive care in advanced non-small cell lung cancer: improved survival without detriment to quality of life. Thorax 2004 59(10): 828-36. NRP

Splinter, P. E. van Schil, G. W. Kramer, J. van Meerbeeck, A. Gregor, P. Rocmans and A. Kirkpatrick. Randomized trial of surgery versus radiotherapy in patients with stage IIIA (N2) non small-cell lung cancer after a response to induction chemotherapy. EORTC 08941. Clin Lung Cancer 2000 2(1): 69-72; discussion 73. NRP

Spych, L. Gottwald, M. Klonowicz, M. Biegala, R. Bibik and J. Fijuth. The analysis of prognostic factors affecting post-radiation acute reaction after conformal radiotherapy for non-small cell lung cancer. Archives of Medical Science 2010 6(5): 756-763. NRO

Srisam-Ang, A. Podhipak, K. Narksawat, P. Supaattagorn and M. Tipayamongkholgul. Survival of patients with advanced non-small-cell lung cancer at Ubon Ratchathani Cancer Center, Thailand. Southeast Asian J Trop Med Public Health 2005 36(4): 994-1006. NRP

Stamatis, W. Eberhardt, G. Stuben, S. Bildat, O. Dahler and L. Hillejan. Preoperative chemoradiotherapy and surgery for selected non-small cell lung cancer IIIB subgroups: long-term results. Ann Thorac Surg 1999 68(4): 1144-9. NRP

Stathopoulos, N. Malamos, D. Antonadou, N. Throuvalas, N. Thalassinos and M. Zoitopoulos. Comparison of effectiveness between chemotherapy alone versus chemo-radiotherapy in stage III non-small cell lung cancer. Oncol Rep 1997 4(1): 119-22. NRP

Stathopoulos, P. Papakostas, N. Malamos, G. Samelis and N. Moschopoulos. Chemo-radiotherapy versus chemo-surgery in stage IIIA non-small cell lung cancer. Oncol Rep 1996 3(4): 673-6. NRP

Stathopoulos, U. G. Dafni, N. A. Malamos, S. Rigatos, G. Kouvatseas and N. Moschopoulos. Induction chemotherapy in non small cell lung cancer stage IIIa-b and IV and second-line treatment. Anticancer Res 1999 19(4C): 3543-8. NRP

Stauder, O. K. Macdonald, K. R. Olivier, J. A. Call, K. Lafata, C. S. Mayo, R. C. Miller, P. D. Brown, H. J. Bauer and Y. I. Garces. Early pulmonary toxicity following lung stereotactic body radiation therapy delivered in consecutive daily fractions. Radiother Oncol 2011 99(2): 166-71. USD

Stephens, D. J. Girling, P. Hopwood and N. Thatcher. A randomised controlled trial of pre-operative chemotherapy followed, if feasible, by resection versus radiotherapy in patients with inoperable stage T3, N1, M0 or T1-3, N2, M0 non-small cell lung cancer. Lung Cancer 2005 49(3): 395-400. NRP

Stevens and S. D. Begbie. Hypofractionated irradiation for inoperable non-small cell lung cancer. Australas Radiol 1995 39(3): 265-70. NRP

Stevens, G. Stevens, J. Kolbe and B. Cox. Management of stages I and II non-small-cell lung cancer in a New Zealand study: divergence from international practice and recommendations. Intern Med J 2008 38(10): 758-68. NRP

Stinchcombe, C. B. Lee, D. T. Moore, M. P. Rivera, J. Halle, S. Limentani, J. G. Rosenman and M. A. Socinski. Long-term follow-up of a phase I/II trial of dose escalating three-dimensional conformal thoracic radiation therapy with induction and concurrent carboplatin and paclitaxel in unresectable stage IIIA/B non-small cell lung cancer. J Thorac Oncol 2008 3(11): 1279-85. NRP

Stinchcombe, D. E. Morris, C. B. Lee, D. T. Moore, D. N. Hayes, J. S. Halle, M. P. Rivera, J. G. Rosenman and M. A. Socinski. Induction chemotherapy with carboplatin, irinotecan, and paclitaxel followed by high dose three-dimension conformal thoracic radiotherapy (74 Gy) with concurrent carboplatin, paclitaxel, and gefitinib in unresectable stage IIIA and stage IIIB non-small cell lung cancer. J Thorac Oncol 2008 3(3): 250-7. NRP

Stinchcombe, L. Hodgson, J. E. Herndon Ii, M. J. Kelley, M. G. Cicchetti, N. Ramnath, H. B. Niell, J. N. Atkins, W. Akerley, M. R. Green and E. E. Vokes. Treatment outcomes of different prognostic groups of patients on Cancer and Leukemia Group B trial 39801: Induction chemotherapy followed by chemoradiotherapy compared with chemoradiotherapy alone for unresectable stage III non-small cell lung cancer. Journal of Thoracic Oncology 2009 4(9): 1117-1125. NRP

Strand, P. F. Brunsvig, D. C. Johannessen, S. Sundstrom, M. Wang, K. Hornslien, R. M. Bremnes, A. Stensvold, O. Garpestad and J. Norstein. Potentially curative radiotherapy for non-small-cell lung cancer in Norway: a population-based study of survival. Int J Radiat Oncol Biol Phys 2011 80(1): 133-41. NRI

Stupp, M. Mayer, R. Kann, W. Weder, A. Zouhair, D. C. Betticher, A. D. Roth, R. A. Stahel, S. Majno, S. Peters, L. Jost, M. Furrer, S. Thierstein, R. A. Schmid, S. F. Hsu-Schmitz, R. O. Mirimanoff, H. B. Ris and M. Pless. Neoadjuvant chemotherapy and radiotherapy followed by surgery in selected patients with stage IIIB non-small-cell lung cancer: a multicentre phase II trial. Lancet Oncol 2009 10(8): 785-93. NRP

Sugarbaker, J. Herndon, L. J. Kohman, M. J. Krasna and M. R. Green. Results of cancer and leukemia group B protocol 8935. A multiinstitutional phase II trimodality trial for stage IIIA (N2) non-small-cell lung cancer. Cancer and Leukemia Group B Thoracic Surgery Group. J Thorac Cardiovasc Surg 1995 109(3): 473-83; discussion 483-5. NRP

Sulman, R. Komaki, A. H. Klopp, J. D. Cox and J. Y. Chang. Exclusion of elective nodal irradiation is associated with minimal elective nodal failure in non-small cell lung cancer. Radiat Oncol 2009 4(): 5. NRO

Sun, S. W. Leung, C. J. Wang, H. C. Chen, F. M. Fang, E. Y. Huang, H. C. Hsu, S. A. Yeh, C. Hsiung and D. T. Huang. Concomitant boost radiation therapy for inoperable non-small-cell lung cancer: preliminary report of a prospective randomized study. Int J Radiat Oncol Biol Phys 2000 47(2): 413-8. NRI

Sundstrom, R. Bremnes, P. Brunsvig, U. Aasebo, K. Olbjorn, P. M. Fayers and S. Kaasa. Immediate or delayed radiotherapy in advanced non-small cell lung cancer (NSCLC)? Data from a prospective randomised study. Radiother Oncol 2005 75(2): 141-8. NRP

Sundstrom, R. Bremnes, U. Aasebo, S. Aamdal, R. Hatlevoll, P. Brunsvig, D. C. Johannessen, O. Klepp, P. M. Fayers and S. Kaasa. Hypofractionated palliative radiotherapy (17 Gy per two fractions) in advanced non-small-cell lung carcinoma is comparable to standard fractionation for symptom control and survival: a national phase III trial. J Clin Oncol 2004 22(5): 801-10. NRP

Sundstrom, R. M. Bremnes, P. Brunsvig, U. Aasebo and S. Kaasa. Palliative thoracic radiotherapy in locally advanced non-small cell lung cancer: can quality-of-life assessments help in selection of patients for short- or long-course radiotherapy?. J Thorac Oncol 2006 1(8): 816-24. NRP

Sunyach, L. Falchero, P. Pommier, M. Perol, D. Arpin, M. Vincent, D. Boutry, P. Rebatu, C. Ginestet, I. Martel-Lafay, D. Perol and C. Carrie. Prospective evaluation of early lung toxicity following three-dimensional conformal radiation therapy in non-small-cell lung cancer: preliminary results. Int J Radiat Oncol Biol Phys 2000 48(2): 459-63. NRP

Sur, S. N. Ahmed, B. Donde, R. Morar, G. Mohamed, M. Sur, J. A. Pacella, D. Van der Merwe and C. Feldman. Brachytherapy boost vs teletherapy boost in palliation of symptomatic, locally advanced non-small cell lung cancer: Preliminary analysis of a randomized, prospective study. Journal of Brachytherapy International 2001 17(4): 309-315. NRD

Sura, E. Yorke, A. Jackson and K. E. Rosenzweig. High-dose radiotherapy for the treatment of inoperable non-small cell lung cancer. Cancer J 2007 13(4): 238-42. NRP

Sura, V. Gupta, E. Yorke, A. Jackson, H. Amols and K. E. Rosenzweig. Intensity-modulated radiation therapy (IMRT) for inoperable non-small cell lung cancer: the Memorial Sloan-Kettering Cancer Center (MSKCC) experience. Radiother Oncol 2008 87(1): 17-23. USD

Surmont, E. F. Smit, M. de Jonge, J. G. Aerts, K. Nackaerts, R. Vernhout, J. Gras, A. Van Wijk, E. C. Phernambucq, J. P. van Meerbeeck, S. Senan, C. J. Kraaij, N. Chouaki, J. Praag and R. J. van Klaveren. Pemetrexed and cisplatin with concurrent radiotherapy for locally advanced non-small cell and limited disease small cell lung cancer: results from 2 phase I studies. Lung Cancer 2010 69(3): 302-6. NRP

Tada, K. Minakuchi, K. Matsui, H. Kin, T. Nishiguchi and H. Fukuda. A single institutional subset analysis of the WJLCG study comparing concurrent and sequential chemoradiotherapy for stage III non-small-cell lung cancer. Radiat Med 2004 22(3): 163-7. NRP

Tada, Y. Chiba, K. Tsujino, H. Fukuda, Y. Nishimura, M. Kokubo, S. Negoro, S. Kudoh, M. Fukuoka, K. Nakagawa and Y. Nakanishi. A Phase I Study of Chemoradiotherapy with Use of Involved-Field Conformal Radiotherapy and Accelerated Hyperfractionation for Stage III Non-Small-Cell Lung Cancer: WJTOG 3305. Int J Radiat Oncol Biol Phys 2011 (): . NRP

Takamori, T. Rikimaru, A. Hayashi, K. Tayama, M. Mitsuoka, K. Fujimoto, M. Horiuchi, N. Hayabuchi, K. Oizumi and K. Shirouzu. A preoperative alternating chemotherapy and radiotherapy program for patients with stage IIIA (N2) non-small cell lung cancer. Lung Cancer 2000 29(1): 49-56. NRP

Takata, H. Ueoka, K. Kiura, M. Tabata, N. Takigawa, H. Katayama, M. Takemoto, Y. Hiraki, M. Harada and M. Tanimoto. Daily low-dose cisplatin and concurrent thoracic irradiation for poor-risk patients with unresectable non-small-cell lung cancer. Acta Med Okayama 2002 56(5): 261-6. FLA

Takeda, E. Kunieda, T. Ohashi, Y. Aoki, Y. Oku, T. Enomoto, K. Nomura and M. Sugiura. Severe COPD is correlated with mild radiation pneumonitis following stereotactic body radiotherapy. Chest 2011 (): . NRP

Takeda, K. Nemoto, H. Saito, Y. Ogawa, Y. Takai and S. Yamada. Dosimetric correlations of acute esophagitis in lung cancer patients treated with radiotherapy. Int J Radiat Oncol Biol Phys 2005 62(3): 626-9. NRP

Takeda, S. Negoro, M. Tanaka, H. Fukuda, K. Nakagawa, M. Kawahara, H. Semba, S. Kudoh, T. Sawa, N. Saijo and M. Fukuoka. A phase II study of cisplatin and irinotecan as induction chemotherapy followed by concomitant thoracic radiotherapy with weekly low-dose irinotecan in unresectable, stage III, non-small cell lung cancer: JCOG 9706. Jpn J Clin Oncol 2011 41(1): 25-31. NRP

Takeda, S. Negoro, S. Kudoh, K. Okishio, N. Masuda, M. Takada, M. Tanaka, T. Nakajima, T. Tada and M. Fukuoka. Phase I/II study of weekly irinotecan and concurrent radiation therapy for locally advanced non-small cell lung cancer. Br J Cancer 1999 79(9-10): 1462-7. NRP

Takigawa, K. Kiura, K. Hotta, S. Hosokawa, N. Nogami, K. Aoe, K. Gemba, K. Fujiwara, S. Harita, M. Takemoto, K. Himei, T. Shinkai, Y. Fujiwara, S. Takata, M. Tabata, S. Kanazawa and M. Tanimoto. A phase I study of S-1 with concurrent thoracic radiotherapy in elderly patients with localized advanced non-small cell lung cancer. Lung Cancer 2011 71(1): 60-4. NRP

Takigawa, K. Kiura, Y. Segawa, K. Hotta, A. Tamaoki, Y. Tokuda, T. Nagata, K. Watanabe, K. Gemba, T. Moritaka, N. Horita, H. Takeda, N. Okimoto, M. Takemoto, K. Matsuo, T. Shinkai, M. Tabata, H. Ueoka, S. Kanazawa and M. Tanimoto. Benefits and adverse events among elderly patients receiving concurrent chemoradiotherapy for locally advanced non-small cell lung cancer: analysis of the Okayama Lung Cancer Study Group trial 0007. J Thorac Oncol 2011 6(6): 1087-91. NRP

Takiguchi, R. Uruma, Y. Asaka-Amano, K. Kurosu, Y. Kasahara, N. Tanabe, K. Tatsumi, T. Uno, H. Itoh and T. Kuriyama. Phase I study of cisplatin and irinotecan combined with concurrent hyperfractionated accelerated thoracic radiotherapy for locally advanced non-small cell lung carcinoma. Int J Clin Oncol 2005 10(6): 418-24. NRP

Takita and K. H. Shin. Radiation induced chemotherapy sensitization in trimodality therapy of stage III non small cell lung cancer. A preliminary report. J Exp Clin Cancer Res 2000 19(4): 413-6. NRP

Takita, K. H. Shin, A. Y. Soh, W. S. Yi and G. Wilding. Induction therapy of loco-regional non-small-cell lung cancer with reliable response and low toxicity (low dose radiotherapy sensitizes tumor to subsequent chemotherapy?). 2009 63(): 387-92. NRI

Tan, J. Wee, P. T. Ang, K. W. Fong, S. S. Leong, K. S. Khoo, T. Tan, K. S. Lee, P. Eng, A. Hsu, Y. K. Tan, E. J. Chua and Y. Y. Ong. Induction chemotherapy followed by concurrent chemoradiotherapy in stage III unresectable non-small cell lung cancer. Acta Oncol 1999 38(8): 1005-9. NRP

Tanabe, T. Koizumi, K. Tsushima, M. Ito, S. Kanda, T. Kobayashi, M. Yasuo, Y. Yamazaki, K. Kubo, T. Honda, R. Kondo and K. Yoshida. Comparative study of three different catheters for CT imaging-bronchoscopy-guided radiofrequency ablation as a potential and novel interventional therapy for lung cancer. Chest 2010 137(4): 890-7. NRI

Tanaka, I. Okamoto, N. Yamamoto, Y. Hattori, N. Masuda, M. Nishio, K. Takeda, T. Seto, Y. Nishimura and K. Nakagawa. Phase 2 study of nimotuzumab in combination with concurrent chemoradiotherapy (CRT) in patients with locally advanced non-small cell lung cancer (NSCLC). European Journal of Cancer 2011 47(): S605. NRD

Tannehill, M. P. Mehta, M. Larson, B. Storer, J. Pellet, T. J. Kinsella and J. H. Schiller. Effect of amifostine on toxicities associated with sequential chemotherapy and radiation therapy for unresectable non-small-cell lung cancer: results of a phase II trial. J Clin Oncol 1997 15(8): 2850-7. NRP

Tawfik, H. Taha Ael and G. A. Attia. Induction Docetaxel and Cisplatin Followed by Weekly Docetaxel and Cisplatin with Concurrent Radiotherapy in Locally Advanced Stage III Non Small Cell Lung Cancer (LA-NSCLC)- A Phase II Study. J Egypt Natl Canc Inst 2007 19(1): 15-20. NRP

Taylor, Z. X. Liao, J. D. Cox, C. Stevens, J. Roth, G. Walsh, J. Y. Chang, T. Guerrero, M. Jeter, J. Putnam, Jr., F. V. Fossella, P. Allen and R. Komaki. Equivalent outcome of patients with clinical Stage IIIA non-small-cell lung cancer treated with concurrent chemoradiation compared with induction chemotherapy followed by surgical resection. Int J Radiat Oncol Biol Phys 2004 58(1): 204-12. NRP

Tejedor, J. J. Valerdi, R. Lopez, M. A. Dominguez, F. Arias, J. J. Illarramendi and E. Martinez. Mitomycin, cisplatin, and vindesine followed by radiotherapy combined with cisplatin in stage III nonsmall cell lung cancer: long-term results. Int J Radiat Oncol Biol Phys 1995 31(4): 813-8. NRP

Tell, C. Sederholm, C. Klintenberg, L. Franksson, E. Branden, G. Hillerdal, U. Lonn, C. J. Linden, S. B. Ewers, K. Lamberg, E. Mrazek, B. Loden, A. Sjogren, T. Linne, S. Friesland and F. Sirzen. Multicentre phase II trial of paclitaxel and carboplatin with concurrent radiotherapy in locally advanced non-small cell lung cancer. Anticancer Res 2008 28(5B): 2851-7. NRP

Testolin, C. Baiocchi, S. Galuppo, M. S. Favretto, S. Schiavon and P. Morandi. Stage i non small cell lung cancer (NSCLC) in patients aged >80 years - Clinical outcomes after stereotactic radiotherapy using real time tumour tracking. European Journal of Cancer 2011 47(): S273-S274. NRD

Thammakumpee. Clinical manifestation and survival of patients with non-small cell lung cancer. J Med Assoc Thai 2004 87(5): 503-7. USD

Thanos, S. Mylona, N. Ptohis, S. Tsiouris, E. Sotiropoulou, A. Pomoni and M. Pomoni. Percutaneous radiofrequency thermal ablation in the management of lung tumors: presentation of clinical experience on a series of 35 patients. Diagn Interv Radiol 2009 15(4): 290-6. USD

Thirion, O. Holmberg, C. D. Collins, C. O'Shea, M. Moriarty, M. Pomeroy, C. O'Sullivan, S. Buckney and J. Armstrong. Escalated dose for non-small-cell lung cancer with accelerated hypofractionated three-dimensional conformal radiation therapy. Radiother Oncol 2004 71(2): 163-6. NRP

Thomas, C. Rube, M. Semik, M. von Eiff, L. Freitag, H. N. Macha, W. Wagner, F. Klinke, H. H. Scheld, N. Willich, W. E. Berdel and K. Junker. Impact of preoperative bimodality induction including twice-daily radiation on tumor regression and survival in stage III non-small-cell lung cancer. J Clin Oncol 1999 17(4): 1185. NRP

Thomas, C. Rube, P. Hoffknecht, H. N. Macha, L. Freitag, A. Linder, N. Willich, M. Hamm, G. W. Sybrecht, D. Ukena, K. M. Deppermann, C. Droge, D. Riesenbeck, A. Heinecke, C. Sauerland, K. Junker, W. E. Berdel and M. Semik. Effect of preoperative chemoradiation in addition to preoperative chemotherapy: a randomised trial in stage III non-small-cell lung cancer. Lancet Oncol 2008 9(7): 636-48. NRP

Thomas, J. P. Kleisbauer, G. Robinet, J. Clavier, R. Poirier, A. Vernenegre, F. Bonnaud, A. Taytard, D. Paillotin, P. Pommier De Santi, J. R. Barriere and T. Pignon. Carboplatin as radiosensitizer in non-small cell lung cancer after cisplatin containing chemotherapy. A phase I study of a groupe francais de pneumo-cancerologie (G.F.P.C.). Lung Cancer 1997 18(1): 71-81. NRP

Timmerman, L. Papiez, R. McGarry, L. Likes, C. DesRosiers, S. Frost and M. Williams. Extracranial stereotactic radioablation: results of a phase I study in medically inoperable stage I non-small cell lung cancer. Chest 2003 124(5): 1946-55. NRI, USD

Timmerman, R. McGarry, C. Yiannoutsos, L. Papiez, K. Tudor, J. DeLuca, M. Ewing, R. Abdulrahman, C. DesRosiers, M. Williams and J. Fletcher. Excessive toxicity when treating central tumors in a phase II study of stereotactic body radiation therapy for medically inoperable early-stage lung cancer. J Clin Oncol 2006 24(30): 4833-9. NRI, USD

Timmerman, R. Paulus, J. Galvin, J. Michalski, W. Straube, J. Bradley, A. Fakiris, A. Bezjak, G. Videtic, D. Johnstone, J. Fowler, E. Gore and H. Choy. Stereotactic body radiation therapy for inoperable early stage lung cancer. JAMA 2010 303(11): 1070-6. NRI, USD

Tiwana, H. N. Lee, M. Gupta, S. Kumar, S. K. Verma and S. Saini. Where do we stand in the multidisciplinary approach to non-small cell lung cancer (NSCLC) - A retrospective single institution experience from rural india. European Journal of Cancer 2011 47(): S600-S601. NRD

Tokuda, N. Takigawa, T. Kozuki, H. Kamei, A. Bessho, A. Tada, K. Hotta, K. Katsui, S. Kanazawa, M. Tanimoto and K. Kiura. Long-term follow-up of phase II trial of docetaxel and cisplatin with concurrent thoracic radiation therapy for locally advanced non-small cell lung cancer. Acta Oncol 2011 (): . NRP

Tombolini, A. Bonanni, V. Donato, N. Raffetto, M. Santarelli, M. Valeriani and R. M. Enrici. Radiotherapy alone in elderly patients with medically inoperable stage IIIA and IIIB non-small cell lung cancer. Anticancer Res 2000 20(6C): 4829-33. NRP

Tomirotti, B. Galassi, M. Dambrosio, V. Fossati, G. Gramegna, F. Colombo, R. Rovej and A. Scanni. Cis/carboplatin + vinorelbine +/- radiotherapy in stage III and IV non small cell lung carcinoma. J Chemother 1997 9(1): 62-5. NRP

Topczewska-Bruns, D. Hempel, B. Pancewicz-Janczuk, E. Sierko, T. Filipowski and M. Wojtukiewicz. 3-year overall survival for inoperable non-small cell lung carcinoma patients treated with radiochemotherapy-single-institution retrospective analysis. Radiotherapy and Oncology 2011 99(): S340. NRD

Treat, R. Gonin, M. A. Socinski, M. J. Edelman, R. B. Catalano, D. M. Marinucci, R. Ansari, H. H. Gillenwater, K. M. Rowland, R. L. Comis, C. K. Obasaju and C. P. Belani. A randomized, phase III multicenter trial of gemcitabine in combination with carboplatin or paclitaxel versus paclitaxel plus carboplatin in patients with advanced or metastatic non-small-cell lung cancer. Annals of Oncology 2010 21(3): 540-547. NRP

Trodella, F. De Marinis, R. M. D'Angelillo, S. Ramella, A. Cesario, S. Valente, F. Nelli, M. R. Migliorino, S. Margaritora, G. M. Corbo, V. Porziella, M. Ciresa, F. Cellini, S. Bonassi, P. Russo, E. Cortesi and P. Granone. Induction cisplatin-gemcitabine-paclitaxel plus concurrent radiotherapy and gemcitabine in the multimodality treatment of unresectable stage IIIB non-small cell lung cancer. Lung Cancer 2006 54(3): 331-8. NRP

Trodella, N. Cellini, A. Picciocchi, P. Marano, M. Balducci, G. Mantini, A. Turriziani, G. M. Corbo, S. Valente, V. Valentini, T. Pirronti, P. Granone and R. R. Dobelbower. Phase I-II trial of concomitant continuous carboplatin (CBDCA) infusion and radiotherapy in advanced nonsmall cell lung cancer with evaluation for surgery: final report. Int J Radiat Oncol Biol Phys 1997 37(1): 93-101. NRP

Trodella, P. Granone, S. Valente, A. Turriziani, G. Macis, G. M. Corbo, S. Margaritora, A. Cesario, R. M. D'Angelillo, G. Gualano, S. Ramella, D. Galetta and N. Cellini. Phase I trial of weekly gemcitabine and concurrent radiotherapy in patients with inoperable non-small-cell lung cancer. J Clin Oncol 2002 20(3): 804-10. NRP

Trodella, P. Granone, S. Valente, S. Margaritora, G. Macis, A. Cesario, R. M. D'Angelillo, V. Valentini, G. M. Corbo, V. Porziella, S. Ramella, G. Tonini, D. Galetta, M. Ciresa, B. Vincenzi and N. Cellini. Neoadjuvant concurrent radiochemotherapy in locally advanced (IIIA-IIIB) non-small-cell lung cancer: long-term results according to downstaging. Ann Oncol 2004 15(3): 389-98. NRP

Trovo, A. Linda, I. El Naqa, C. Javidan-Nejad and J. Bradley. Early and late lung radiographic injury following stereotactic body radiation therapy (SBRT). Lung Cancer 2010 69(1): 77-85. NRP

Tsao, D. Liu, J. J. Lee, M. Spitz and W. K. Hong. Smoking affects treatment outcome in patients with advanced nonsmall cell lung cancer. Cancer 2006 106(11): 2428-36. NRP

Tselis, K. Ferentinos, C. Kolotas, J. Schirren, D. Baltas, A. Antonakakis, H. Ackermann and N. Zamboglou. Computed tomography-guided interstitial high-dose-rate brachytherapy in the local treatment of primary and secondary intrathoracic malignancies. J Thorac Oncol 2011 6(3): 545-52. NRI

Tsoutsou, M. E. Froudarakis, D. Bouros and M. I. Koukourakis. Hypofractionated/accelerated radiotherapy with cytoprotection (HypoARC) combined with vinorelbine and liposomal doxorubicin for locally advanced non-small cell lung cancer (NSCLC). Anticancer Res 2008 28(2B): 1349-54. NRP

Tsuchiya, Y. Ohe, T. Sugiura, N. Fuwa, Y. Kitamoto, K. Mori, H. Kobayashi, K. Nakata, T. Sawa, K. Hirai, T. Etoh, H. Saka, A. Saito, H. Fukuda, N. Ishizuka, N. Saijo and S. Japan Clinical Oncology Group. Randomized phase I study of standard-fractionated or accelerated-hyperfractionated radiotherapy with concurrent cisplatin and vindesine for unresectable non-small cell lung cancer: a report of Japan Clinical Oncology Group Study (JCOG 9601). 2001 31(): 488-94. NRP

Uematsu, A. Shioda, A. Suda, T. Fukui, Y. Ozeki, Y. Hama, J. R. Wong and S. Kusano. Computed tomography-guided frameless stereotactic radiotherapy for stage I non-small cell lung cancer: a 5-year experience. Int J Radiat Oncol Biol Phys 2001 51(3): 666-70. NRI

Uitterhoeve, J. S. Belderbos, M. G. Koolen, P. J. van der Vaart, P. T. Rodrigus, J. Benraadt, C. C. Koning, D. Gonzalez Gonzalez and H. Bartelink. Toxicity of high-dose radiotherapy combined with daily cisplatin in non-small cell lung cancer: results of the EORTC 08912 phase I/II study. European Organization for Research and Treatment of Cancer. Eur J Cancer 2000 36(5): 592-600. NRP

Uitterhoeve, M. G. Koolen, R. M. van Os, K. Koedooder, M. van de Kar, B. R. Pieters and C. C. Koning. Accelerated high-dose radiotherapy alone or combined with either concomitant or sequential chemotherapy; treatments of choice in patients with Non-Small Cell Lung Cancer. Radiat Oncol 2007 2(): 27. USD

Ukena, M. Leutz, P. Schlimmer, H. Huwer, H. J. SchÃ¤fers and G. Sybrecht. Non-small cell lung cancer (NSCLC) stage IIIA/IIIB. A pilot study of neoadjuvant chemotherapy with paclitaxel and carboplatin. 1997 92 Suppl 5(): 49-53. FLA

Ulutin, M. Guden, K. Oysul, S. Surenkok and Y. Pak. Split-course radiotherapy with or without concurrent or sequential chemotherapy in non-small cell lung cancer. Radiat Med 2000 18(2): 93-6. NRP

Unlu, G. Diniz, B. Komurcuoglu, M. Gayaf, T. Gokce, I. Karadogan and C. Akcay. Comparison of curative and palliative radiotherapy efficacy in unresectable advanced non-small cell lung cancer patients with or without metastasis. Saudi Med J 2006 27(6): 849-53. NRP

Urbanic, A. T. Turrisi, 3rd, A. K. Sharma, G. A. Silvestri, T. E. Williams, K. N. Vanek and C. A. Sherman. Conformal high dose external radiation therapy, 80.5 Gy, alone for medically inoperable non-small cell lung cancer: a retrospective analysis. J Thorac Oncol 2006 1(2): 112-9. NRP

Uy, G. Darling, W. Xu, Q. L. Yi, M. De Perrot, A. F. Pierre, T. K. Waddell, M. R. Johnston, A. Bezjak, F. A. Shepherd and S. Keshavjee. Improved results of induction chemoradiation before surgical intervention for selected patients with stage IIIA-N2 non-small cell lung cancer. J Thorac Cardiovasc Surg 2007 134(1): 188-93. NRP

Valerio, A. Russo, M. A. Latteri, G. Modica, G. Gulotta, M. G. Armata, E. Bajardi, G. Cicero, G. Pantuso, N. Grassi, G. Agosta and N. Gebbia. Weekly docetaxel as II line therapy in non-small cell lung cancer: an interim analysis of a phase II study. Lung Cancer 2001 34 Suppl 4(): S31-5. NRI

van Baardwijk, G. Bosmans, L. Boersma, S. Wanders, A. Dekker, A. M. Dingemans, G. Bootsma, W. Geraedts, C. Pitz, J. Simons, P. Lambin and D. De Ruysscher. Individualized radical radiotherapy of non-small-cell lung cancer based on normal tissue dose constraints: a feasibility study. Int J Radiat Oncol Biol Phys 2008 71(5): 1394-401. NRP

van Baardwijk, S. Wanders, L. Boersma, J. Borger, M. Ollers, A. M. Dingemans, G. Bootsma, W. Geraedts, C. Pitz, R. Lunde, P. Lambin and D. De Ruysscher. Mature results of an individualized radiation dose prescription study based on normal tissue constraints in stages I to III non-small-cell lung cancer. J Clin Oncol 2010 28(8): 1380-6. USD

Van den Brande, D. De Ruysscher, J. Vansteenkiste, P. Spaas, P. Specenier and M. Demedts. Sequential treatment with vindesine-ifosfamide-platinum (VIP) chemotherapy followed by platinum sensitized radiotherapy in stage IIIB non-small cell lung cancer: a phase II trial. Lung Cancer 1998 22(1): 45-53. NRP

van der Voort van Zyp, B. van der Holt, R. J. van Klaveren, P. Pattynama, A. Maat and J. J. Nuyttens. Stereotactic body radiotherapy using real-time tumor tracking in octogenarians with non-small cell lung cancer. Lung Cancer 2010 69(3): 296-301. OPP

van der Voort van Zyp, J. B. Prevost, B. van der Holt, C. Braat, R. J. van Klaveren, P. M. Pattynama, P. C. Levendag and J. J. Nuyttens. Quality of life after stereotactic radiotherapy for stage I non-small-cell lung cancer. Int J Radiat Oncol Biol Phys 2010 77(1): 31-7. USD

van Dijck, J. Festen, E. M. de Kleijn, G. W. Kramer, V. C. Tjan-Heijnen and A. L. Verbeek. Treatment and survival of patients with non-small cell lung cancer Stage IIIA diagnosed in 1989-1994: a study in the region of the Comprehensive Cancer Centre East, The Netherlands. Lung Cancer 2001 34(1): 19-27. NRP

Van Kooten, M. Rosenberg, M. Orlando, J. Morero, M. Vilanova, O. Rojas, H. Vicente, C. Bagnes, C. Silva and R. D. Chacon. Neoadjuvant chemotherapy with gemcitabine and cisplatin in stage IIIA/B non-small cell lung cancer. Invest New Drugs 2002 20(4): 439-46. NRP van Loon, J. Grutters, R. Wanders, L. Boersma, M. Oellers, A. M. Dingemans, G. Bootsma, W. Geraedts, C. Pitz, J. Simons, S. A. Fatah, G. Snoep, M. Hochstenbag, P. Lambin and D. De Ruysscher. Follow-up with 18FDG-PET-CT after radical radiotherapy with or without chemotherapy allows the detection of potentially curable progressive disease in non-small cell lung cancer patients: a prospective study. Eur J Cancer 2009 45(4): 588-95. NRI

van Meerbeeck, G. W. Kramer, P. E. Van Schil, C. Legrand, E. F. Smit, F. Schramel, V. C. Tjan-Heijnen, B. Biesma, C. Debruyne, N. van Zandwijk, T. A. Splinter and G. Giaccone. Randomized controlled trial of resection versus radiotherapy after induction chemotherapy in stage IIIA-N2 non-small-cell lung cancer. J Natl Cancer Inst 2007 99(6): 442-50. NRP

van Putten, A. Price, A. H. van der Leest, A. Gregor, F. A. Little and H. J. Groen. A Phase I study of gemcitabine with concurrent radiotherapy in stage III, locally advanced non-small cell lung cancer. Clin Cancer Res 2003 9(7): 2472-7. NRP

Van Zandwijk, E. F. Smit, G. W. Kramer, F. Schramel, S. Gans, J. Festen, A. Termeer, N. J. Schlosser, C. Debruyne, D. Curran and G. Giaccone. Gemcitabine and cisplatin as induction regimen for patients with biopsy-proven stage IIIA N2 non-small-cell lung cancer: a phase II study of the European Organization for Research and Treatment of Cancer Lung Cancer Cooperative Group (EORTC 08955). J Clin Oncol 2000 18(14): 2658-64. NRP

Vansteenkiste, P. R. De Leyn, G. J. Deneffe, Y. N. Lievens, K. L. Nackaerts, D. E. Van Raemdonck, E. van der Schueren, T. E. Lerut and M. G. Demedts. Vindesine-ifosfamide-platinum (VIP) induction chemotherapy in surgically staged IIIA-N2 non-small-cell lung cancer: a prospective study. Leuven Lung Cancer Group. Ann Oncol 1998 9(3): 261-7. NRP

Vansteenkiste, S. G. Stroobants, P. R. De Leyn, P. J. Dupont and E. K. Verbeken. Potential use of FDG-PET scan after induction chemotherapy in surgically staged IIIa-N2 non-small-cell lung cancer: a prospective pilot study. The Leuven Lung Cancer Group. Ann Oncol 1998 9(11): 1193-8. NRP

Varveris, M. Mazonakis, M. Vlachaki, S. Kachris, E. Lyraraki, O. Zoras, T. Maris, M. Froudarakis, J. Velegrakis, C. Perysinakis, J. Damilakis and G. Samonis. A phase I trial of weekly docetaxel and cisplatinum combined to concurrent hyperfractionated radiotherapy for non-small cell lung cancer and squamous cell carcinoma of head and neck. Oncol Rep 2003 10(1): 185-95. NRP

Vergnenegre, C. Daniel, H. Lena, P. Fournel, J. P. Kleisbauer, H. Le Caer, J. Letreut, D. Paillotin, M. Perol, E. Bouchaert, P. M. Preux and G. Robinet. Docetaxel and concurrent radiotherapy after two cycles of induction chemotherapy with cisplatin and vinorelbine in patients with locally advanced non-small-cell lung cancer. A phase II trial conducted by the Groupe Francais de Pneumo-Cancerologie (GFPC). Lung Cancer 2005 47(3): 395-404. NRP

Verstegen, F. J. Lagerwaard, C. J. A. Haasbeek, B. J. Slotman and S. Senan. Outcomes of stereotactic ablative radiotherapy following a clinical diagnosis of stage i NSCLC: Comparison with a contemporaneous cohort with pathologically proven disease. Radiotherapy and Oncology 2011 101(2): 250-254. USD

Viallet, M. A. Brassard, L. Souhami, J. Ayoub, P. Del Vecchio, H. Kreisman, J. Guerra, J. Gruber, A. Langleben, J. Hohneker and P. Rousseau. A phase I/II trial of neoadjuvant chemotherapy with cisplatin and vinorelbine followed by accelerated irradiation for patients with inoperable nonsmall cell lung carcinoma. Cancer 1999 85(12): 2562-9. NRP

Vogt, C. Kolotas, T. Martin, L. V. Schneider, A. Neeb, P. S. Mitrou, K. Diergarten, W. Dornoff and N. Zamboglou. Simultaneous radiochemotherapy with paclitaxel in non-small cell lung cancer: a clinical phase I study. Semin Oncol 1996 23(6 Suppl 15): 26-30. NRP

Vogt, C. Kolotas, T. Martin, L. V. Schneider, R. Goes-Schmieder, K. Diergarten and N. Zamboglou. Concurrent paclitaxel/radiotherapy in locally advanced stage IIIA/B non- small cell lung cancer: Results of a clinical phase I study. Seminars in Radiation Oncology 1997 7(2 SUPPL. 1): S1-19-S1-24. NRP

Vogt, C. Kolotas, T. Martin, L. V. Schneider, R. Goes-Schmieder, P. S. Mitrou, K. Diergarten, B. Kober and N. Zamboglou. Paclitaxel and simultaneous radiation in locally advanced stage IIIA/B non-small cell lung cancer: a clinical phase I study. Semin Oncol 1996 23(6 Suppl 16): 120-3. NRP

Vokes, D. J. Haraf, L. C. Drinkard, P. C. Hoffman, M. K. Ferguson, N. J. Vogelzang, S. Watson, N. J. Lane and H. M. Golomb. A phase I trial of concomitant chemoradiotherapy with cisplatin dose intensification and granulocyte-colony stimulating factor support for advanced malignancies of the chest. Cancer Chemother Pharmacol 1995 35(4): 304-12. NRP

Vokes, J. E. Herndon, 2nd, J. Crawford, K. A. Leopold, M. C. Perry, A. A. Miller and M. R. Green. Randomized phase II study of cisplatin with gemcitabine or paclitaxel or vinorelbine as induction chemotherapy followed by concomitant chemoradiotherapy for stage IIIB non-small-cell lung cancer: cancer and leukemia group B study 9431. J Clin Oncol 2002 20(20): 4191-8. NRP

Vokes, J. E. Herndon, 2nd, M. J. Kelley, M. G. Cicchetti, N. Ramnath, H. Neill, J. N. Atkins, D. M. Watson, W. Akerley and M. R. Green. Induction chemotherapy followed by chemoradiotherapy compared with chemoradiotherapy alone for regionally advanced unresectable stage III Non-small-cell lung cancer: Cancer and Leukemia Group B. J Clin Oncol 2007 25(13): 1698-704. NRP

Voltolini, L. Luzzi, C. Ghiribelli, P. Paladini, M. Di Bisceglie and G. Gotti. Results of induction chemotherapy followed by surgical resection in patients with stage IIIA (N2) non-small cell lung cancer: the importance of the nodal down-staging after chemotherapy. Eur J Cardiothorac Surg 2001 20(6): 1106-12. NRP

Vora, B. D. Daly, L. Blaszkowsky, J. J. McGrath, M. Bankoff, S. Supran and T. A. Dipetrillo. High dose radiation therapy and chemotherapy as induction treatment for stage III nonsmall cell lung carcinoma. Cancer 2000 89(9): 1946-52. NRP

Voroney, A. Hope, M. R. Dahele, T. G. Purdie, K. N. Franks, S. Pearson, J. B. Cho, A. Sun, D. G. Payne, J. P. Bissonnette, A. Bezjak and A. M. Brade. Chest wall pain and rib fracture after stereotactic radiotherapy for peripheral non-small cell lung cancer. J Thorac Oncol 2009 4(8): 1035-7. NRD

Vyas, U. Suryanarayana, S. Dixit, S. Singhal, D. C. Bhavsar, J. P. Neema and H. A. Baboo. Inoperable non-small cell lung cancer: palliative radiotherapy with two weekly fractions. Indian J Chest Dis Allied Sci 1998 40(3): 171-4. NRP

Wagner, M. von Eiff, F. Klinke, O. Micke, C. Rübe and N. Willich. Neoadjuvant radiochemotherapy in locally advanced non-small cell bronchial carcinoma. Initial results of a prospective multicenter study. 1995 171(): 390-7. FLA

Wanders, J. Steevens, A. Botterweck, A. M. Dingemans, B. Reymen, A. Baardwijk, J. Borger, G. Bootsma, C. Pitz, R. Lunde, W. Geraedts, P. Lambin and D. De Ruysscher. Treatment with curative intent of stage III non-small cell lung cancer patients of 75years: A prospective population-based study. Eur J Cancer 2011 47(18): 2691-7. NRP

Wang, C. R. Correa, L. Zhao, J. Hayman, G. P. Kalemkerian, S. Lyons, K. Cease, D. Brenner and F. M. Kong. The effect of radiation dose and chemotherapy on overall survival in 237 patients with Stage III non-small-cell lung cancer. Int J Radiat Oncol Biol Phys 2009 73(5): 1383-90. NRP

Wang, J. Lu, T. Liu, K. M. Chen, G. Huang and F. J. Liu. CT-guided interstitial brachytherapy of inoperable non-small cell lung cancer. Lung Cancer 2011 74(2): 253-7. NRP

Wang, M. Song, H. Xu and Y. Fang. Prospective trial of combined hyperfractionated radiotherapy and bronchial arterial infusion of chemotherapy for locally advanced nonsmall cell lung cancer. Int J Radiat Oncol Biol Phys 1996 34(2): 309-13. NRP

Wang, N. Wu, M. D. Cham and Y. Song. Tumor response in patients with advanced non-small cell lung cancer: perfusion CT evaluation of chemotherapy and radiation therapy. AJR Am J Roentgenol 2009 193(4): 1090-6. NRP

Wang, S. Y. Wang, S. Yang, Y. Ding and Y. Shang. Late course three-dimensional conformal radiotherapy in patients with stage III non-small cell lung cancer. 2005 25(): 726-8. FLA

Wang, T. Y. Xia, Y. J. Wang, H. Q. Li, P. Li, J. D. Wang, D. S. Chang, L. Y. Liu, Y. P. Di, X. Wang and W. Z. Wu. Prospective study of epidermal growth factor receptor tyrosine kinase inhibitors concurrent with individualized radiotherapy for patients with locally advanced or metastatic non-small-cell lung cancer. Int J Radiat Oncol Biol Phys 2011 81(3): e59-65. NRP

Wang, X. B. Huang, Y. Ding, K. L. Mo and S. Yang. Three-dimensional conformal radiotherapy combined with stereotactic radiotherapy for locally advanced non-small cell lung cancer: efficacy and complications. 2008 28(): 1996-8. FLA

Waters, B. Dingle, G. Rodrigues, M. Vincent, R. Ash, R. Dar, R. Inculet, W. Kocha, R. Malthaner, M. Sanatani, L. Stitt, B. Yaremko, J. Younus and E. Yu. Analysis of a novel protocol of combined induction chemotherapy and concurrent chemoradiation in unresected non-small-cell lung cancer: a ten-year experience with vinblastine, Cisplatin, and radiation therapy. Clin Lung Cancer 2010 11(4): 243-50. NRP

Watkins, A. E. Wahlquist, A. J. Zauls, E. C. Fields, E. Garrett-Mayer, E. G. Aguero, G. A. Silvestri and A. K. Sharma. High-dose fractionated radiotherapy to 80 Gy for stage I-II medically inoperable non-small-cell lung cancer. J Med Imaging Radiat Oncol 2010 54(6): 554-61. NRP

Weitberg, L. Liu, J. Yashar and A. S. Glicksman. Twelve-year follow-up of trimodality therapy for stage IIIA non-small cell lung cancer. J Exp Clin Cancer Res 2001 20(3): 335-40. NRP

Werner-Wasik, E. Pequignot, D. Leeper, W. Hauck and W. Curran. Predictors of severe esophagitis include use of concurrent chemotherapy, but not the length of irradiated esophagus: a multivariate analysis of patients with lung cancer treated with nonoperative therapy. Int J Radiat Oncol Biol Phys 2000 48(3): 689-96. NRD

Werner-Wasik, R. Paulus, W. J. Curran, Jr. and R. Byhardt. Acute esophagitis and late lung toxicity in concurrent chemoradiotherapy trials in patients with locally advanced non-small-cell lung cancer: analysis of the radiation therapy oncology group (RTOG) database. Clin Lung Cancer 2011 12(4): 245-51. NRP

Widder, D. Postmus, J. F. Ubbels, E. M. Wiegman and J. A. Langendijk. Survival and quality of life after stereotactic or 3D-conformal radiotherapy for inoperable early-stage lung cancer. International Journal of Radiation Oncology Biology Physics 2011 81(4): e291-e297. USD

Willers, F. Wurschmidt, H. Bunemann and H. P. Heilmann. High-dose radiation therapy alone for inoperable non-small cell lung cancer--experience with prolonged overall treatment times. Acta Oncol 1998 37(1): 101-5. NRP

Willner, M. Schmidt, J. Kirschner, S. Lang, A. Borgmeier, R. M. Huber and M. Flentje. Sequential chemo- and radiochemotherapy with weekly paclitaxel (Taxol) and 3D-conformal radiotherapy of stage III inoperable non-small cell lung cancer. Results of a dose escalation study. Lung Cancer 2001 32(2): 163-71. NRP

Winterhalder, S. Deschler-Marini, C. Landmann, R. Kann, J. Passweg, R. Herrmann and M. Pless. Vinorelbine plus low-dose cisplatinum with concomitant radiotherapy for the treatment of locally advanced or inoperable non-metastasized non-small-cell lung cancer (stage I-IIIB): a phase II study. Radiother Oncol 2004 73(3): 321-4. NRP

Wirth, J. Lucca, P. Ostler, P. Fidias, C. Lynch, P. A. Janne, R. S. Herbst, B. E. Johnson, D. J. Sugarbaker, D. J. Mathisen, J. M. Lukanich, N. C. Choi, S. M. Berman and A. T. Skarin. Induction docetaxel and carboplatin followed by weekly docetaxel and carboplatin with concurrent radiotherapy, then surgery in stage III non-small cell lung cancer: a Phase I study. Clin Cancer Res 2003 9(5): 1698-704. NRP

Wisnivesky, E. Halm, M. Bonomi, C. Powell and E. Bagiella. Effectiveness of radiation therapy for elderly patients with unresected stage I and II non-small cell lung cancer. Am J Respir Crit Care Med 2010 181(3): 264-9. NRP

Wisnivesky, M. Bonomi, C. Henschke, M. Iannuzzi and T. McGinn. Radiation therapy for the treatment of unresected stage I-II non-small cell lung cancer. Chest 2005 128(3): 1461-7. NRP

Wolf, C. Faoro, C. Goerg, R. Pfab, K. Havemann and H. Kettner. Paclitaxel and simultaneous radiation in the treatment of stage IIIA/B non-small cell lung cancer. Semin Oncol 1996 23(6 Suppl 16): 108-12. NRP

Wolski, A. Bhatnagar, J. C. Flickinger, C. P. Belani, S. Ramalingam and J. S. Greenberger. Multivariate analysis of survival, local control, and time to distant metastases in patients with unresectable non-small-cell lung carcinoma treated with 3-dimensional conformal radiation therapy with or without concurrent chemotherapy. Clin Lung Cancer 2005 7(2): 100-6. NRP

Wu, G. L. Jiang, Y. Liao, H. Qian, L. J. Wang, X. L. Fu and S. Zhao. Three-dimensional conformal radiation therapy for non-small-cell lung cancer: a phase I/II dose escalation clinical trial. Int J Radiat Oncol Biol Phys 2003 57(5): 1336-44. NRP

Wu, H. Zhu, H. Tang, C. Li and F. Xu. Clinical Analysis of stereotactic body radiation therapy using extracranial gamma knife for patients with mainly bulky inoperable early stage non-small cell lung carcinoma. Radiation Oncology 2011 6(1): . NRI

Wu, Y. J. Bang, E. K. Choi, Y. C. Ahn, Y. W. Kim, T. H. Lim, C. Suh, K. Park and C. I. Park. Phase I study of weekly docetaxel and cisplatin concurrent with thoracic radiotherapy in Stage III non-small-cell lung cancer. Int J Radiat Oncol Biol Phys 2002 52(1): 75-80. NRP

Wu, Z. Xie, Z. N. Wang, L. P. Feng and Z. X. Yang. Efficacy of concurrent radio-chemotherapy and chemotherapy alone in the treatment of locally advanced non-small-cell lung cancer. 2005 27(): 502-4. FLA

Wulf, U. Haedinger, U. Oppitz, W. Thiele, G. Mueller and M. Flentje. Stereotactic radiotherapy for primary lung cancer and pulmonary metastases: a noninvasive treatment approach in medically inoperable patients. Int J Radiat Oncol Biol Phys 2004 60(1): 186-96. NRP

Wurstbauer, H. Deutschmann, P. Kopp, M. Kranzinger, F. Merz, O. Nairz, M. Studnicka and F. Sedlmayer. Nonresected non-small-cell lung cancer in Stages I through IIIB: accelerated, twice-daily, high-dose radiotherapy--a prospective Phase I/II trial with long-term follow-up. Int J Radiat Oncol Biol Phys 2010 77(5): 1345-51. NRP

Wurstbauer, H. Weise, H. Deutschmann, P. Kopp, F. Merz, M. Studnicka, O. Nairz and F. Sedlmayer. Non-small cell lung cancer in stages I-IIIB: Long-term results of definitive radiotherapy with doses >/= 80 Gy in standard fractionation. Strahlenther Onkol 2010 186(10): 551-7. NRP

Xia, H. Li, Q. Sun, Y. Wang, N. Fan, Y. Yu, P. Li and J. Y. Chang. Promising clinical outcome of stereotactic body radiation therapy for patients with inoperable Stage I/II non-small-cell lung cancer. Int J Radiat Oncol Biol Phys 2006 66(1): 117-25. USD

Xu, J. Wang, Y. Shen, H. Zhang and Q. Zhou. Phase I/II study of gemcitabine and oxaliplatin chemotherapy in combination with concurrent 3-D conformal radiotherapy for locally advanced non-small cell lung cancer. Zhongguo Fei Ai Za Zhi 2006 9(4): 362-8. NRP

Yalman, A. Arican, O. Karakoyun, I. Karadogan, V. Yurut Denizli, M. Esassolak and A. Haydaroglu. Radical radiotherapy in advanced-stage non-small cell lung cancer: Evaluation of 332 cases. Journal of B.U.ON. 1999 4(4): 383-387. NRP

Yamada, S. Kudoh, H. Fukuda, K. Nakagawa, N. Yamamoto, Y. Nishimura, S. Negoro, K. Takeda, M. Tanaka and M. Fukuoka. Dose-escalation study of weekly irinotecan and daily carboplatin with concurrent thoracic radiotherapy for unresectable stage III non-small cell lung cancer. Br J Cancer 2002 87(3): 258-63. NRP

Yamada, T. Soejima, Y. Ota, R. Sasaki, E. Yoden, N. Kanaoka, T. Maruta and K. Sugimura. Radiotherapy for medically inoperable non-small cell lung cancer at clinical stage I and II. Tumori 2003 89(1): 75-9. NRI

Yamamoto, K. Nakagawa, Y. Nishimura, K. Tsujino, M. Satouchi, S. Kudo, T. Hida, M. Kawahara, K. Takeda, N. Katakami, T. Sawa, S. Yokota, T. Seto, F. Imamura, H. Saka, Y. Iwamoto, H. Semba, Y. Chiba, H. Uejima and M. Fukuoka. Phase III study comparing second- and third-generation regimens with concurrent thoracic radiotherapy in patients with unresectable stage III non-small-cell lung cancer: West Japan Thoracic Oncology Group WJTOG0105. J Clin Oncol 2010 28(23): 3739-45. NRP

Yamamoto, Y. Nishimura, K. Nakagawa, K. Matsui and M. Fukuoka. Phase I/II study of weekly docetaxel dose escalation in combination with fixed weekly cisplatin and concurrent thoracic radiotherapy in locally advanced non-small cell lung cancer. Cancer Chemother Pharmacol 2006 58(3): 285-91. NRP

Yang, C. M. Tsai, L. S. Wang, Y. C. Lee, C. J. Chang, L. T. Lui, S. H. Yen, C. Hsu, A. L. Cheng, M. Y. Liu, S. C. Chiang, Y. M. Chen, K. T. Luh, M. H. Huang, P. C. Yang and R. P. Perng. Gemcitabine and cisplatin in a multimodality treatment for locally advanced non-small cell lung cancer. Br J Cancer 2002 86(2): 190-5. NRP

Yang, X. W. Fan, G. Q. Zhang and L. Shan. Efficacy and safety of chemotherapy combined with interstitial (125)I seed implantation brachytherapy in unresectable stage IIIa/IIIb non-small cell lung cancer. 2010 32(): 626-9. FLA

Yano, H. Yokoyama, I. Yoshino, K. Tayama, H. Asoh, K. Hata and Y. Ichinose. Results of a limited resection for compromised or poor-risk patients with clinical stage I non-small cell carcinoma of the lung. J Am Coll Surg 1995 181(1): 33-7. NRI

Yap, W. T. Lim, K. F. Foo, S. W. Hee, S. S. Leong, K. W. Fong, P. Eng, A. A. Hsu, J. Wee, T. Agasthian, H. N. Koong and E. H. Tan. Induction concurrent chemoradiotherapy using Paclitaxel and Carboplatin combination followed by surgery in locoregionally advanced non-small cell lung cancer--Asian experience. Ann Acad Med Singapore 2008 37(5): 377-82. NRP

Yendamuri, R. R. Komaki, A. M. Correa, P. Allen, B. Wynn, S. Blackmon, W. L. Hofstetter, D. C. Rice, J. A. Roth, S. G. Swisher, A. A. Vaporciyan, G. L. Walsh and R. J. Mehran. Comparison of limited surgery and three-dimensional conformal radiation in high-risk patients with stage I non-small cell lung cancer. J Thorac Oncol 2007 2(11): 1022-8. NRP

Yeo, M. J. Cho, S. Y. Kim, S. P. Lim, K. H. Kim and J. S. Kim. Treatment outcomes of three-dimensional conformal radiotherapy for stage III non-small cell lung cancer. Cancer Res Treat 2005 37(5): 273-8. NRP

Yokoyama, Y. Kurita, N. Saijo, T. Tamura, K. Noda, K. Shimokata and T. Matsuda. Dose-finding study of irinotecan and cisplatin plus concurrent radiotherapy for unresectable stage III non-small-cell lung cancer [seecomments]. Br J Cancer 1998 78(2): 257-62. NRP

Yom, Z. Liao, H. H. Liu, S. L. Tucker, C. S. Hu, X. Wei, X. Wang, S. Wang, R. Mohan, J. D. Cox and R. Komaki. Initial evaluation of treatment-related pneumonitis in advanced-stage non-small-cell lung cancer patients treated with concurrent chemotherapy and intensity-modulated radiotherapy. Int J Radiat Oncol Biol Phys 2007 68(1): 94-102. NRP

Yoo, D. E. Dupuy, S. L. Hillman, H. C. Fernando, W. S. Rilling, J. A. Shepard and B. A. Siegel. Radiofrequency ablation of medically inoperable stage IA non-small cell lung cancer: are early posttreatment PET findings predictive of treatment outcome?. AJR Am J Roentgenol 2011 197(2): 334-40. NRO

Yoon, Y. C. Hong, H. J. Park, J. E. Lee, S. Y. Kim, J. H. Kim, S. W. Lee, S. Y. Park, J. S. Lee and E. K. Choi. The polymorphism and haplotypes of XRCC1 and survival of non-small-cell lung cancer after radiotherapy. Int J Radiat Oncol Biol Phys 2005 63(3): 885-91. NRP

Yoshizawa, J. Tanaka, H. Kagamu, Y. Maruyama, H. Miyao, K. Ito, T. Sato, A. Iwashima, E. Suzuki and F. Gejyo. Phase I/II study of daily carboplatin, 5-fluorouracil and concurrent radiation therapy for locally advanced non-small-cell lung cancer. Br J Cancer 2003 89(5): 803-7. NRP

Yu, X. D. Sun, M. H. Li, J. D. Zhang, C. P. Yao, S. Liu and Z. Zhang. Involved-field three-dimensional conformal radiation treatment for stage III non-small-cell lung. 2006 28(): 526-9. FLA

Yu, Y. F. Liu, J. M. Yu, J. Liu, Y. Zhao and M. Hou. Involved-field radiotherapy is effective for patients 70 years old or more with early stage non-small cell lung cancer. Radiother Oncol 2008 87(1): 29-34. NRP

Yuan, X. Sun, M. Li, J. Yu, R. Ren, Y. Yu, J. Li, X. Liu, R. Wang, B. Li, L. Kong and Y. Yin. A randomized study of involved-field irradiation versus elective nodal irradiation in combination with concurrent chemotherapy for inoperable stage III nonsmall cell lung cancer. Am J Clin Oncol 2007 30(3): 239-44. NRP

Zaric, B. Perin, A. Jovelic, N. Lalic, N. Secen, I. Kopitovic and M. Antonic. Clinical risk factors for early complications after high-dose-rate endobronchial brachytherapy in the palliative treatment of lung cancer. Clin Lung Cancer 2010 11(3): 182-6. USD

Zarogoulidis, T. Kontakiotis, P. Hatziapostolou, E. Fachantidou, D. Delis, J. Goutsikas, T. C. Constantinidis, A. Athanasiadis and D. Patakas. A Phase II study of docetaxel and carboplatin in the treatment of non-small cell lung cancer. Lung Cancer 2001 32(3): 281-7. NRP

Zatloukal, L. Petruzelka, M. Zemanova, L. Havel, F. Janku, L. Judas, A. Kubik, E. Krepela, P. Fiala and L. Pecen. Concurrent versus sequential chemoradiotherapy with cisplatin and vinorelbine in locally advanced non-small cell lung cancer: a randomized study. Lung Cancer 2004 46(1): 87-98. NRP

Zemlyak, W. H. Moore and T. V. Bilfinger. Comparison of survival after sublobar resections and ablative therapies for stage I non-small cell lung cancer. J Am Coll Surg 2010 211(1): 68-72. USD

Zhang, J. M. Yu, X. Meng, J. B. Yue, R. Feng and L. Ma. Prognostic value of serial [18F]fluorodeoxyglucose PET-CT uptake in stage III patients with non-small cell lung cancer treated by concurrent chemoradiotherapy. Eur J Radiol 2011 77(1): 92-6. NRP

Zhang, Y. Zheng, P. Yu, F. Yu, Q. Zhang, Y. Lv, X. Xie and Y. Gao. The combined treatment of CT-guided percutaneous 125I seed implantation and chemotherapy for non-small-cell lung cancer. J Cancer Res Clin Oncol 2011 137(12): 1813-22. NRP

Zhao, B. T. West, J. A. Hayman, S. Lyons, K. Cease and F. M. Kong. High radiation dose may reduce the negative effect of large gross tumor volume in patients with medically inoperable early-stage non-small cell lung cancer. Int J Radiat Oncol Biol Phys 2007 68(1): 103-10. NRI

Zhao, L. Wang, W. Ji, X. Wang, X. Zhu, J. A. Hayman, G. P. Kalemkerian, W. Yang, D. Brenner, T. S. Lawrence and F. M. Kong. Elevation of plasma TGF-beta1 during radiation therapy predicts radiation-induced lung toxicity in patients with non-small-cell lung cancer: a combined analysis from Beijing and Michigan. Int J Radiat Oncol Biol Phys 2009 74(5): 1385-90. NRP

Zhao, W. Ji, L. Zhang, G. Ou, Q. Feng, Z. Zhou, M. Lei, W. Yang and L. Wang. Changes of circulating transforming growth factor-beta1 level during radiation therapy are correlated with the prognosis of locally advanced non-small cell lung cancer. J Thorac Oncol 2010 5(4): 521-5. NRP

Zhou and J. X. Zheng. Hyperfractionated radiation therapy combined with concomitant chemotherapy for inoperable stage III non-small cell lung cancer: clinical analysis of 70 cases. 2004 24(): 841-2, 844. FLA

Zhu and R. Wu. Sequential and concurrent radiochemotherapy for stage III non-small cell lung cancer. Chinese Journal of Cancer Prevention and Treatment 2009 16(14): 1105-1107. FLA

Zhu, M. Fan, K. L. Wu, K. L. Zhao, H. J. Yang, G. Y. Chen, G. L. Jiang, L. J. Wang, S. Zhao and X. L. Fu. A phase II trial of accelerated hypofractionated three-dimensional conformal radiation therapy in locally advanced non-small cell lung cancer. Radiother Oncol 2011 98(3): 304-8. NRP

Zhu, T. D. Yan, D. Glenn and D. L. Morris. Radiofrequency Ablation of Lung Tumors: Feasibility and Safety. Annals of Thoracic Surgery 2009 87(4): 1023-1028. NRP

Zierhut, C. Bettscheider, K. Schubert, M. van Kampen and M. Wannenmacher. Radiation therapy of stage I and II non-small cell lung cancer (NSCLC). Lung Cancer 2001 34 Suppl 3(): S39-43. NRI

Zimmermann, H. Geinitz, S. Schill, A. Grosu, U. Schratzenstaller, M. Molls and B. Jeremic. Stereotactic hypofractionated radiation therapy for stage I non-small cell lung cancer. Lung Cancer 2005 48(1): 107-14. OPP

Zimmermann, H. Geinitz, S. Schill, R. Thamm, C. Nieder, U. Schratzenstaller and M. Molls. Stereotactic hypofractionated radiotherapy in stage I (T1-2 N0 M0) non-small-cell lung cancer (NSCLC). Acta Oncol 2006 45(7): 796-801. OPP

Zinner, R. Komaki, J. D. Cox, B. S. Glisson, K. M. Pisters, R. S. Herbst, M. Kies, Z. Liao, W. K. Hong and F. V. Fossella. Dose escalation of gemcitabine is possible with concurrent chest three-dimensional rather than two-dimensional radiotherapy: a phase I trial in patients with stage III non-small-cell lung cancer. Int J Radiat Oncol Biol Phys 2009 73(1): 119-27. NRP

Zwitter, V. Kovac, U. Smrdel and P. Strojan. Gemcitabine, cisplatin, and hyperfractionated accelerated radiotherapy for locally advanced non-small cell lung cancer. J Thorac Oncol 2006 1(7): 662-6. NRP

Appendix C. Evidence Tables

Appendix Table C1. Description of studies that address Key Question 1

Study	Study design, enrollment numbers and lost to FU/excluded	Inclusion/exclusion criteria	Stage Distribution	Tumor/Obstruction Location & Histopathology	Patient Characteristics
Andratschke-2011, Germany, #132	**Study design:** RET, SAS **Patients enrolled:** 92 (100%) **Lost to FU/excluded/missing:** 0	**Inclusion criteria:** 1. Histologically proven NSCLC stage 1 not suitable for surgery for medical or functional reasons **Exclusion criteria:** 1. Patients with mediastinal lymph node metastases	**Stage I:** 92 (100%)	**Location:** Central: 24 (26%) Peripheral: 68 (74%) **Histopathology:** AC: 35 (38%) SCC: 49 (53%) BAC: 2 (2%) NOS: 6 (7%)	**Age (years):** 75 (53-93) **Women:** 28 (30%) **Race:** NR **Comorbidities:** COPD: 76 (83%) CVD: 37 (40%) **Performance status:** KPS: 70 (60–100) ≤70: 16 (17%) 70: 50 (54%) >70: 26 (28%)
Baumann-2006, Sweden, Denmark, #271	**Study design:** RET, SAS **Patients enrolled:** Total: 141 (100%) Medically inoperable: 136 (96%) Refused surgery: 5 (4%) **Lost to FU/excluded/missing:** Lost to follow up: 3 (2%) (Baseline data based on 141 Patients, outcome data based on 138 Patients)	**Inclusion criteria:** NR **Exclusion criteria:** NR	**Stage I:** 141 (100%)	**Location:** NR **Histopathology:** AC: 44(31%) SCC: 39(28%) BAC: 3 (2%) NOS: 21 (15%) Unknown: 31 (24%)	**Age (years):** 74 (56-90) **Women:** 72 (51%) **Race:** NR **Comorbidities:** COPD: 78(55%) CVD: 25 (18%) COPD + CVD: 21(15%) Other malignancies: 14(10%) Other compromising disease: 3 (2%) **Performance status:** NR
Baumann-2009, Sweden, Norway,	**Study design:** RET, SAS	**Inclusion criteria:** 1. Stage 1 Peripherally located NSCLC.	**Stage I (T1):** 37 (65%) **Stage I (T2):** 20 (35%)	**Location:** Superior: 37 (65%) Inferior: 16 (28%)	**Age (years):** 75 (59-87)

Study	Study design, enrollment numbers and lost to FU/excluded	Inclusion/exclusion criteria	Stage Distribution	Tumor/Obstruction Location & Histopathology	Patient Characteristics
Denmark, #270	**Patients enrolled:** SBRT Total: 60 (100%) Medically inoperable: 56 (99%) Refused surgery: 1 (2%) **Lost to FU/excluded/missing:** Lost to follow-up: 1 (2%) Excluded due to being given inadequate doses: 2 (4%)	2. Consent **Exclusion criteria:** 1. Central tumor growth adjacent to trachea, main bronchus, or esophagus 2. Prior malignancy within the past 5 years		**Middle:** 4 (7%) **Histopathology:** AC: 19 (33%) SCC: 8 (14%) LCC: 1 (2%) NOS: 10 (18%) Unknown: 19 (33%)	**Women:** 31 (54%) **Race:** NR **Comorbidities:** COPD: 40 (70%) CVD: 14 (26%) COPD & CVD: 8 (14%) Lung Fibrosis: 1 (2%) Advanced Age (years) + joint disease: 1 (2%) Mean FEV1%: 64 (20-162) **Performance status:** KPS: 80 (70-90) 70: 4 (7%) 80: 36 (63%) 90: 17 (30%)
Bogart-2010, USA, #382	**Study design:** PRO, SAS **Patients enrolled:** 39 (100%) **Lost to FU/excluded/missing:** Declined treatment: 1	**Inclusion criteria:** 1. A histologic or cytologic diagnosis of stage IA or IB NSCLC with a solitary parenchymal lung lesion measuring ≤4 cm 2. Patients at high risk for complications after standard lobectomy, as defined by pulmonary dysfunction 3. Have high-risk features of comorbid medical illness making them unsuitable for surgical resection 4. ECOG performance status of 0 to 2 5. Weight loss less than 10% in the 6 months before protocol entry **Exclusion criteria:** 1. Prior chemotherapy for lung cancer 2. Prior radiotherapy to the chest	**Stage I:** 39 (100%)	**Location:** NR **Histopathology:** NOS: 39 (100%)	**Age (years):** 75 (48-87) **Women:** 21 (53%) **Race:** NR **Comorbidities:** (N=38) Median FEV1:0.96 95% CI: (0.83 to 1.31) Eleven (28%) of 39 patients required supplemental oxygen, between 2 and 4 L nasal canula, before the start of therapy. **Performance status:** ECOG: 0: 2 (5%) 1: 26 (67%) 2: 11 (28%)
Bollineni-2012, Netherlands,	**Study design:** RET, SAS	**Inclusion criteria:** Patients not suitable for surgery	**Stage I:** 132 (100%)	**Location:** Not stated	**Age (years):** 75 (46-90)

Study	Study design, enrollment numbers and lost to FU/excluded	Inclusion/exclusion criteria	Stage Distribution	Tumor/Obstruction Location & Histopathology	Patient Characteristics
#4548	**Patients enrolled:** 132 (100%) **Lost to FU/excluded/missing:** 0	for medical or functional reasons with a solitary FDG-PET positive lesion in the lung **Exclusion criteria:** Not stated		**Histopathology:** NSCLC not stated Pathological confirmation: 40 (30%)	**Women:** 37 (28%) **Race:** NR **Comorbidities:** Median CCI: 4 (2-12) **Performance status:** WHO 0-1: 106 (80%) 2-3: 26 (20%)
Bradley-2003, USA, #445	**Study design:** PRO, SAS **Patients enrolled:** 56 (100%) **Lost to FU/excluded/missing:** NR	**Inclusion criteria:** 1. Histologically proven NSCLC **Exclusion criteria:** 1. Patients treated with only palliative intent (≤ 60 Gy)	**Stage I:** 56 (100%)	**Location:** Upper lobe: 35 (62%) Middle or lower lobe: 21 (38%) **Histopathology:** AC: 14 (25%) SCC: 25 (44%) LCC: 6 (11%) NOS: 11 (20%)	**Age (years):** 73 (52-90) **Women:** 32 (57%) **Race:** White: 43 (77%) Black: 13 (23%) **Comorbidities:** KFI Comorbidity Score: 0: 10 (18%) 1: 19 (32%) 2: 14 (25%) 3: 13 (23%) **Performance status:** KPS: ≥ 70: 49 (88%) < 70: 7 (12%)
Burdick-2010, USA, #521	**Study design:** RET, SAS **Patients enrolled:** 72 (100%) **Lost to FU/excluded/missing:** NR	**Inclusion criteria:** 1. Patients without histologic diagnosis were treated only after signs of progression on serial CT and PET/CT studies **Exclusion criteria:** 1. Patients with recurrent tumors	**Stage I:** 72 (100%)	**Location:** NR **Histopathology:** NOS: 49 (68%)	**Age (years):** 73 (52-90) **Women:** NR **Race:** NR **Comorbidities:** Inadequate predicted pulmonary reserve after resection; CVD;

Study	Study design, enrollment numbers and lost to FU/excluded	Inclusion/exclusion criteria	Stage Distribution	Tumor/Obstruction Location & Histopathology	Patient Characteristics
					cerebrovascular disease (Proportions NR) **Performance status:** KPS: 80 (40-100)
Bush-2004, USA, #535	**Study design:** PRO, SAS **Patients enrolled:** Total: 68 (100%) Medically inoperable: 63 (93%) Refused surgery: 5 (7%) **Lost to FU/excluded/missing:** NR	**Inclusion criteria:** 1. Histologic diagnosis of NSCLC 2. Clinical stage 1 disease 3. consent **Exclusion criteria:** NR	**Stage I:** 68 (100%)	**Location:** NR **Histopathology:** NR	**Age (years):** Mean: 72 (52-87) **Women:** 38 (56%) **Race:** NR **Comorbidities:** FEV1 Mean (L) 1.15 (0.4-2.1) **Performance status:** KPS Mean: 65 (50-90)
Campeau-2009, Australia, #565	**Study design:** RET, SAS **Patients enrolled:** 34 (100%) **Lost to FU/excluded/missing:** (See comments)	**Inclusion criteria:** 1. UICC Stage I histologically or cytologically proven NSCLC treated with or without concomitant chemotherapy. **Exclusion criteria:** 1. Previous diagnosis of lung cancer 2. Prior treatment for NSCLC 3. Surgery forming part of the initial treatment 4. Evidence of recurrence from a previous cancer.	**Stage I:** 34 (100%)	**Location:** NR **Histopathology:** AC: 13 (38%) SCC: 12 (35%) LCC: 2 (6%) NOS: 7 (21%)	**Age (years):** 81 (54-88) **Women:** 14 (41%) **Race:** NR **Comorbidities:** SCS: <9: 12 (35%) >9: 21 (62%) NA: 1 (3%) **Performance status:** ECOG: 0: 3 (9%) 1: 6 (18%) 2: 9 (26%) 3: 2 (6%) NA: 14 (41%)
Coon-2008, USA, #803	**Study design:** RET, SAS **Patients enrolled:** Total: 26(100%)	**Inclusion criteria:** 1. Stage I NSCLC, or residual/recurrent lung cancer after previous treatment, or solitary lung metastases	**Stage I:** 26 (100%)	**Location:** Upper: 18 (69%) Middle: 1 (4%) Lower: 6 (23%) Other: 1 (4%)	**Age (years):** Median: 76.5 **Women:** NR

Study	Study design, enrollment numbers and lost to FU/excluded	Inclusion/exclusion criteria	Stage Distribution	Tumor/Obstruction Location & Histopathology	Patient Characteristics
	Medically inoperable: 24 (92%) Refused surgery: 2 (8%) **Lost to FU/excluded/missing:** NR	**Exclusion criteria:** NR		**Histopathology:** AC: 12 (46%) SCC: 3 (12%) Atypical: 1 (4%) Unknown: 10 (38%)	**Race:** NR **Comorbidities:** Total: 24 (92%) COPD: 15 (62%) OMC: 4 (17%) Previous lung surgery: 5 (21%) **Performance status:** KPS: 65 (60-80)
Dunlap-2010, USA, #1032	**Study design:** RET, SAS **Patients enrolled:** Total: 40(100%) Medically inoperable: 37 (92%) Refused surgery: 3 (8%) **Lost to FU/excluded/missing:** Out of 60, 20 excluded reasons NR.	**Inclusion criteria:** 1. Patients who have a medically inoperable condition or refused surgery. **Exclusion criteria:** 1. Patients with abnormal fluorodeoxyglucose (FDG) uptake (maximum standardized uptake value [SUV]>2.5) in the mediastinum	**Stage I:** 40 (100%)	**Location:** NR **Histopathology:** NR	**Age (years):** 73 (54-87) **Women:** NR **Race:** NR **Comorbidities:** Total: 34 (100%) Poor pulmonary reserve: 26 (76%) CAD: 3 (9%) Cardiac dysfunction (ejection fraction < 30%): 5 (15%) **Performance status:** KPS < 70%: 3 (8%)
Fritz-2008, Germany, #1238	**Study design:** RET, SAS **Patients enrolled:** Total: 40 (100%) Medically inoperable: 37 (92%) Refused surgery: 3 (8%) **Lost to FU/excluded/missing:** NR	**Inclusion criteria:** 1. Patients had only one target and no signs of local lymph node metastases or of remote metastases. 2. Karnofsky performance ≥60% and FEV1 > 0.5 L/s (no permanent need of supplemental oxygen). 3. Histological confirmation of NSCLC 4. In case of previous chemotherapy, the time period between chemotherapy and	**Stage I:** 40 (100%)	**Location:** Peripheral: 40 (100%) **Histopathology:** AC: 17(43%) SCC: 8(20%) LCC: 13(32%) NOS: 2 (5%)	**Age (years):** 74 (59-82) **Women:** 8 (20%) **Race:** NR **Comorbidities:** MI: 7 (18%) CAD: 5 (13%) CHF: 3(8%) CPD: 22(60%)

Study	Study design, enrollment numbers and lost to FU/excluded	Inclusion/exclusion criteria	Stage Distribution	Tumor/Obstruction Location & Histopathology	Patient Characteristics
		SBRT had to be more than 6 weeks. 5. With reference to stage T2 tumors: tumor size ≤10 cm (largest focus), no involvement of main bronchus, no atelectasis or obstructive pneumonitis, no chest wall involvement **Exclusion criteria:** 1. Concurrent or adjuvant chemotherapy given			PVD: 2 (5%) Diabetes: 4 (10%) Renal disease: 2 (5%) FEV1: 0.66—2.93(median: 1.4 L/s; five patients < 1.0 L/s) **Performance status:** KPS: 80 % (60%-100%)
Graham-2006, Australia, #1403	**Study design:** RET, SAS **Patients enrolled:** Total: 39 (100%) Medically inoperable: 36 (92%) Refused surgery or unknown: 3 (8%) **Lost to FU/excluded/missing:** 0	**Inclusion criteria:** 1. Hst confirmed primary clinical stage I NSCLC 2. Medically inoperable or refused surgery **Exclusion criteria:** NR	**Stage I:** 39 (100%)	**Location:** NR **Histopathology:** SCC: 17 (43%)	**Age (years):** Mean: 72 (53-84) **Women:** 15 (38%) **Race:** NR **Comorbidities:** Respiratory inadequacy: 25 (64%) (FEV 1 < 1.3: 18/25 (72%)) CVD: 6 (15%) >80 years: 2 (5%) **Performance status:** ECOG > 1: 5 (13%)
Iwata-2010, Japan, # 1747	**Study design:** NRCS, NR whether data collection was RET or PRO **Patients enrolled:** Total: 57 (100%) PBRT 80Gy: 20 (35%) PBRT 60 Gy: 37 (65%) Medically Inoperable: Total: 28 (49%) PBRT 80Gy: 10 (34%) PBRT 60 Gy: 19 (66%) Refused surgery: Total: 29 (51%)	**Inclusion criteria:** 1. Hst confirmed primary NSCLC staged IA or IB 2. Medical inoperability or refusal of surgical resection; 3. WHO performance status ≤2; 4. No history of previous LC; 5. No prior chest RT or chemotherapy;	Total: 57 (100%) Stage 1A: 27(47%) Stage 1B: 30 (57%) PBRT 80Gy: 20 (100%) Stage 1A: 6 (30%) Stage 1B: 14(70%) PBRT 60 Gy: 37 (100%) Stage 1A: 21 (57%) Stage 1B: 16 (43%)	**Location:** NR **Histopathology:** Total: 57 (100%) AC: 32 (56%) SCC: 23 (40%) Others: 2 (4%) PBRT 80Gy: 20 (100%) AC: 11 (55%) SCC: 8 (40%) Others: 1 (5%) PBRT 60 Gy: 37 (100%) AC: 21 (57%)	**Age:** Total: 76 (48-89) PBRT 80Gy: 75 (48-87) PBRT 60 Gy: 78 (57-87) **Women:** Total: 23 (29%) PBRT 80Gy: 7 (36%) PBRT 60 Gy: 7 (19%) **Race:** NR **Co-morbidities:** Total: 28 (100%) Pulmonary: 13 (46%)

Study	Study design, enrollment numbers and lost to FU/excluded	Inclusion/exclusion criteria	Stage Distribution	Tumor/Obstruction Location & Histopathology	Patient Characteristics
	PBRT 80Gy: 10 (34%) PBRT 60 Gy: 19 (66%) **Lost to FU/excluded/missing:** None	**Exclusion criteria:** NR		SCC: 15 (41%) Others: 1 (3%)	CVD: 9 (32%) Severe DM: 5 (18%) Age: 2 (7%) Others: 2 (7%) PBRT 80Gy: 10 (100%) Pulmonary: 7 (70%) CVD: 3 (30%) Severe DM: 1 (10%) Age: 0 Others: 0 PBRT 60 Gy: 18 (100%) Pulmonary: 6 (33%) CVD: 6 (33%) Severe DM: 4 (22%) Age: 2 (11%) Others: 2 (11%) **Performance status:** NR
Jimenez-2010, Spain, #1842	**Study design:** RET, SAS **Patients enrolled:** 47 (100%) **Lost to FU/excluded/missing:** 0	**Inclusion criteria:** 1. HSt confirmed primary clinical stage I NSCLC 2. Medically inoperable 3. Moderate to good lung function (a forced expiratory volume in 1 s (FEV1) ≥ 30% of predicted value and a carbon monoxide diffusing capacity (DLCO) ≥ 30%). **Exclusion criteria:** 1. Prior chemotherapy or radiotherapy	**Stage I:** 47 (100%)	**Location:** NR **Histopathology:** NOS: 47 (100%)	**Age (years):** Mean 68±10 **Women:** 11 (23%) **Race:** NR **Comorbidities:** Mean FEV1: 54±17% Mean CCI score: 2.4±1.3 **Performance status:** NR
Kopek-2009, Denmark, #2040	**Study design:** PRO, SAS **Patients enrolled:** 88 (100%) **Lost to FU/excluded/missing:** 0	**Inclusion criteria:** 1. HSt confirmed primary clinical stage I NSCLC 2. Medically inoperable 3. Tumor < 6 cm diameter 4. WHO performance status 0-2	**Stage I:** 88 (100%)	**Location:** NR **Histopathology:** ACC: 30 (34%) SCC: 34 (39%) NOS: 24 (27%)	**Age (years):** 73 (47-88) **Women:** 43 (49%) **Race:** NR **Comorbidities:**

Study	Study design, enrollment numbers and lost to FU/excluded	Inclusion/exclusion criteria	Stage Distribution	Tumor/Obstruction Location & Histopathology	Patient Characteristics
		Exclusion criteria: NR			Mean FEV1: 1.06 (0.25-2.60) L CCI score: ≤ 3: 16 (18%) 4: 24 (27%) 5: 25 (28%) ≥6: 23 (26%) **Performance status:** WHO 0: 15 (17%) 1 (51 (58%) 2: 19 (21%) 3: 2 (2%)
Mirri-2009, Italy, #2576	**Study design:** PRO, SAS **Patients enrolled:** 15 (100%) **Lost to FU/excluded/missing:** 0	**Inclusion criteria:** 1. Primary clinical stage I NSCLC 2. Medically inoperable 3. Tumor < 5 cm diameter 4. KPS > 70 **Exclusion criteria:** NR	**Stage I:** 15 (100%)	**Location:** Peripheral: 13 (87%) Central: 2 (13%) **Histopathology:** SCC: 9 (60%) ACC: 2 (13%)	**Age (years):** 76 **Women:** NR **Race:** NR **Comorbidities:** COPD (number NR)
Nakayama-2010, Japan, #2684	**Study design:** RET, SAS **Patients enrolled:** Total: 55 (100%) Medically inoperable: 52 (94%) Refused surgery: 3 (6%) **Lost to FU/excluded/missing:** 0	**Inclusion criteria:** 1. Primary clinical stage I NSCLC 2. EORTC performance status of 1-2 3. Medically inoperable or refused surgery **Exclusion criteria:** 1. Existing pleural effusion 2. NSCLC located close to stomach or esophagus	**Stage I:** 55 (100%)	**Location:** Lesions: 58 Peripheral: 41 (71%) Central: 17 (29%) 3 patients had a second tumor in contralateral lung **Histopathology:** ACC: 31 (53%) SCC: 15 (26%) NOS: 4 (7%) LCC: 1 (2%) Undiagnosed: 7 (12%)	**Performance status:** KPS > 70 (number NR) **Age (years):** 74±9 years **Women:** 14 (26%) **Race:** NR **Comorbidities:** Fletcher-Hugh-Jones criteria: I: 7 (13%) II: 9 (16%) III: 32 (58%) IV: 7 (13%) CVD: 8 (14%)

Study	Study design, enrollment numbers and lost to FU/excluded	Inclusion/exclusion criteria	Stage Distribution	Tumor/Obstruction Location & Histopathology	Patient Characteristics
					Liver/renal: 2 (4%) FEV1 (mL) 818 ± 217 FEV1 (%) 68.2 ± 19.9 **Performance status:** EORTC criteria: 0: 37 (67%) 1: 16 (29%) 2: 2 (4%)
Narayan-2004, USA, #2686	**Study design:** PRO, SAS **Patients enrolled:** 13 (100%) **Lost to FU/excluded/missing:** 0	**Inclusion criteria:** 1. HSt confirmed primary clinical stage I NSCLC 2. Medically inoperable 3. SWOG performance status 0-2 **Exclusion criteria:** 1. Prior thoracic RT	Stage I: 13 (100%)	**Location:** NR **Histopathology:** NOS: 13 (100%)	**Age (years):** Mean 67±18 (calculated) **Women:** 1 (9%) (calculated) **Race:** NR **Comorbidities:** NR **Performance status:** NR
Nyman-2006, Sweden, #2750	**Study design:** PRO, SAS **Patients enrolled:** 45 (100%) **Lost to FU/excluded/missing:** 0	**Inclusion criteria:** 1. Primary clinical stage I NSCLC 2. Medically inoperable **Exclusion criteria:** 1. Tumor diameter > 5 cm 2. Central tumor with extension close to trachea, main bronchus, or esophagus	Stage I: 45 (100%)	**Location:** NR **Histopathology:** SCC: 18 (40%) ACC: 15 (33%) NOS: 3 (7%)	**Age (years):** Mean 74 (58-84) **Women:** 20 (44%) **Race:** NR **Comorbidities:** Mean FEV1: 1.3 (0.7-2.7) Poor lung function: 31 (69%) CVD: 24 (53%) Other serious malignancies: 6 (13%) **Performance status:** KPS: Mean 80 (60-100)
Olsen-2011, USA, #2792	**Study design:** RET, SAS **Patients enrolled:**	**Inclusion criteria:** 1. Primary clinical stage I NSCLC 2. Single lesion	Stage I: 130 (100%)	**Location:** Peripheral: 115 (88%) Central: 15 (12%)	**Age (years):** 75 (31-92) **Women:**

Study	Study design, enrollment numbers and lost to FU/excluded	Inclusion/exclusion criteria	Stage Distribution	Tumor/Obstruction Location & Histopathology	Patient Characteristics
	Total: 130 (100%) Medically inoperable: 117 (90%) Refused surgery: 13 (10%) **Lost to FU/excluded/missing:** 0	3. No prior malignancy for prior 2 years 4. Prescribed SBRT dose: 18Gy in 3, 9 Gy in 5, or 10 Gy in 5 frs 5. FU duration > 3 months **Exclusion criteria:** 1. Nodal or metastatic disease		**Histopathology:** Hst confirmed: 110 (85%) Undiagnosed: 20 (15%) NR	65 (50%) **Race:** NR **Comorbidities:** NR **Performance status:** NR
Palma-2011, Netherlands, #2843	**Study design:** PRO, SAS **Patients enrolled:** Total: 176 Medically inoperable: 169 (96%) Refused surgery or NR: 7 (4%) **Lost to FU/excluded/missing:** 0	**Inclusion criteria:** 1. Primary clinical stage I NSCLC 2. Severe COPD or ventilatory impairment 3. Medically inoperable or refused surgery **Exclusion criteria:** NR	**Stage I:** 176 (100%) (16 Patients had a second primary T1 tumor treated synchronously)	**Location:** NR **Histopathology:** Hst confirmed: 57 (32%) Histology NR	**Age (years):** 70 (47-86) **Women:** 79 (45%) **Race:** NR **Comorbidities:** COPD: GOLD III: 133 (76%) GOLD IV: 43 (24%) FEV1: median 0.94 (0.36 1.99) L CCI score: median 4 (2-9) **Performance status:** NR
Pennathur-2007, USA, #2896	**Study design:** RET, SAS **Patients enrolled:** 19 (100%) **Lost to FU/excluded/missing:** 0	**Inclusion criteria:** 1. Primary clinical stage I NSCLC 2. Medically inoperable 3. Peripheral tumor ≤ 4 cm diameter **Exclusion criteria:** 1. Central tumor	**Stage I:** 19 (100%)	**Location:** Peripheral: 19 (100%) **Histopathology:** SCC: 8 (42%) ACC: 8: (42%) NOS: 3 (16%)	**Age (years):** Median 78 (68-88) **Women:** 11 (58%) **Race:** NR **Comorbidities:** Median CCI: 4 (3-12) Poor pulmonary function: 10 (53%) Increased cardiac risk: 7 (37%) Multiple comorbidities: 8 (42%)

Study	Study design, enrollment numbers and lost to FU/excluded	Inclusion/exclusion criteria	Stage Distribution	Tumor/Obstruction Location & Histopathology	Patient Characteristics
					Mean FEV1: 0.73 ± 0.21 **Performance status:** NR
Pennathur-2009, USA, #2898	**Study design:** RET, SAS **Patients enrolled:** 21 (100%) **Lost to FU/excluded/missing:** 0	**Inclusion criteria:** 1. Primary clinical stage I NSCLC 2. Medically inoperable **Exclusion criteria:** NR	**Stage I:** 21 (100%)	**Location:** NR **Histopathology:** SCC: 8 (38%) ACC: 6 (29%) NOS: 6 (29%) Not determined: 1 (5%)	**Age (years):** 71 (61-85) **Women:** 12 (57%) **Race:** NR **Comorbidities:** Median CCI: 5 (0-10) Median FEV1: 0.67 (0.5 0.86) L Median DLCO: 30% (19 58%) Median CCI: 5 (0-10) Cardiac risk: 6 (29%) Multiple: 8 (38%) **Performance status:** NR
Ricardi-2010, Italy, #3098	**Study design:** PRO, SAS **Patients enrolled:** Total: 62 (100%) Medically inoperable: 56 (90%) Refused surgery: 6 (10%) **Lost to FU/excluded/missing:** 0	**Inclusion criteria:** 1. Primary clinical stage I NSCLC < 5 cm diameter 2. Medically inoperable or refused surgery 3. ECOG performance status < 2 4. No prior RT at site of SBRT **Exclusion criteria:** 1. Lesions located < 2 cm from airways or < 1 cm from major blood vessels	**Stage I:** 62 (100%)	**Location:** NR **Histopathology:** ACC: 13 (20%) SCC: 14 (23%) LCC: 3 (5%) BAC: 1 (2%) NOS: 9 (14%)	**Age (years):** Mean 74 (53-83) **Women:** 10 (16%) **Race:** NR **Comorbidities:** COPD: 31 (50%) CVD: 15 (24%) Elderly: 10 (16%) **Performance status:** ECOG < 2
Scorsetti-2007, Italy, #3362	**Study design:** SAS (unclear if PRO or RET) **Patients enrolled:** 43 (100%) **Lost to FU/excluded/missing:**	**Inclusion criteria:** 1. Primary clinical stage I NSCLC 2. Medically inoperable **Exclusion criteria:** 1. Tumor diameter > 5.5 cm	**Stage I:** 43 (100%)	**Location:** Right upper lobe: 18 (39%) Right lower lobe: 8 (17%) Right hilum: 2 (4%) Left upper lobe: 11 (24%) Left lower lobe: 4 (9%) Left hilum: 3 (7%)	**Age (years):** 76 (52-90) **Women:** 9 (21%) **Race:**

Study	Study design, enrollment numbers and lost to FU/excluded	Inclusion/exclusion criteria	Stage Distribution	Tumor/Obstruction Location & Histopathology	Patient Characteristics
	0	2. Central tumor growth < 2 cm to the trachea, main bronchus or esophagus 3. Prior chemotherapy		**Histopathology:** Lesions: 43 ACC: 9 (21%) SCC: 12 (28%) BAC: 5 (12%) NOS: 14 (33%) Mixed: 1 (2%)	NR **Comorbidities:** COPD: 24 (56%) Age (years)/CVD: 19 (44%) **Performance status:** ECOG 0: 29 (21%) 1: 9 (67%) 2: 5 (12%)
Shibamoto-2012, Japan, #4629	**Study design:** PRO, SAS **Patients enrolled:** Total: 180 (100%) Medically inoperable: 120 (67%) Refused surgery: 60 (33%) **Lost to FU/excluded/missing:** 0	**Inclusion criteria:** Histologically proven NSCLC stage 1 not suitable for surgery for medical or functional reasons **Exclusion criteria:** 1. Tumor > 5 cm in greatest dimension 2. WHO PS < 2 or PS 3 when not due to pulmonary disease 3. Active concurrent cancer 4. FEV1/FVC < 60% or percentage vital capacity < 75%	**Stage I:** 120 (100%)	**Location:** Not stated by operability **Histopathology:** Pathological confirmation: 120 (100%) Not stated by operability	**Age (years):** 77 (29-89) all cases **Women:** 57 (32%) all cases **Race:** NR **Comorbidities:** NR **Performance status:** WHO 0: 87 (48%) 1: 69 (38%) 2: 21 (12%) 3: 3 (2%) all cases
Song-2009, Korea, #3549	**Study design:** PRO, SAS **Patients enrolled:** Total: 32 (100%) Medically inoperable: 31 (97%) Refused surgery: 1 (3%) **Lost to FU/excluded/missing:** 0	**Inclusion criteria:** 1. Pathologically confirmed NSCLC 2. Primary clinical stage I NSCLC 3. Medically inoperable or refused surgery 4. Tumor < 5 cm in diameter 5. ECOG performance status < 2 **Exclusion criteria:** Recurrent or new primary lung cancer with prior history of lung	**Stage I:** 32 (100%)	**Location:** Peripheral: 23 (72%) Central: 9 (28%) **Histopathology:** SCC: 18 (56%) ACC: 11 (34%) NOS: 3 (9%)	**Age (years):** 72 (58-89) **Women:** 6 (19%) **Race:** NR **Comorbidities:** Poor lung function: 20 (62%) (Median FEV1: 1.06 L) Other medical problem: 7 (22%) Age (years) > 80 years: 4

Study	Study design, enrollment numbers and lost to FU/excluded	Inclusion/exclusion criteria	Stage Distribution	Tumor/Obstruction Location & Histopathology	Patient Characteristics
		cancer			(12%) **Performance status:** ECOG 1: 21 (66%) 2: 11 (34%)
Stephans-2009, USA, #3614	**Study design:** RET (registry) **Patients enrolled:** 86 (100%) **Lost to FU/excluded/missing:** 0	**Inclusion criteria:** 1. Primary clinical stage I NSCLC 2. Medically inoperable **Exclusion criteria:** NR	**Stage I patients:** 86 (100%) **Stage I lesions:** 94 (100%)	**Location:** NR **Histopathology:** SCC: 32 (34%) ACC: 15 (16%) PD/other: 14 (15%) No diagnosis: 33 (35%)	**Age (years):** 73 (40-90) **Women:** 48 (56%) **Race:** NR **Comorbidities:** Pulmonary: 69 (73%) Cardiac: 15 (16%) Other/multiple: 10 (11%) CHF: 41 (48%) **Performance status:** KPS: 80 (40-90)
Taremi-2011, Canada, #3732	**Study design:** PRO, SAS **Patients enrolled:** 108 (100%) **Lost to FU/excluded/missing:** 0	**Inclusion criteria:** 1. Primary clinical stage I NSCLC 2. Medically inoperable **Exclusion criteria:** NR	**Stage I:** 108 (100%)	**Location:** 114 lesions Right upper lobe: 38 (33%) Right middle lobe: 10 (9%) Right lower lobe: 18 (16%) Left upper lobe: 31 (27%) Left lower lobe: 17 (15%) **Histopathology:** Lesions: 114 ACC: 34 (30%) SCC: 22 (19%) LCC: 6 (5%) NOS: 19 (17%) Undiagnosed: 33 (29%)	**Age (years):** Mean 73 (48-90) years **Women:** 55 (51%) **Race:** NR **Comorbidities:** NR, medical inoperability assessed by an experienced thoracic surgeon and/or a multidisciplinary tumor board **Performance status:** NR

Study	Study design, enrollment numbers and lost to FU/excluded	Inclusion/exclusion criteria	Stage Distribution	Tumor/Obstruction Location & Histopathology	Patient Characteristics
Takeda-2009, Japan, #3700	**Study design:** RET, SAS **Patients enrolled:** Total: 63 (100%) Medically inoperable: 49 (78%) Refused surgery: 14 (22%) **Lost to FU/excluded/missing:** 0	**Inclusion criteria:** 1. Primary clinical stage I NSCLC 2. WHO performance status ≤ 2 **Exclusion criteria:** 1. Prior radiation to lung or mediastinum	Stage I: 63 (100%)	**Location:** NR **Histopathology:** Hst confirmed: 52 (82%) ACC: 35 (56%) SCC: 14: 22%) NOS: 3 (5%) Undiagnosed: 11 (18%)	**Age:** 78 (56-91) **Women:** 23 (36%) **Race:** NR **Co-morbidities:** COPD, advanced age, other illnesses: 49 (78%) **Performance status:** WHO ≤ 2: 63 (100%)
Turzer-2011, Norway, #3842	**Study design:** RET, SAS **Patients enrolled:** Total: 36 (100%) Medically inoperable: 35 (97%) Refused surgery: 1 (3%) **Lost to FU/excluded/missing:** 0	**Inclusion criteria:** 1. Pathologically confirmed NSCLC or PET positive pulmonary lesion with evidence of growth evaluated by at least 2 consecutive CT scans 2. Primary clinical stage I NSCLC 3. Medically inoperable or refused surgery 4. Tumor < 6 cm diameter 5. Tumor located > 2 cm from main bronchus 6. ECOG performance status 0-4 **Exclusion criteria:** NR	**Stage I:** 35 (100%) (Total of 38 Lesions)	**Location:** NR **Histopathology:** Hst confirmed: 28 lesions (74%) ACC: 17 (45%) SCC: 10 (26%) LCC: 1 (3%) Undiagnosed: 10 (26%)	**Age (years):** 74 (54-85) **Women:** 23 (64%) **Race:** NR **Comorbidities:** Median FEV1: 1.4 (0.4-4.5) CVD: 32 (89%) **Performance status:** ECOG: 0: 3 (8%) 1: 9 (25%) 2: 18 (50%) 3: 8 (22%)
Vahdat-2010, USA, #3864	**Study design:** PRO, SAS **Patients enrolled:** 20 (100%) **Lost to FU/excluded/missing:** 0	**Inclusion criteria:** 1. Hst confirmed primary clinical stage I NSCLC 2. Medically inoperable **Exclusion criteria:** 1. Pure BAC	Stage I: 20 (100%)	**Location:** NR **Histopathology:** ACC: 8 (40%) ACC: 5 (25%) NOS: 7 (35%)	**Age (years):** Mean 75 (64-86) **Women:** 16 (80%) **Race:** NR **Comorbidities:** Mean FEV1: 1.12 (0.53

Study	Study design, enrollment numbers and lost to FU/excluded	Inclusion/exclusion criteria	Stage Distribution	Tumor/Obstruction Location & Histopathology	Patient Characteristics
					2.48) FEV1 < 40% DLCO < 40% **Performance status:** NR
van der Voort van der Zyp-2009, Netherlands, #3885	**Study design:** SAS, unclear if PRO or RET **Patients enrolled:** Total: 70 (100%) Medically inoperable: 65 (93%) Refused surgery: 5 (7%) **Lost to FU/excluded/missing:** 0	**Inclusion criteria:** 1. Primary clinical stage I NSCLC 2. Medically inoperable or refused surgery 3. Peripheral tumor > 2 cm from trachea and main bronchus **Exclusion criteria:** NR	**Stage I:** 70 (100%)	**Location:** NR **Histopathology:** LCC: 16 (44%) SCC: 11 (31%) ACC: 7 (19%) NOS: 2 (6%) Unknown: 34 (49%)	**Age (years):** 76 (54-90) **Women:** NR **Race:** NR **Comorbidities:** CCI score: ≥4: 5 (7%) 3-4: 31 (44%) 1-2: 32 (46%) 0: 2 (3%) Median FEV1: 1.38 (0.81 3.81) **Performance status:** NR
Videtic-2010, USA, #3958	**Study design:** RET, SAS **Patients enrolled:** 26 (100%) **Lost to FU/excluded/missing:** 0	**Inclusion criteria:** 1. Primary clinical stage I NSCLC 2. Medically inoperable **Exclusion criteria:** NR	**Stage I:** 26 (100%)	**Location:** Peripheral: 25 (89%) Central: 3 (11%) **Histopathology:** Lesions: 28 NOS: 20 (71%)	**Age (years):** 74 (49-88) **Women:** 13 (50%) **Race:** NR **Comorbidities:** Median FEV1: 1.26 (0.62 2.41) Median Charlson score: 3 (0-8) Pulmonary: 20 (77%) Cardiac: 4 (15%) Multiple: 2 (8%) **Performance status:** Median KPS: 70 (40-100)

Values are presented as median (range) unless otherwise noted.

Appendix Table C2. Outcomes and interventions of studies that address Key Question 1

Study	Study Outcomes	Interventions
Andratschke 2011, #132	**Study Objective:** To report patterns of failure of SBRT in inoperable patients with histologically confirmed stage I NSCLC **Primary outcome:** NR **Definition:** NA **Secondary outcome(s):** NR **Definitions:** NA **List of Outcome(s):** OS, CSS, LCT, Toxicity **Cause of death:** Dead: 59 (64%) Dead due to LC: 25 (42%) Dead due to concurrent disease: 29 (49%) Cause of death NR: 5 (8%) **Length of FU:** 21 (3-87) months	**Intervention name:** SBRT **Vendor name:** NR **Dose/frequency/details:** Hypofractionated SBRT Total dose: 24-45 Gy to 60% isodose line of PTV in 3-5 frs for 5-12 days Total dose given at 60% isodose line (Gy): 37.5 (24-45) Dose given per fraction (Gy): 12.5 (5-15) No. of frs given: 3 (3-7) **Technical details:** None **Treatment Intention:** Curative **Follow-up and Evaluation Criteria:** • All time intervals were calculated from the last day of SBRT • During Rx, Patients monitored daily for acute Rx toxicity. Thereafter, follow-up visits at 4–6 weeks and 4, 7, and 12 months and then at 6 month intervals. • FU investigations included lung function test and CT thorax. • Acute toxicity: CTCAE v3.0 criteria during and up to 3 months after RT. • Late toxicity: RTOG/EORTC criteria.
Baumann-2006, #271	**Study Objective:** To review results of SBRT treatment of 138 Patients with medically inoperable stage I NSCLC treated during 1996 - 2003 at five different centers in Sweden and Denmark. **Primary outcome:** NR **Definition:** NA **Secondary outcome(s):** NR **Definitions:** NA **List of Outcomes:** LCT, OS, CSS, Toxicity **Cause of death:** Dead: 91 (66%)	**Intervention name:** SBRT **Vendor name:** NR **Dose/frequency/details:** 10 to 20 Gy X 2-4 frs given 2 to 3 days apart. Total dose: 30-48 Gy, 65% isodose at the periphery of PTV **Technical details:** 3D planning Linear accelerator delivered at 6-MV **Treatment Intention:** Curative **Follow-up and Evaluation Criteria:** • Response is based on CT-scans performed in a period of 0.5–89.3 months (median 16.3) post therapy, and should therefore be regarded as "best

Study	Study Outcomes	Interventions

Dead due to concurrent disease: 55 (60%)
Cause of death NR: 36 (40%)

response."
• Toxicity evaluated according to RTOC criteria

Length of FU:
33 (1-107) months

Baumann-2009, #270

Study Objective:
To evaluate the impact of COPD and CVD on Patients treated in this phase II study, subjective toxicity data were registered during follow-up and compared to the objective data of spirometry evaluations, CT-scans and dosimetric data (#269).

Intervention name:
SBRT

Vendor name:
NR

Dose/frequency/details:
15 Gy in 3 frs (total dose of 45 Gy) at the 67% isodose of the PTV. BED: 112 Gy. Rx was given every second day.

Technical details:
3DCT planning
Linear accelerator delivered at 6-MV

Treatment Intention:
Curative

Primary outcome:
Progression-free survival at 36 months
Definition:
NR

Secondary outcome(s):
LCT, OS, Toxicity
Definitions:
NR

Follow-up and Evaluation Criteria:
• Clinical, pulmonary and radiological evaluations- 6 weeks, 3, 6, 9, 12, 18, and 36 months post SBRT.
• Median FU time was calculated from date of registration to date of last visit
• Toxicity CTCAE version 2
• Radiation-related pulmonary fibrosis >90 days post-Rx, RTOG/EORTC Late Radiation Morbidity Scoring Scheme-Lung was used
• FEV1 was graded according to the GOLD criteria
• Early toxicity defined as ≤ 18 months. Late toxicity defined as > 18 months

Cause of death:
Dead: 27 (47%)
Dead due to LC: 7 (26%)
Dead due to concurrent disease: 18 (67%)
Cause of death unknown: 2 (7%)

Length of FU:
Median: 35 months (4-47)

Bogart-2010, #382

Study Objective:
To define the maximally accelerated course of conformal radiotherapy and to describe the short-term and long-term toxicity of therapy.

Intervention name:
3DRT

Vendor name:
NR

Dose/frequency/details:
Daily radiation fraction size was escalated and the number of frs reduced. Total nominal radiotherapy dose maintained at 70 Gy throughout each course. Treatment administered on consecutive weekdays.
Range N of frs: (17 – 29)
Range fraction size (Gy): (2.41-4.11)
Range N of weeks: (3.4 – 5.8)

Technical details:
3D planning

Primary outcome:
NR
Definition:
NA

Secondary outcome(s):
NR
Definitions:
NA

List of outcomes:
OS, LCT, Toxicity

Study	Study Outcomes	Interventions
	Cause of death: NA **Length of FU:** 53 (35-61) months	**Beam energy:** (4 -25) MV 83% treated with 6MV photons **Treatment Intention:** NR **Follow-up and Evaluation Criteria:** • Overall survival was defined as the time between protocol registration and death • Toxicity was assessed using the NCI CTC (version 2.0) • Patients were assessed weekly during therapy. Patients were assessed 3 weeks, 6 weeks, and 3 months after the completion of therapy, then at least every 3 months for 2 years, and then every 6 months for 3 years. • Evaluation by a thoracic surgeon (for suitability for lobectomy) was mandated if criteria for pulmonary dysfunction were not met,
Bollineni-2012, #4548	**Study Objective:** To investigate the prognostic value of FDG-PET uptake at 12 weeks after SBRT for stage I NSCLC **Primary outcome:** NR **Definition:** NA **Secondary outcome(s):** NR **Definitions:** NA **List of Outcome(s):** OS, CSS, LCT **Cause of death:** Dead: 29 (22%) Dead due to LC: 13 (45%) Dead due to concurrent disease: 16 (55%)	**Intervention name:** SBRT **Vendor name:** Novalis-BrainLAB system (Westchester, IL) **Dose/frequency/details:** Hypofractionated SBRT Total dose: 60 Gy to 90% isodose line of PTV in 3-8 frs for 5-12 days **Technical details:** 4-D CT planning **Treatment Intention:** Curative **Follow-up and Evaluation Criteria:** NR
Bradley-2003, #445	**Length of FU:** 17 (3-40) months **Study Objective:** To review the outcome for 56 Stage I non-small-cell lung cancer treated definitively with three dimensional conformal radiotherapy (3D-CRT) and to investigate the value of elective nodal irradiation in this patient population. **Primary outcome:** NR **Definition:** NA **Secondary outcome(s):** NR	**Intervention name:** 3DRT **Vendor name:** NR **Dose/frequency/details:** 60–69 Gy: 7 (13%) 70 Gy: 23 (42%) >70 Gy: 25 (45%) Median isocenter dose: 70 Gy (59.94 - 83.85), frs of 1.8 or 2 Gy, given 5 days weekly within 6 – 8 weeks.

Study	Study Outcomes	Interventions
		Twenty-two patients received RT directed to elective regional lymphatics in doses of 45–50 Gy
	Definitions: NA	**Technical details:** 3D planning
	List of outcomes: OS, LCT, Toxicity	**Treatment Intention:** Curative
	Cause of death: NA	**Follow-up and Evaluation Criteria:**
	Length of FU: 20 (6 – 72) months	• RTOG criteria used to evaluate toxicity grade 1-5 patients were followed at 3-month intervals for the first 2 years and at 6-month intervals thereafter. • Evaluations at the time of follow-up consisted of a history and physical examination. Chest radiographs were done at 3- or 6-month intervals for the first 2 years. CT scans of the chest were typically done 6 and 12 Months after treatment completion and thereafter only when clinically indicated. • Patients who had an initial radiographic response to treatment and a stable mass at each follow-up visit were considered to have local control. • Patients were considered to have local failure only if clinical, radiographic, or biopsy evidence of progression was observed
Burdick-2010, #521	**Study Objective:** To determine whether the pretreatment SUVmax from the staging FDG PET/CT could predict for mediastinal failure, distant metastases, and OS in medically inoperable patients treated with SBRT for early-stage NSCLC. To "define the maximal accelerated course of therapy"	**Intervention name:** SBRT
		Vendor name: Novalis-BrainLAB system (Westchester, IL)
	Primary outcome: NR	**Dose/frequency/details:** Total dose: 60 Gy (20 Gy X 3): 26 (36%) 50 Gy (10 Gy X 5): 40 (56%) 50 Gy (5 Gy X 10): 8 (11%)
	Definition: NA	
	Secondary outcome(s): NR	**Technical details:** 3D planning 6-MV photons
	Definitions: NA	**Treatment Intention:** NR
	List of outcomes: OS, LCT	**Follow-up and Evaluation Criteria:**
	Cause of death: Dead: 30 (42%) Dead due to LC: 13 (43%) Dead due to concurrent disease: 14 (47%) Causes of death unknown: 3 (10%)	• Patients were followed every 3 Months with clinical examination and CT scan of the chest. Pulmonary function testing was done at 6-month intervals. Post-treatment PET scans were only performed to evaluate possible recurrences and are not included in this analysis. • Local failure was dated from the initial CT abnormality. Local failure was defined as increasing lesion size on two consecutive CT scans, confirmed by serial PET imaging with or without positive biopsy for carcinoma.
	Length of FU: 16.9 (0.1 – 37.9) months	
Bush-2004, #535	**Study Objective:**	**Intervention name:**

Study	Study Outcomes	Interventions
	To determine the efficacy and toxicity of high-dose hypofractionated PBRT for Patients with clinical stage I lung cancer.	PBRT
		Vendor name: NR
	Primary outcome: NR	**Dose/frequency/details:** 51 CGE in 10 equally divided frs over 2-weeks: 22 (32%) 60 CGE in 10 frs over 2-weeks: 46 (68%)
	Definition: NA	
		Technical details: Hypofractionated 3D planning Linear accelerator delivered at 6-MV
	Secondary outcome(s): NR	
	Definitions: NA	**Treatment Intention:** NR
	List of Outcomes: CSS, LCT, OS, Acute Toxicity	**Follow-up and Evaluation Criteria:**
		• Patients received clinical evaluation every 3 months for the first year, then every 6 months, then annually after the fifth year.
	Cause of death: NR	• Chest CT scans to determine tumor status were done at 3-month intervals up to 1 year after treatment, then every 6 months, and annually after the fifth year of follow-up.
	Length of FU: Median: 30 months	• Patients were monitored weekly for acute toxicity during treatment.
Campeau-2009, #565	**Study Objective:** To review retrospectively disease control and survival in patients with Stage I NSCLC patients who were treated with chemoradiotherapy or RT between 2000 and 2005.	**Intervention name:** 3DRT
		Vendor name: NR
	Primary outcome: OS	**Dose/frequency/details:** 60 Gy X 30 frs over 6 weeks: 23 (68%) Hypofractionated dose: 50-55 Gy X 20 frs over 4 weeks: 11 (32%)
	Definition: OS was measured from treatment starting date to the date of death, regardless of the cause of death	The hypofractionated regimen was used only in cases in which the mediastinum and spinal cord were not included in the treatment volume.
		Technical details: ≥6-MV photons
	Secondary outcome(s): LCT, Distant LCT, and PFS	
	Definitions: NR for LCT	**Treatment Intention:** NR
	List of outcomes: OS, LCT	**Follow-up and Evaluation Criteria:**
		• Patients were seen every 3 months after completion of treatment for the first 2 years. The interval was usually increased to every 6 months provided there was no evidence of recurrence.
	Cause of death: NR	• Chest X-ray or CT scan of the chest and upper abdomen were performed before each visit in most cases. An F-18 FDG PET scan was performed in case of equivocal CT scan results
	Length of FU: NR	

Study	Study Outcomes	Interventions
		• Local progression of (LCT) was defined per the RECIST criteria • Local PFS was not censored by distant progression
Coon-2008, #803	**Study Objective:** To assess the outcomes of Patients treated with stereotactic body radiation therapy (SBRT) in Patients with primary, recurrent, or metastatic lung lesions, with a focus on positron emission tomography (PET)/computed tomography (CT)–based management. **Primary outcome:** NR **Definition:** NA **Secondary outcome(s):** NR **Definitions:** NA **List of Outcomes:** LCT, OS **Cause of death:** NR **Length of FU:** Median: 12 months	**Intervention name:** SBRT **Vendor name:** NR **Dose/frequency/details:** 60 Gy X 3 frs prescribed to the 80% isodose line **Technical details:** CyberKnife® Robotic Radiosurgery System with Synchrony™ Linear accelerator delivered at 6-MV **Treatment Intention:** NR **Follow-up and Evaluation Criteria:** • All Patients received regularly scheduled follow-up with planned CT or PET-CT imaging per standard protocol. • Local control was defined in our study as the lack of disease progression or reduction of standardized uptake value (SUV) at the site treated on follow-up imaging.
Dunlap-2010, #1032	**Study Objective:** The purpose of this study was to compare the outcomes and local control rates of Patients with peripheral T1 and T2 non–small-cell lung cancer treated with stereotactic body radiation therapy. **Primary outcome:** NR **Definition:** NA **Secondary outcome(s):** NR **Definitions:** NA **List of Outcomes:** LCT, OS, Toxicity **Cause of death:** No treatment related deaths occurred **Length of FU:** 12.5 (2-35) months	**Intervention name:** SBRT **Vendor name:** NR **Dose/frequency/details:** Median prescribed dose: 60 Gy (30-60 Gy) in 3 to 5 frs Median BED: 150 Gy (78-180 Gy) **Technical details:** 3D planning **Treatment Intention:** NR **Follow-up and Evaluation Criteria:** • After SBRT, followup was performed approximately 4 to 8 weeks after treatment and approximately every 3 months thereafter. CT of the chest was routinely obtained at 3-month intervals from the completion of radiotherapy. PET–CT was not routinely obtained before the initiation of therapy. • Toxicity was graded using CTCAE version 3.0 • Local tumor recurrence was defined as a 20% increase in the largest tumor

Study	Study Outcomes	Interventions
		diameter on successive follow-up imaging at 3-month intervals based on RECIST. • Local recurrences were demonstrated by an increase in abnormal FDG uptake required to correspond to an enlarging CT abnormality. • Follow-up was determined from the date of the final SBRT treatment. • Guidelines for inoperability were determined by the thoracic surgeon and typically included a predicted postoperative forced expiratory volume in 1 second of less than 30%, severely reduced diffusion capacity greater 40% predicted, a performance status of 3 or greater, or severe cardiac disease.
Fritz-2008, #1238	**Study Objective:** To review response rates, local control, survival and side effects after nonfractionated stereotactic high single-dose body radiation therapy for lung tumors. **Primary outcome:** NR **Definition:** NA **Secondary outcome(s):** NR **Definitions:** NA **List of Outcomes:** LCT, OS, Lung function, Toxicity **Cause of death:** Dead: 18 (45%) Dead due to LC: 13 (72%) Dead due to concurrent disease: 5 (28%) **Length of FU:** 20 (6-61.5) months	**Intervention name:** SBRT **Vendor name:** NR **Dose/frequency/details:** BED 90% isodose: 99.9 Gy **Technical details:** 4D Planning **Treatment Intention:** NR **Follow-up and Evaluation Criteria:** • All of the Patients were checked using high-resolution helical CT scans of the entire lung at 6 and 12 weeks after the single-dose radiation treatment. For all Patients further CT scan follow-up examinations then took place in 3-month intervals. • The follow-up periods for overall and lung cancer specific survival were defined as the time between irradiation and the last contact (censored) or death. No patient dropped out of follow-up. This means all Patients could be observed until the date of evaluation or the occurrence of an event. • RTOG criteria used to evaluate toxicity
Graham-2006, #1403	**Study Objective:** To review results of radical radiotherapy with 3DRT in Sydney to inform Patients contemplating treatment options for early stage NSCLC. **Primary outcome:** NR **Definition:** NA **Secondary outcome(s):** NR	**Intervention name:** 3DRT **Vendor name:** NR **Dose/frequency/details:** Prescribed dose: 65 Gy 35 frs using concurrent end-phase boost 5 weeks **Technical details:** 3D Planning Delivered: 45 Gy in 25 frs plus 20 Gy in 10 frs concurrently during the last 2

Study	Study Outcomes	Interventions

Study Outcomes column / Interventions column content:

Interventions:

weeks of treatment, with a 6-hour interfraction interval

Treatment Intention:
Curative

Follow-up and Evaluation Criteria:
NR

Iwata-2010, #1747

Study Outcomes

Definitions:
NA

List of outcomes:
OS, CSS, toxicity

Cause of death:
Dead: 22 (56%)
Dead due to LC: 12 (55%)
Dead due to concurrent disease: 10 (45%)

Length of FU:
Mean 40 (11-88) months

Study Objective: To analyzed the safety and efficacy of high-dose proton therapy and carbon-ion therapy applied to stage I NSCLC

Primary outcome: NR

Definition: NA

Secondary outcome(s): NR

Definitions: NA

List of Outcome(s): OS, DSS, Local control, Toxicity

Cause of death: NR

Length of FU: All patients observed for a minimum of 1.5 years or until death. Median duration of follow-up was 35.5 (18-66) months for living pts & 30.5 (4-66) months for all pts.

Interventions

Intervention name:
PBRT

Vendor name:
Synchrotron (Mitsubishi Electric Corporation, Kobe, Japan
3-D Rx planning system ((FOCUS-M, CMS, St. Louis, Mo and Mitsubishi Electric Corporation)

Dose/frequency/details:
PBRT 80Gy:
    20 fractions,
    BED 10(Gy): 112

PBRT 60 Gy:
    10 fractions
    BED 10(Gy): 96

Technical details: Pts were treated with 150-MeV proton beams

Treatment Intention: NR

Follow-up and Evaluation Criteria:
- After Rx, pts FU at 1.5, 3, 4.5, 6, 9, and 12 months during the 1st yr, at intervals of 3 months in the 2nd yr, and at 6-month intervals in the 3rd yr.
- CT, tumor marker, Brain MRI and FDG-PET were used to monitor tumor progression.
- Local responses was assessed according to the modified WHO response evaluation criteria.
- Toxicities were evaluated with the CTCAE version 3.0.
- Medically inoperability defined as pts with poor pulmonary function (vital capacity <75% or ratio of FEV 1 to forced vital capacity <60%), a history of major CVD, severe DM, advanced age (80 years old), or other debilitating conditions that preclude surgery.

Jimenez-2010, #1842

Study Objective:
To assess clinical outcomes of high-dose accelerated 3DRT in medically

Intervention name:
3DRT

Study	Study Outcomes	Interventions
	inoperable patients with primary stage I NSCLC	**Vendor name:** XiO treatment planning system, Computer Medical System, Inc. Linear accelerator: Elekta SL15, Elekta, Crawley, OK, or Siemens Oncor, Siemens Medical Solutions, Concord, CA
	Primary outcome: NR	
	Definition: NA	**Dose/frequency/details:** Individual dose-escalation scheme to maximal allowed total tumor dose of 79Gy in twice daily (BID) frs of 1.8 Gy with interfraction interval of at least 8 hours
	Secondary outcome(s): NR	
	Definition: NA	**Technical details:** 3D planning Beam energy NR
	List of outcomes: OS	**Treatment Intention:** Curative
	Cause of death: NR	**Follow-up and Evaluation Criteria:** • Survival status of the patients (alive or dead by any cause) was evaluated in July 2009 in both series of cases • Follow-up was done by the Pulmonologist and/or Radiation Oncologist according to the national guidelines. Survival was updated using the "Gemeentelijke Basis Administratie" system, a decentralized population registration system containing information about all inhabitants of The Netherlands. • During radiation treatment, patients were seen weekly by the Radiation Oncologist to treat the radiation-related complaints. (Details of complaints not specified)
	Length of FU: 36 months	
Kopek-2009, #2040	**Study Objective:** To determine the prognostic role of co-morbidity in medically inoperable patients with stage I NSCLC treated with SBRT	**Intervention name:** SBRT
	Primary outcome: NR	**Vendor name:** Treatment planning system: MDS_Nordion, Freiburg, GermanyHelax-TMS CadPlan Plus/Eclipse, Varian Medical Systems, Palo, Alto, CA
	Definition: NA	**Linear accelerator:** Siemens Primus, Siemens Medical Solutions, Concord, CA Varian Clinac 2100/2300
	Secondary outcome(s): NR	
	Definition: NA	**Dose/frequency/details:** Prescribed dose: 45 or 68 Gy to PTV 95% isodose line 3 frs 5-8 days
	List of outcomes: OS, CSS, LCT, toxicity	**Technical details:** Beam energy 6- or 8-MeV
	Cause of death: NR	**Treatment Intention:**

Study	Study Outcomes	Interventions
	Length of FU: 44 (2-96) months	Curative **Follow-up and Evaluation Criteria:** • Clinical FU and CT scan at 3, 6, 9, 12, 24 months then annually after SBRT • Toxicity assessed according to CTCAE v.3.0 criteria; Only deteriorations from baseline were registered as adverse events.
Mirri-2009, #2576	**Study Objective:** To report on the clinical outcome of hypofractionated conformal radiotherapy for medically inoperable stage I NSCLC < 5 cm in diameter **Primary outcome:** NR **Definition:** NA **Secondary outcome(s):** NR **Definition:** NA **List of outcomes:** OS, LCT, toxicity **Cause of death:** Dead: 7 (47%) **Length of FU:** 25 (4-46) months	**Intervention name:** 3DRT **Vendor name:** Treatment planning system: ECLIPSE.v.6.2, Varian Associates, Palo Alto, CA Pinnacle. V.7.4f, Philips Medical System, Best, Netherlands **Dose/frequency/details:** Prescribed dose: 40 Gy to the PTV 95% isodose line BED: 72 Gy 5 frs 2.5 weeks **Technical details:** Beam energy 6-MeV **Treatment Intention:** Curative
Nakayama-2010, #2684	**Study Objective:** To evaluate the role of PBT for Patients with medically inoperable stage I NSCLC **Primary outcome:** NR **Definition:** NA **Secondary outcome(s):** NR **Definition:** NA **List of outcomes:**	**Follow-up and Evaluation Criteria:** • CT scan at 4 months after 3DRT, then every 4 months thereafter • Acute toxicity assessed according to RTOG criteria Late toxicity assessed according to EORTC and CTCAE v.2.0 Data also evaluated by ECOG CTC criteria (both late and acute) **Intervention name:** PBT **Vendor name:** PROBEAT, Hitachi, Tokyo **Dose/frequency/details:** Central Lesions: 73 GyE in 22 frs: 17 (29%) Peripheral Lesions: 66 GyE in 10 frs: 41 (71%) BED: 1.1 **Technical details:** Beam energies 155-250 MeV **Treatment Intention:** Curative

Study	Study Outcomes	Interventions
	OS, LCT, toxicity	**Follow-up and Evaluation Criteria:** • Monthly at completion of PBT for 6 months • Chest CT every 3 months for 2 years after PBT Spirometry • Toxicity scored according to CTCAE v3.0 • The local control rate for 58 tumors was calculated to the date of tumor size increase of >20%. • Survival rates were calculated from the first day of treatment with PBT
	Cause of death: Dead due to LC: 0 Dead due to concurrent disease: 2 (4%) **Length of FU:** 18 (1.4-53) months	
Narayan-2004, #2686	**Study Objective:** To evaluate clinical outcomes of dose escalated 3DRT in medically inoperable patients with NSCLC	**Intervention name:** 3DRT
	Primary outcome: NR	**Vendor name:** NR
	Definition: NA	**Dose/frequency/details:** Prescribed dose: 92 (N=7 (54%)) or 103 Gy (N=6 (46%)) to PTV 95% isodose line 2.1 Gy fraction daily Once per day, 5 days per week
	Secondary outcome(s): NR	**Technical details:** Beamenergy NR
	Definition: NA	**Treatment Intention:** Curative
	List of outcomes: OS, CSS	**Follow-up and Evaluation Criteria:** • 1 month after 3DRT, every 3 months for 2 years, every 4 months for the third year, every 6 months for the next 2 years, then annually • Chest Xray every visit, CT scan every 6 months • Toxicity assessed according to SWOG criteria • Patients with disease visualized on bronchoscopy at diagnosis underwent repeat bronchoscopy at 6 months to evaluate local control. • Overall survival (OS) was calculated from the date of the initiation of radiation to the date of death or last follow-up • Deaths due to causes other than lung cancer were censored to determine cause specific survival (CSS)
	Cause of death: Dead: 12 (80%) Dead due to LC: 4 (33%) Dead due to concurrent disease: 8 (67%) **Length of FU:** NR	
Nyman-2006, #2750	**Study Objective:** To determine clinical outcomes with SBRT in the treatment of stage I NSCLC in medically inoperable patients	**Intervention name:** SBRT
	Primary outcome: NR	**Vendor name:** CadPlan Treatment Planning System, Varian
	Definition: NA	**Dose/frequency/details:** Prescribed dose: 45 Gy to the PTV 100% isodose line 3 frs 1 week
	Secondary outcome(s): NA	**Technical details:**

Study	Study Outcomes	Interventions
	Definition: NA **List of outcomes:** OS, CSS, toxicity **Cause of death:** Dead: 24 (53%) Dead due to LC: 15 (62%) Dead due to concurrent disease: 9 (38%) **Length of FU:** 43 (24-74) months	6-MeV beam energy **Treatment Intention:** Curative **Follow-up and Evaluation Criteria:** • 6 weeks, 3 months, 6 months, every 6 months thereafter • Physical exam, performance status, toxicity assessed • CT scan at all time points except 6 weeks • Acute and late toxicity assessed according to EORTC/RTOG scoring system. The acute toxicity was registered during treatment or at the 6-week follow-up visit. • Nine patients who died without tumor progression or metastases were censored at the time of deaths.
Olsen-2011, #2792	**Study Objective:** To compare the efficacy of three lung SBRT regimens in a large institutional cohort **Primary outcome:** NR **Definition:** NA **Secondary outcome(s):** NR **Definition:** NA **List of outcomes:** OS, LCT, toxicity **Cause of death:** NR **Length of FU:** Median: 11, 13, 16 months for 3 dose groups	**Intervention name:** SBRT **Vendor name:** Pinnacle3 treatment planning system, Philips Medical **Dose/frequency/details:** Three prescribed dose regimens: Peripheral: 18 Gy X 3 frs = 54 Gy (N=111), Central: 9 Gy X 5 frs = 45 Gy (N=8) OR 10 Gy X 5 frs = 50 Gy (N=11) 5 Patients received: 5 frs at incremental doses of 9, 10, 11, and 12 Gy 9 Patients received: 9-10 Gy X 5 frs **Technical details:** 4D Planning 6-MV photons 8–11 beams **Treatment Intention:** Curative **Follow-up and Evaluation Criteria:** • Duration NR • CT imaging and physician visits • Toxicity scored according to CTCAE v.3.0
Palma 2012, #2843	**Study Objective:** To evaluate outcomes after SBRT in Patients with severe COPD **Primary outcome:** NR	**Intervention name:** SBRT **Vendor name:** Brainscan v.5.2 treatment planning system, BrainLab, Feldkirchen, Germany

Study	Study Outcomes	Interventions
		RapidArc linear accelerator, Varian, Palo Alto, CA
	Definition: NA	**Dose/frequency/details:** Prescribed dose: BrainLab:3 x 20 Gy, 5 x 12 Gy, or 8 x 7.5 Gy RapdArc: 3 x 18 Gy, 5 x 11 Gy, or 8 x 7.5 Gy
	Secondary outcome(s): NR	80% PTV isodose line
	Definitions: NA	**Technical details:** 6-MV photons 8–12 noncoplanar static beams
	List of outcomes: OS, LCT, toxicity	**Treatment Intention:** Curative
	Cause of death: Total: 62 (35%) Cause NR	**Follow-up and Evaluation Criteria:** • Outpatient assessments at 3-6 month intervals post-SBRT • Diagnostic CT scan at each visit • Toxicity assessed according to CTCAE v.3.0 • Late toxicity defined as >6 weeks after treatment
	Length of FU: Median: 21 months	
Pennathur-2007, #2896	**Study Objective:** To evaluate CT-guided RFA as an alternative treatment option for high-risk medically inoperable patients with stage I NSCLC	**Intervention name:** RFA
	Primary outcome: NR	**Vendor name:** Generator: RF3000, Boston Scientific, Boston, MA RITA Starburst XL, RITA Medical Systems
	Definition: NA	Needle electrodes: LeVeen, Radiotherapeutics Corporation, Sunnyvale, CA Starburst XL, RITA Medial Systems
	Secondary outcome(s): NR	**Dose/frequency/details:** RF3000: power 5-10W increments until system impedance > 400 ohm RITA: power 35-50 W, target temperature 90 degrees C
	Definition: NA	**Technical details:** With both systems, electrode was repositioned as many times as needed to encompass the target tissue and a small rim of about 0.5-1.0 cm nondiseased tissue
	List of outcomes: OS, complications	**Treatment Intention:** Curative
	Cause of death: Dead: 6 (33%) Dead due to LC: 3 (50%) Dead due to concurrent disease: 2 (33%) Causes of death unknown: 1 (17%)	**Follow-up and Evaluation Criteria:** • 3-month intervals
	Length of FU:	

Study	Study Outcomes	Interventions
	28 (9-52) months	• Clinical examination, CT and selective FDG PET scans • Modified RECIST criteria were used to assess initial response to treatment at 3 to 5 months • The time to progression was calculated from the treatment date.
Pennathur-2009, #2898	**Study Objective:** To determine the outcomes of SRS in the treatment of stage I NSCLC.	**Intervention name:** SBRT
	Primary outcome: NR	**Vendor name:** Cyberknife, Accuray, Sunnyvale, CA
	Definition: NA	**Dose/frequency/details:** Hypofractionated Prescribed dose: 20-60 Gy to the 80% PTV isodose line BED: 60-70 Gy 1-3 frs
	Secondary outcome(s): NR	
	Definition: NA	**Technical details:** 6-MeV beam energy
	List of outcomes: OS, complications	**Treatment Intention:** Curative
	Cause of death: Total: 10 (48%) cause not specified	**Follow-up and Evaluation Criteria:** • 3-month intervals with CT and FDG PET scans • Modified RECIST criteria were used to assess initial response to treatment at 3 months • The time to progression was calculated from the treatment date after censoring data from patients who died without progression.
	Length of FU: 21 (12-43) months	
Ricardi-2010, #3098	**Study Objective:** To evaluate clinical outcomes and toxicity of SBRT in Patients with stage I NSCLC who were medically inoperable or refused surgery	**Intervention name:** SBRT
	Primary outcome: LCT	**Vendor name:** Oncentra OTP 3D treatment planning system, Nucletron, Netherlands Elekta Precise linear accelerator, Elekta, Netherlands
	Definition: LCT defined as absence of local failure, diagnosed as tumor growth or re-growth after initial shrinkage	**Dose/frequency/details:** Prescribed dose: (15 Gy x3) 45 Gy to 80% PTV isodose line BED: 124 Gy 3 frs 1 week
	Secondary outcome(s): OS, CSS, toxicity	**Technical details:** 6-10 MV photons 6-8 noncoplanar static beams Average time for a single session was approximately 45 min
	Definitions: OS defined as death from any cause after SBRT CSS defined as death due to cancer after SBRT	**Treatment Intention:** Curative
	List of outcomes:	

Study	Study Outcomes	Interventions
	OS, CSS, LCT, toxicity	**Follow-up and Evaluation Criteria:**
	Cause of death: Dead: 20 (32%) Dead due to LC: 12 (60%) Dead due to concurrent disease: 8 (40%)	• 6 weeks, then every 3 months after SBRT • Clinical examination and CT scans • Acute and late toxicity assessed according to RTOG criteria • Late toxicity defined as: events occurring after day 90 • Acute toxicity defined as: events occurring between day 1 and day 90 from the start of radiation treatment
	Length of FU: 28 (9-61) months	• RECIST criteria used to evaluate tumor response • Local tumor control was defined as absence of local failure, diagnosed as tumor growth or re-growth after initial shrinkage.
		Overall survival started from time of SBRT until death from any cause
Scorsetti-2007, #3362	**Study Objective:** To determine clinical outcomes with SBRT in the treatment of stage I NSCLC in medically inoperable patients	**Intervention name:** SBRT
	Primary outcome: NR	**Vendor name:** Ergo TPS treatment planning system
	Definition: NA	**Dose/frequency/details:** Prescribed dose: 20-32 Gy BED: 40-117 Gy 7-10 Gy per fraction 2-4 frs
	Secondary outcome(s): NR	
	Definition: NA	**Technical details:** Beam strength NR
	List of outcomes: OS, LCT, toxicity	**Treatment Intention:** Curative
		Follow-up and Evaluation Criteria:
	Cause of death: Dead: 10 (23%) Dead due to LC: 2 (20%) Dead due to concurrent disease: 8 (80%)	• 45 days, then every 3 months after SBRT • CT scans, spirometry • Toxicity assessed according to RTOG/EORTC criteria • 3 months= acute toxicity after radiotherapy and after 3 months =late toxicity. • Local progression defined as: increase of tumor volume of more than 25% in volume in CT scan and/or increased uptake in PET
	Length of FU: 14 (6-36) months	
Shibamoto -2012, #4629	**Study Objective:** To report a multi-institutional study of SBRT in inoperable and operable patients with histologically confirmed stage I NSCLC	**Intervention name:** SBRT
	Primary outcome: LC at 3-years follow-up	**Vendor name:** Novalis image-guided system (Varian Medical Systems, Palo Alto, CA) CLINAC 23EX or 21 EXS (Varian)
	Definition: Calculated from the start of SBRT	
	Secondary outcome(s): OS, CSS	Eclipse v.7.5.14.3 (Varian)

Study	Study Outcomes	Interventions
	Definitions: Calculated from the start of SBRT	BRAINSCAN v.5.31 (BrainLAB, Feldkirchen, Germany) Pinnacle3 (Philips, Madison, WI)
	List of Outcome(s): OS, CSS, LCT, Toxicity	**Dose/frequency/details:** Hypofractionated SBRT Total dose: 44-52 Gy to 90% of the isodose line of PTV in 4 frs for 9-21 days
	Cause of death: Dead: 65 (36%) NR by operability	**Technical details:** 6-MV photons
		Treatment Intention: Curative
	Length of FU: 36 months NR by operability	**Follow-up and Evaluation Criteria:** • All time intervals were calculated from the start of SBRT • CT scans of chest and upper abdomen at 2-months intervals up to 6 months, every 2-4 months thereafter • Toxicity: CTCAE v3.0 criteria during and up to 3 months after RT
Song-2009, #3549	**Study Objective:** To evaluate clinical outcomes and toxicity of SBRT as treatment for Patients with primary Stage I NSCLC adjacent to central large bronchus and who are medically inoperable or refuse surgery	**Intervention name:** SBRT
	Primary outcome: NR	**Vendor name:** Render 3-D treatment planning system, Elekta Oncology, Netherlands Eclipse treatment planning system, Varian USA
	Definition: NA	**Dose/frequency/details:** Prescribed dose: 40-60 Gy to 85% PTV isodose line 3-4 frs 10-20 Gy per fraction 3-4 consecutive days
	Secondary outcome(s): NR	
	Definitions: NA	**Technical details:** 3D Planning Beam energy NR
	List of outcomes: OS, LCT, toxicity	**Treatment Intention:** Curative
	Cause of death: NR	**Follow-up and Evaluation Criteria:** • 1, 6, 12 months after SBRT • Chest CT • Pulmonary toxicity scored by NCI-CTC v. 2.0 • Local tumor control was defined as a tumor response of stable disease (SD) or better. • Radiation-induced bronchial stricture was initially determined on scheduled follow-up CT scans or simple Chest X-ray by narrowing of bronchus or secondary collapsed lung parenchyma. Some Patients were observed with only follow-up CT scans without additional examination if the radiation-induced stricture was stable.
	Length of FU: 26 (5-92) months	

Study	Study Outcomes	Interventions
Stephans-2009, #3614	**Study Objective:** To assess the impact of fractionation upon tumor control and toxicity in medically inoperable early stage lung cancer patients treated with SBRT **Primary outcome:** NR **Definition:** NA **Secondary outcome(s):** NR **Definition:** NA **List of outcomes:** OS, LCT, toxicity **Cause of death:** Dead: 25 (29%) **Length of FU:** 15 (2-48) months	**Intervention name:** SBRT **Vendor name:** BrainScan 5.31 treatment planning system, BrainLAB, Feldkirchen, Germany Novalis linear accelerator, BrainLAB **Dose/frequency/details:** Two fractionation schemes: 60 Gy to 81-90% isodose line 3 frs 8-14 days 50 Gy to 97-100% isodose line 5 frs 5 days **Technical details:** 6-MeV beam energy **Treatment Intention:** Curative **Follow-up and Evaluation Criteria:** • 6-8 weeks after SBRT, every 3 months thereafter with CT and pulmonary function test twice annually • Toxicity assessed according to CTCAE v.3.0
Taremi-2011, #3732	**Study Objective:** To present the results of SBRT for medically inoperable patients with stage I NSCLC and contrast outcomes in patients with and without a pathologic diagnosis **Primary outcome:** NR **Definition:** NA **Secondary outcome(s):** NR **Definition:** NA **List of outcomes:**	**Intervention name:** SBRT **Vendor name:** Pinnacle treatment planning system, Philips, Madison, WI Linear accelerator NR **Dose/frequency/details:** Prescribed dose: 48-60 Gy to the PTV 90% isodose line 3-10 frs Daily fractionation for some regimens, duration NR for all regimens **Technical details:** Beam energy NR **Treatment Intention:** Curative

Study	Study Outcomes	Interventions
	OS, CSS, LCT, toxicity	**Follow-up and Evaluation Criteria:**
		• 6 weeks after SBRT, then every 3 months for first year, every 6 months in second year, annually thereafter
		• FDG PET at 3 months after SBRT
		• CT at 6 and 12 months after SBRT, every 6-12 months thereafter
	Cause of death:	• CTCAE v 3.0
	Dead: 45 (42%)	
	Dead due to LC: 17 (38%)	
	Dead due to concurrent disease: 28 (62%)	
	Length of FU:	
	19 (1-56) months	
Takeda-2009, #3700	**Study Objective:** To analyze clinical outcomes of SBRT for patients with stages IA and IB NSCLC	**Intervention name:** SBRT
	Primary outcome: NR	**Vendor name:** XiO treatment planning system, V.4.2 or v.4.3, CMS, St. Louis, MO
		Linear accelerator NR
	Definition: NA	**Dose/frequency/details:** Prescribed dose: 50 Gy to the 80% isodose line
	Secondary outcome(s): NR	10 Gy per fraction
		5 fractions
	Definitions: NA	**Technical details:** Beam energy NR
	List of outcomes: OS, CSS, LCT, toxicity	**Treatment Intention:** Curative
	Cause of death: NR	**Follow-up and Evaluation Criteria:** • Monthly for first 6 mos, with chest X-ray
		• CT scans at 1 and 3 mos after SBRT, then at 3-mos intervals during first 2 years
	Length of FU: 31 (10-72) mos	• FU interviews and CT scans at 4-6 mos intervals after 2 years
		• Toxicity assessed according to CTCAE v.3.0
Turzer-2011, #3842	**Study Objective:** To assess SBRT results and toxicity for stage I NSCLC Patients with low performance status and severe comorbidity	**Intervention name:** SBRT
	Primary outcome: NR	**Vendor name:** Elekta Synergy linear accelerator, Elekta AB
	Definition: NA	**Dose/frequency/details:** Prescribed dose: 45 Gy to PTV 100% isodose line
		3 frs
	Secondary outcome(s): NR	1 week
		Technical details: Beam energy NR
	Definitions: NA	**Treatment Intention:**

Study	Study Outcomes	Interventions
		Curative
	List of outcomes: OS, LCT, toxicity	**Follow-up and Evaluation Criteria:** • 6 weeks, 3, 6 months after SBRT. Every 6 months thereafter • Physical examination and chest CT every visit, FDG PET twice annually • Toxicity assessed according to CTCAE v.3.0 criteria
	Cause of death: Dead: 1 (3%)	
	Length of FU: 14 (0-21) months	
Vahdat-2010, #3864	**Study Objective:** To report serial FGD PET/CT tumor response following Cyberknife radiosurgery for stage IA NSCLC in inoperable patients	**Intervention name:** SBRT
		Vendor name: Cyberknife, Accuray
	Primary outcome: NR	**Dose/frequency/details:** Prescribed dose: 42-60 Gy to PTV 95% isodose line 3 frs
	Definition: NA	**Technical details:** Beam energy NR
	Secondary outcome(s): NR **Definition:** NA	**Treatment Intention:** Curative
	List of outcomes: OS, LCT	**Follow-up and Evaluation Criteria:** • FDG PET at 3-6, 9-15, 18-24 months after SBRT
	Cause of death: Dead: 3 (15%) Dead due to concurrent disease: 3 (100%)	
	Length of FU: 43 months	
van der Voort van Zyp-2009, #3885	**Study Objective:** To report the clinical outcome of treatment using real-time tumor tracking for 70 Patients with inoperable stage I NSCLC	**Intervention name:** SBRT
		Vendor name: On Target treatment planning system, v.3.4.1, Accuray, Sunnyvale, CA Cyberknife Synchrony RTS linear accelerator, Accuray
	Primary outcome: LCT, OS, CSS	**Dose/frequency/details:** Prescribed dose: 36-60 Gy to the PTV 70-85% isodose line 3 frs Duration NR
	Definition: LCT: Calculated from first day of treatment until diagnosis of local recurrence OS: measured from start of SBRT until death from any cause CSS: measured from start of SBRT until death from lung cancer	**Technical details:** Beam energy NR
	Secondary outcome(s): NR	**Treatment Intention:**

Study	Study Outcomes	Interventions
	Definitions: NA	Curative
		Follow-up and Evaluation Criteria: • Clinical examination and chest CT 3 weeks, 2-3, 6, 9, 12, 18, 24, 30 months thereafter • Toxicity assessed according to CTCAE v.3.0 criteria • Toxicity was acute if it occurred within 4 months and late if it occurred thereafter
	List of outcomes: OS, CSS, LCT	
	Cause of death: Dead: 19 (27%) Dead due to LC: 6 (32%) Dead due to concurrent disease: 13: (68%)	
	Length of FU: Median 15 months	
Videtic-2010, #3958	**Study Objective:** To validate the use of SBRT using IMRT beams for medically inoperable stage I NSCLC	**Intervention name:** SBRT with IMRT beams
		Vendor name: Novalis-BrainLAB treatment system
	Primary outcome: OS, LCT	**Dose/frequency/details:** Prescribed dose: 50 Gy to the 95% isodose line 5 frs 5 days
	Definition: Measured from time of diagnosis until death or last patient contact	
	Secondary outcome(s): NR	**Technical details:** Beam energy NR
	Definition: NA	**Treatment Intention:** Curative
	List of outcomes: OS, LCT, toxicity	**Follow-up and Evaluation Criteria:** • Initially 6-8 weeks after SBRT, every 3 months for 2 years thereafter • Chest CT scan at each visit with same-day pulmonary function test twice annually • Toxicity assessed according to CTCAE v.3.0 criteria
	Cause of death: Dead: 14 (54%) Dead due to LC: 8 (57%) Dead due to concurrent disease: 6 (43%)	
	Length of FU: 31 (10-51) months	

Appendix Table C3. Survival and local control outcomes of studies that address Key Question 1

Study	Survival Outcomes for Intervention Group 1	Survival Outcomes for Intervention Group 2	Local Control Outcomes for Intervention Group 1	Local Control Outcomes for Intervention Group 2	Arm
Andratschke 2011, #132	SBRT: **Overall survival:** Median 29 months 1-year: 79% 3-years: 38% 5-years: 17% **Cancer/disease specific survival:** Median 46 months 1-year: 93% 3-years: 64% 5-years: 48%	**Overall survival:** NA **Cancer/disease specific survival:** NA	SBRT **Local control:** 1-year: 89% 3-years: 83% 5-years: 83%	**Local control:** NA	No
Baumann 2006, #271	SBRT **Overall survival:** 3-year: 52% 5-year: 26% **Cancer/disease specific survival:** 3-year: 66% 5-year: 40%	**Overall survival:** NA **Cancer/disease specific survival:** NA	SBRT **Local control:** 88% Time to failure: 17.8 (10-49) months	**Local control:** NA	No
Baumann 2009, #270	SBRT **Overall survival:** Median: 40.6 months 1-year: 68% 2-years:65% 3-years:60% **Cancer/disease specific survival:** 1-year: 93% 2-years:88% 3-years:88%	**Overall survival:** NA **Cancer/disease specific survival:** NA	SBRT **Local control:** 3-years: 92%	**Local control:** NA	No
Bogart-2010, #382	3DRT **Overall survival:** Median: 38.5 months (95% CI: 22.4 to 58.7) **Cancer/disease specific survival:** NR	**Overall survival:** NA **Cancer/disease specific survival:** NA	3DRT **Local control:** 93%	**Local control:** NA	No
Bollineni-2012, #4548	SBRT: **Overall survival:**	**Overall survival:** NA	SBRT **Local control:**	**Local control:** NA	No

C-36

Study	Survival Outcomes for Intervention Group 1	Survival Outcomes for Intervention Group 2	Local Control Outcomes for Intervention Group 1	Local Control Outcomes for Intervention Group 2	Arm
	Median NR 2-years high SUV: 62% 2-years low SUV: 81% **Cancer/disease specific survival:** Median NR 2-years high SUV: 74% 2-years low SUV: 90%		2-years: 96%		
Bradley-2003, #445	3DRT **Overall survival:** 1-year: 73% 2-year: 51% 3-year: 34% **Cancer/disease specific survival:** 1-year: 82% 2-year: 67% 3-year: 51%	3DRT **Overall survival:** NA **Cancer/disease specific survival:** NA	3DRT **Local control:** 1-year: 88% 2-year: 69% 3-year: 63%	**Local control:** NA	No
Burdick-2010, #521	SBRT **Overall survival:** 2-year: 33% (95% CI: 18%-51%) **Cancer/disease specific survival:** NR	SBRT **Overall survival:** NA **Cancer/disease specific survival:** NA	SBRT **Local control:** 2-year: 94%	**Local control:** NA	No
Bush-2004, #535	PBRT **Overall survival:** Total 3-year: 44% Rx 51 CGE, 3-year: 27% Rx: 60 CGE, 3-year: 55% (p=0.03) **Cancer/disease specific survival:** 3-year: 72%	PBRT **Overall survival:** NA **Cancer/disease specific survival:** NA	PBRT **Local control:** 3-year:74%	**Local control:** NA	No
Campeau 2009, #565	3DRT **Overall survival:** 2-year: 61.3% **Cancer/disease specific survival:** NR	3DRT **Overall survival:** NA **Cancer/disease specific survival:** NA	3DRT **Local control:** 2-year: 85%	**Local control:** NA	No
Coon-2008, #803	SBRT **Overall survival:**	SBRT **Overall survival:** NA	SBRT **Local control:**	**Local control:** NA	No

Study	Survival Outcomes for Intervention Group 1	Survival Outcomes for Intervention Group 2	Local Control Outcomes for Intervention Group 1	Local Control Outcomes for Intervention Group 2	Arm
	11 months: 81% Cancer/disease specific survival: NR	Cancer/disease specific survival: NA	11 months: 85%		
Dunlap-2010, #1032	SBRT **Overall survival:** Median: 20.1 months (95% CI: 18.7-28.4) 1-year: 85% 2-year:45% **Cancer/disease specific survival:** 3-year: 82%	SBRT **Overall survival:** NA **Cancer/disease specific survival:** NA	SBRT **Local control:** 2-year: 83% Stage IA, 2-years:90% Stage IB, 2-years: 70% (p=0.035)	**Local control:** NA	No
Fritz-2008, #1238	SBRT **Overall survival:** Median:37 months 2-year: 66% 3-year:53% **Cancer/disease specific survival:** 2-year:71% 3-year:57%	**Overall survival:** NA **Cancer/disease specific survival:** NA	SBRT **Local control:** 3-year: 81%	**Local control:** NA	No
Graham-2006, #1403	3DRT **Overall survival:** Median 43 months 5-years: 30% (95% CI: 13-48%) **Cancer/disease specific survival:** 5-years: 53% (95% CI: 28-72%)	**Overall survival:** NA **Cancer/disease specific survival:** NA	3DRT **Local control:** NA	**Local control:** NA	No
Iwata-2010, # 1747	**Overall survival:** 3-years: 65% **Cancer/disease specific survival:** NR	**Overall survival:** NA **Cancer/disease specific survival:** NA	**Local control:** NR	**Local control:** NA	Yes
Jimenez-2010, #1842	3DRT **Overall survival:** 3-years: 44% (95% CI: 28-58%) **Cancer/disease specific survival:** NR	3DRT **Overall survival:** NA **Cancer/disease specific survival:** NA	3DRT **Local control:** NR	**Local control:** NA	No

Study	Survival Outcomes for Intervention Group 1	Survival Outcomes for Intervention Group 2	Local Control Outcomes for Intervention Group 1	Local Control Outcomes for Intervention Group 2	Arm
Kopek-2009, #2040	SBRT **Overall survival:** Median 22 months 1-year: 67% 2-years: 49% 3-years: 36% 4-years: 24% 5-years: 21% **Cancer/disease specific survival:** Median 61 months	SBRT **Overall survival:** NA **Cancer/disease specific survival:** NA	SBRT **Local control:** 4-years: 89%	**Local control:** NA	No
Mirri-2009, #2576	3DRT **Overall survival:** 1-year: 81% 3-years: 61% **Cancer/disease specific survival:** NR	3DRT **Overall survival:** NA **Cancer/disease specific survival:** NA	3DRT **Local control:** 1-year: 88% 3-years: 72%	**Local control:** NA	No
Nakayama 2010, #2684	PBRT **Overall survival:** 2-years: 98% (95% CI, 94-102%) **Cancer/disease specific survival:** 2-years: 100%	PBRT **Overall survival:** NA **Cancer/disease specific survival:** NA	PBRT **Local control:** 2-years: 97% (95% CI, 91-103%)	**Local control:** NA	No
Narayan-2004, #2686	3DRT **Overall survival:** 2-years: 54% 3-years: 33% **Cancer/disease specific survival:** 2-years: 76% 3-years: 48%	3DRT **Overall survival:** NA **Cancer/disease specific survival:** NA	3DRT **Local control:** 77%	**Local control:** NA	No
Nyman-2006, #2750	SBRT **Overall survival:** Median: 39 months 1-year: 80% 2-years: 71% 3-years: 55% 5-years: 30% **Cancer/disease specific survival:** Median: 55 months 1-year: 88%	SBRT **Overall survival:** NA **Cancer/disease specific survival:** NA	SBRT **Local control:** 80%	**Local control:** NA	No

Study	Survival Outcomes for Intervention Group 1	Survival Outcomes for Intervention Group 2	Local Control Outcomes for Intervention Group 1	Local Control Outcomes for Intervention Group 2	Arm
Olsen-2011, #2792	2-years: 83% 3-years: 67% 5-years: 41% SBRT **Overall survival:** Median overall : 14 months (not reached) Median 34 months for each dose group **Cancer/disease specific survival:** NR	**Overall survival:** NA **Cancer/disease specific survival:** NA	SBRT **Local control:** 45 Gy: 1-year: 75% 2-years: 50% 50 Gy: 1-year: 100% 2-years: 100% 54 Gy: 1-year: 99% 2-years: 91%	**Local control:** NA	No
Palma 2012, #2843	SBRT **Overall survival:** Median: 32 months 1-year: 79% 3-years: 47% 5-years: 28% **Cancer/disease specific survival:** NR	**Overall survival:** NA **Cancer/disease specific survival:** NA	SBRT **Local control:** 3-years: 89%	**Local control:** NA	No
Pennathur 2007, #2896	RFA **Overall survival:** Median not reached Probability at 1-year: 95% (95% CI, 85-100%) Probability at 2-years: 68% (95% CI, 49-96%) **Cancer/disease specific survival:** NR	**Overall survival:** NA **Cancer/disease specific survival:** NA	RFA **Local control:** 58%	**Local control:** NA	No
Pennathur 2009, #2898	SBRT **Overall survival:** Median 26.4 (68% CI, 19.6-not reached) months 1-year: 81% (68% CI, 73-90%) **Cancer/disease specific survival:** NR	**Overall survival:** NA **Cancer/disease specific survival:** NA	SBRT **Local control:** 58%	**Local control:** NA	No
Ricardi-2010, #3098	SBRT **Overall survival:** Median not reached	**Overall survival:** NA	SBRT **Local control:** 3-years: 88%	**Local control:** NA	No

Study	Survival Outcomes for Intervention Group 1	Survival Outcomes for Intervention Group 2	Local Control Outcomes for Intervention Group 1	Local Control Outcomes for Intervention Group 2	Arm
	2-years: 69% 3-years: 57% **Cancer/disease specific survival:** 2-years: 79% 3-years: 72%	**Cancer/disease specific survival:** NA			
Scorsetti-2007, Italy, #3362	SBRT **Overall survival:** 1-year: 93±5% 2-years: 53±11% **Cancer/disease specific survival:** NR	**Overall survival:** NA **Cancer/disease specific survival:** NA	SBRT **Local control:** NR	**Local control:** NA	No
Shibamoto 2012, #4629	SBRT: **Overall survival:** Median ~52 months 3-years: 59% 5-years: 44% **Cancer/disease specific survival:** NR by operability	**Overall survival:** NA **Cancer/disease specific survival:** NA	SBRT **Local control:** NR by operability	**Local control:** NA	No
Song-2009, #3549	SBRT **Overall survival:** 1-year: 71% 2-years: 38% **Cancer/disease specific survival:** NR	**Overall survival:** NA **Cancer/disease specific survival:** NA	SBRT **Local control:** 1-year: 85% 2-years: 85%	**Local control:** NA	No
Stephans 2009, #3614	SBRT **Overall survival:** 1-year: 81% (all patients) 1.5-years: 75% (all patients) 1-year: 83% (50 Gy) 1-year: 77% (60 Gy) **Cancer/disease specific survival:** NR	**Overall survival:** NA **Cancer/disease specific survival:** NA	SBRT **Local control:** 6-months:100% (all patients) 1-year: 98% (all patients) 1.5-years: 95% (all patients) 1-year: 97% (50 Gy) 1-year: 100% (60 Gy)	**Local control:** NA	No
Taremi-2011, Canada, #3732	SBRT **Overall survival:**	**Overall survival:** NA	SBRT **Local control:**	**Local control:** NA	No

Study	Survival Outcomes for Intervention Group 1	Survival Outcomes for Intervention Group 2	Local Control Outcomes for Intervention Group 1	Local Control Outcomes for Intervention Group 2	Arm
	All patients 1-year: 84% (95% CI, 76-90%) 4-years: 30% (95% CI, 15-46%) Cancer/disease specific survival: All patients 1-year: 92% (95% CI, 87-98%) 4-years: 77% (95% CI, 64-89%)	Cancer/disease specific survival: NA	All patients 1-year: 92% (95% CI, 86-97%) 4-years: 89% (95% CI, 81-96%) Biopsy-proven 1-year: 93% (95% CI, 87-98%) Nonbiopsy-proven 1-year: 87% (95% CI, 76-99%) p = 0.41 versus biopsy-proven		
Takeda-2009, #3700	SBRT Overall survival: 3-years: 90% (stage IA) 3-years: 63% (stage IB) p = 0.09 3-years: 77% (inoperable) p = 0.31 Cancer/disease specific survival: 3-years: 100% (stage IA) 3-years: 81% (stage IB) p = 0.10 3-years: 94% (inoperable) p = 0.66	SBRT Overall survival: NA Cancer/disease specific survival: NA	SBRT Local control: 3-years: 93% (stage IA) 3-years: 96% (stage IB) p = 0.86	Local control: NA	No
Turzer-2011, #3842	SBRT Overall survival: 97% (calculated) Cancer/disease specific survival: NR	SBRT Overall survival: NA Cancer/disease specific survival: NA	SBRT Local control: 1.5 years: 100%	Local control: NA	No
Vahdat-2010, #3864	SBRT Overall survival: 2-years: 90% Cancer/disease specific survival: 85% (calculated)	SBRT Overall survival: NA Cancer/disease specific survival: NA	SBRT Local control: 2-years: 95%	Local control: NA	No
van der Voort van Zyp-2009, #3885	SBRT Overall survival: 1-year: 83% (95% CI, 71-90%) 2-years: 62% (95% CI, 45-75%) Cancer/disease specific survival: 1-year: 94% 2-years: 86%	SBRT Overall survival: NA Cancer/disease specific survival: NA	SBRT Local control: 60 Gy 2-years: 78% (95% CI, 84-99%) 45 Gy 2-years: 78% (95% CI, 37-94%)	Local control: NA	No

Study	Survival Outcomes for Intervention Group 1	Survival Outcomes for Intervention Group 2	Local Control Outcomes for Intervention Group 1	Local Control Outcomes for Intervention Group 2	Arm
Videtic-2010, #3958	SBRT **Overall survival:** Median 38 months 3-years: 52% **Cancer/disease specific survival:** SBRT 69% (calculated)	**Overall survival:** NA **Cancer/disease specific survival:** NA	SBRT **Local control:** 3-years: 94%	**Local control:** NA	No

Appendix Table C4. Miscellaneous outcomes of studies that address Key Question 1

Study	Intervention Group 1	Intervention Group 2
Andratschke-2011, #132	SBRT: **Lung function:** NR **Obstructive symptoms:** NR **Quality of life:** NR **Performance status:** NR **Others:** NR	**Lung function:** NA **Obstructive symptoms:** NA **Quality of life:** NA **Performance status:** NA **Others:** NA
Baumann 2008, #270	SBRT **Lung function:** Baseline FEV1%: 49.0 (20.0-162.0) Post Rx FEV1% (at 14.3 months [3.0-33.4]): 52.5 (19.0-167.0) **Obstructive symptoms:** NR **Quality of life:** NR **Performance status:** NR **Others:** NA	**Lung function:** NA **Obstructive symptoms:** NA **Quality of life:** NA **Performance status:** NA **Others:** NA
Baumann-2006, #271	SBRT **Lung function:** NR **Obstructive symptoms:** NR **Quality of life:** NR **Performance status:** NR **Others:** NA	**Lung function:** NA **Obstructive symptoms:** NA **Quality of life:** NA **Performance status:** NA **Others:** NA

Study	Intervention Group 1	Intervention Group 2
Bogart-2010, #382	3DRT **Lung function:** A significant trend for changes in pulmonary function was not observed.	**Lung function:** NA
		Obstructive symptoms: NA
	Obstructive symptoms: NR	**Quality of life:** NA
	Quality of life: NR	**Performance status:** NA
	Performance status: NR	**Others:** NA
	Others: NR	
Bollineni-2012, #4548	SBRT: **Lung function:** NR	**Lung function:** NA
		Obstructive symptoms: NA
	Obstructive symptoms: NR	**Quality of life:** NA
	Quality of life: NR	**Performance status:** NA
	Performance status: NR	**Others:** NA
	Others: NR	
Bradley-2003, #445	3DRT **Lung function:** NR	**Lung function:** NA
		Obstructive symptoms: NA
	Obstructive symptoms: NR	**Quality of life:** NA
	Quality of life: NR	**Performance status:** NA
	Performance status: NR	**Others:** NA
	Others: NR	
Burdick-2010, #521	SBRT **Lung function:** NR	**Lung function:** NA
	Obstructive symptoms:	**Obstructive symptoms:**

Study	Intervention Group 1	Intervention Group 2
	Obstructive symptoms: NR **Quality of life:** NR **Performance status:** NR **Others:** NA	NA **Quality of life:** NA **Performance status:** NA **Others:** NA
Bush-2004, #535	PBRT **Lung function:** NR **Obstructive symptoms:** NR **Quality of life:** NR **Performance status:** NR **Others:** NA	**Lung function:** NA **Obstructive symptoms:** NA **Quality of life:** NA **Performance status:** NA **Others:** NA
Campeau-2009, #565	3DRT **Lung function:** NR **Obstructive symptoms:** NR **Quality of life:** NR **Performance status:** NR **Others:** NA	**Lung function:** NA **Obstructive symptoms:** NA **Quality of life:** NA **Performance status:** NA **Others:** NA

Study	Intervention Group 1	Intervention Group 2
Coon-2008, #803	SBRT **Lung function:** NR **Obstructive symptoms:** NR **Quality of life:** NR **Performance status:** NR **Others:** NA	**Lung function:** NA **Obstructive symptoms:** NA **Quality of life:** NA **Performance status:** NA **Others:** NA
Dunlap-2010, #1032	SBRT **Lung function:** NR **Obstructive symptoms:** NR **Quality of life:** NR **Performance status:** NR **Others:** NA	**Lung function:** NA **Obstructive symptoms:** NA **Quality of life:** NA **Performance status:** NA **Others:** NA
Fritz-2008, #1238	SBRT **Lung function:** Pre:0.66-2.93 Post (1-year):0.6-2.5 Post (2-years):0.8-2.1 Post (3-years): 1.1-1.9 **Obstructive symptoms:** NR **Quality of life:** NR **Performance status:** NR **Others:** NA	**Lung function:** NA **Obstructive symptoms:** NA **Quality of life:** NA **Performance status:** NA **Others:** NA
Graham-2006,	3DRT	3DRT

Study	Intervention Group 1	Intervention Group 2
#1403	**Lung function:** NR **Obstructive symptoms:** NR **Quality of life:** NR **Performance status:** NR **Others:** NR	**Lung function:** NA **Obstructive symptoms:** NA **Quality of life:** NA **Performance status:** NA **Others:** NA
Iwata-2010, # 1747	PBRT **Lung function:** NR **Obstructive symptoms:** NR **Quality of life:** NR **Performance status:** NR **Others:** NR	PBRT **Lung function:** NA **Obstructive symptoms:** NA **Quality of life:** NA **Performance status:** NA **Others:** NA
Jimenez-2010, #1842	3DRT **Lung function:** NR **Obstructive symptoms:** NR **Quality of life:** NR **Performance status:** NR **Others:** NR	3DRT **Lung function:** NA **Obstructive symptoms:** NA **Quality of life:** NA **Performance status:** NA **Others:** NA
Kopek-2009, #2040	SBRT **Lung function:** NR **Obstructive symptoms:**	SBRT **Lung function:** NA **Obstructive symptoms:**

Study	Intervention Group 1	Intervention Group 2
	NR	NA
	Quality of life: NR	**Quality of life:** NA
	Performance status: ≥ 3 performance status decline from baseline: 4 (5%)	**Performance status:** NA
	Others: NR	**Others:** NA
Mirri-2009, #2576	3DRT **Lung function:** NR	3DRT **Lung function:** NA
	Obstructive symptoms: NR	**Obstructive symptoms:** NA
	Quality of life: NR	**Quality of life:** NA
	Performance status: NR	**Performance status:** NA
	Others: NR	**Others:** NA
Nakayama 2010, #2684	PBT **Lung function:** Fletcher-Hugh-Jones criteria: Decline: 2 (4%)	PBT **Lung function:** NA
	Obstructive symptoms: NR	**Obstructive symptoms:** NA
	Quality of life: NR	**Quality of life:** NA
	Performance status: NR	**Performance status:** NA
	Others: NR	**Others:** NA
Narayan-2004, #2686	3DRT **Lung function:** NR	3DRT **Lung function:** NA
	Obstructive symptoms: NR	**Obstructive symptoms:** NA
	Quality of life:	**Quality of life:**

Study	Intervention Group 1	Intervention Group 2
	NR	NA
	Performance status: NR	**Performance status:** NA
	Others: NR	**Others:** NA
Nyman-2006, #2750	SBRT	SBRT
	Lung function: NR	**Lung function:** NA
	Obstructive symptoms: NR	**Obstructive symptoms:** NA
	Quality of life: NR	**Quality of life:** NA
	Performance status: NR	**Performance status:** NA
	Others: NR	**Others:** NA
Olsen-2011, #2792	SBRT	SBRT
	Lung function: NR	**Lung function:** NA
	Obstructive symptoms: NR	**Obstructive symptoms:** NA
	Quality of life: NR	**Quality of life:** NA
	Performance status: NR	**Performance status:** NA
	Others: NR	**Others:** NA
Palma 2012, #2843	SBRT	SBRT
	Lung function: NR	**Lung function:** NA
	Obstructive symptoms: NR	**Obstructive symptoms:** NA
	Quality of life: NR	**Quality of life:** NA
	Performance status: NR	**Performance status:** NA

Study	Intervention Group 1	Intervention Group 2
	Others: NR	**Others:** NA
Pennathur-2007, #2896	RFA **Lung function:** NR	RFA **Lung function:** NA
	Obstructive symptoms: NR	**Obstructive symptoms:** NA
	Quality of life: NR	**Quality of life:** NA
	Performance status: NR	**Performance status:** NA
	Others: NR	**Others:** NA
Pennathur-2009, #2898	SBRT **Lung function:** NR	SBRT **Lung function:** NA
	Obstructive symptoms: NR	**Obstructive symptoms:** NA
	Quality of life: NR	**Quality of life:** NA
	Performance status: NR	**Performance status:** NA
	Others: NR	**Others:** NA
Ricardi-2010, #3098	SBRT **Lung function:** NR	SBRT **Lung function:** NA
	Obstructive symptoms: NR	**Obstructive symptoms:** NA
	Quality of life: NR	**Quality of life:** NA
	Performance status: NR	**Performance status:** NA
	Others: NR	**Others:** NA
Scorsetti-2007,	SBRT	SBRT

Study	Intervention Group 1	Intervention Group 2
#3362	**Lung function:** NR	**Lung function:** NA
	Obstructive symptoms: NR	**Obstructive symptoms:** NA
	Quality of life: NR	**Quality of life:** NA
	Performance status: NR	**Performance status:** NA
	Others: NR	**Others:** NA
Shibamoto-2012, #4629	SBRT: **Lung function:** NR	**Lung function:** NA
	Obstructive symptoms: NR	**Obstructive symptoms:** NA
	Quality of life: NR	**Quality of life:** NA
	Performance status: NR	**Performance status:** NA
	Others: NR	**Others:** NA
Song-2009, #3549	SBRT **Lung function:** NR	SBRT **Lung function:** NA
	Obstructive symptoms: NR	**Obstructive symptoms:** NA
	Quality of life: NR	**Quality of life:** NA
	Performance status: NR	**Performance status:** NA
	Others: NR	**Others:** NA
Stephans-2009, #3614	SBRT **Lung function:** NR	SBRT **Lung function:** NA
	Obstructive symptoms:	**Obstructive symptoms:**

Study	Intervention Group 1	Intervention Group 2
	NR Quality of life: NR Performance status: NR Others: NR	NA Quality of life: NA Performance status: NA Others: NA
Taremi-2011, #3732	SBRT Lung function: NR Obstructive symptoms: NR Quality of life: NR Performance status: NR Others: NR	SBRT Lung function: NA Obstructive symptoms: NA Quality of life: NA Performance status: NA Others: NA
Takeda-2009, #3700	SBRT Lung function: NR Obstructive symptoms: NR Quality of life: NR Performance status: NR Others: NR	SBRT Lung function: NA Obstructive symptoms: NA Quality of life: NA Performance status: NA Others: NA
Turzer-2011, #3842	SBRT Lung function: NR Obstructive symptoms: NR Quality of life: NR	SBRT Lung function: NA Obstructive symptoms: NA Quality of life: NA

Study	Intervention Group 1	Intervention Group 2
	Performance status: NR	**Performance status:** NA
	Others: NR	**Others:** NA
Vahdat-2010, #3864	SBRT **Lung function:** NR	SBRT **Lung function:** NA
	Obstructive symptoms: NR	**Obstructive symptoms:** NA
	Quality of life: NR	**Quality of life:** NA
	Performance status: NR	**Performance status:** NA
	Others: NR	**Others:** NA
van der Voort van Zyp-2009, #3885	SBRT **Lung function:** NR	SBRT **Lung function:** NA
	Obstructive symptoms: NR	**Obstructive symptoms:** NA
	Quality of life: NR	**Quality of life:** NA
	Performance status: NR	**Performance status:** NA
	Others: NR	**Others:** NA
Videtic-2010, #3958	SBRT **Lung function:** Median post-treatment FEV1: 1.17 (range NR)	SBRT **Lung function:** NA
	Obstructive symptoms: NR	**Obstructive symptoms:** NA
	Quality of life: NR	**Quality of life:** NA
	Performance status: NR	**Performance status:** NA
	Others:	**Others:**

Study	Intervention Group 1	Intervention Group 2
	NR	NA

Appendix Table C5. Toxicity outcomes of studies that address Key Question 1

Study	Intervention Group 1	Intervention Group 2
Andratschke 2011, #132	SBRT: Hemoptysis: 2 (2%) Grade 2 pneumonitis: 12 (13%) Grade 3 pneumonitis: 2 (2%). Grade 3 dyspnea: 7 (8%) Grade 4 dyspnea: 4 (4%) Grade 2 thoracic wall pain: 4 (4%) Grade 3 fatigue (late): 1 (1%) Rib fractures: 3 (3%) Benign pleural effusion: 4 (4%) Atelectasis: 2 (2%)	NA

Study	Intervention Group 1	Intervention Group 2

Baumann-2006, #271	SBRT
	Toxicities Total: 83 (60%)
	Grade 3-4:
	    Thoracic pain: 4 (3%)
	    Lung atelectasis: 2 (1%)
	    Rib fracture: 2 (1%)
	    Decreased Lung function: 2 (1%)
	    Decreased Performance status: 2(1%)
	    Pneumonitis: 1 (0.7%)
	    Pneumonia: 1 (0.7%)
	< Grade 3:
	    Lung Fibrosis: 21 (15%)
	    Skin rash: 12 (9%)
	    Lung atelectasis: 8 (6%)
	    Esophagitis: 5 (4%)
	    Pleural exudates: 4 (3%)
	    Thoracic Pain: 2 (1%)
	    Nausea: 1(0.7%)
		NA

Baumann-2009, #270	SBRT
	Grade 3 (≤18 months):
	    Dyspnea: 4 (7%)
	    Cough: 1 (2%)
	    Pneumonia: 1 (2%)
	    Fibrosis: 2 (4%)
	    Atelectasis: 1 (2%)
	    Pleural effusion: 2 (4%)
	    Heart disorder: 1 (2%)
	    Rib fracture: 1 (2%)
	    Pain: 2(4%)
	    Fatigue: 1 (2%)
	Grade 3 (>18 months):
	    Rib fracture: 1 (2%)
	    Heart failure: 1 (2%)
	    Fibrosis: 1 (2%)
	Grade 4 at 36 months:
	    Dyspnea: 1(2%)
		NA

Bogart-2010, #382	3DRT Grade 3 hematological toxicity: 1 (3%) Grade 3 dyspnea: 1 (3%) Grade 3 pain: 1 (3%)	NA
Bollineni-2012, #4548	SBRT NR	NA
Bradley-2003, #445	3DRT Grade 3-4 Esophagitis: 2 (4%) Grade 3 Pneumonitis: 1 (2%) Grade 4 Pneumonitis: 1 (2%) Acute: Grade 1-2: Esophagitis: 14 (25%)	NA

Study	Intervention Group 1	Intervention Group 2
	Grade 1-2: Pneumonitis: 3 (5%) Late: Grade 1-2: Esophagitis: 2 (4%) Grade 1-2: Pneumonitis: 19 (34%)	
Burdick-2010, #521	SBRT NR	NA
Bush-2004, #535	PBRT Acute toxicities were limited to mild fatigue and radiation dermatitis that was seen as mild-to-moderate erythema. These required no specific medical treatment. No cases of clinical acute radiation pneumonitis were identified. No patient required steroids or anti-inflammatory therapy. No cases of acute or late esophageal or cardiac toxicity were identified.	NA
Campeau-2009, #565	3DRT 3 patients did not complete treatment due to treatment related toxicities. Details of toxicities not reported	NA
Coon-2008, #803	SBRT Grade 2: Pneumonitis: 1 (1 %)	NA
Dunlap-2010, #1032	SBRT Grade 2: Pneumonitis: 1 (3%) Grade 3: Pneumonitis: 1 (3%) Rib fracture: 2 (5%) Chest wall pain: 9 (23%)	NA
Fritz-2008, #1238	SBRT Grade 4: rib fracture: 2 (5%)	NA
Graham-2006, #1403	3DRT Grade 2 pneumonitis: 3 (8%)	NA

Iwata-2010, # 1747	PBRT 60 Gy:
	  RP Grade 2: 4 (10.8%)
	  RP Grade 3: 0
	  Dermatitis Grade 2: 4 (10.8%)
	  Dermatitis Grade 3: 0
	  Rib fracture Grade 2: 6 (16.2%)
	  Soft Tissue Grade 2: 2 (5.4%)
	
	PBRT 80Gy: To be extracted
	  RP Grade 2: 3 (15.0%)
	  RP Grade 3: 1 (5.0%)
	  Dermatitis Grade 2: 4 (20.0%)
	  Dermatitis Grade 3: 3 (15.0%)
	  Rib fracture Grade 2: 9 (45.0)
	  Soft Tissue Grade 2: 2 (10.0%)
		NA

Jimenez-2010, #1842	3DRT NR	NA
Kopek-2009,	SBRT	NA

Study	Intervention Group 1	Intervention Group 2

#2040	Grade 2:
	    Esophagitis: 1 (1%)
	    Pain: 9 (10%)
	    Analgesia: 5 (6%)
	    Dyspnea: 9 (10%)
	    Pulmonary fibrosis: 2 (2%)
	    Pneumonitis: 1 (1%)
	    Pleural effusion: 2 (2%)
	    Skin hyperpigmentation: 2 (2%)
	    Skin erythema: 1 (1%)
	
	≥ 3 grade point worsening in analgesia use from baseline: 7 (8%)
	Grade ≥3:
	    Dyspnea: 11 (%)
	    Analgesia: 9 (10%)
	    Pain: 2 (2%)
	    Cough: 1 (1%)
	
	Rib fracture: 7 (8%)	

Mirri-2009, #2576	3DRT Late Grade 2 pulmonary: 2 (13%) *One patient, affected by dilated cardiomyopathy, developed pericardial effusion 3 months after the end of radiotherapy. However, because of the previous cardiac problems, it was difficult to assess whether this was radiation related.	NA
Nakayama 2010, #2684	PBT Grade 2 pneumonitis: 2 (4%) Grade 3 pneumonitis: 2 (4%) Grade 3 pulmonary dysfunction: 1 (2%) Rib fracture: 1 (2%)	NA
Narayan-2004, #2686	3DRT Grade 2 esophagitis: 1 (9%) No patient developed Grade 2 or higher pneumonitis	NA

Nyman-2006, #2750	SBRT
	23 (51%) did not experience any acute toxicity.
	No Grade 2 or greater pneumonitis reported
	Late:
	    Rib fractures: 2 (4%)
	    Atelectasis: 3 (7%)
		NA

Olsen-2011, #2792	SBRT Chest wall pain requiring analgesia: 21 (16%) Grade 2 radiation pneumonitis: 4 (3%) No Grade 3 or greater toxicities reported	NA
Palma 2012, #2843	SBRT Acute Grade 3 pneumonitis: 1 (< 1%) Late Grade 3 pneumonitis: 2 (1%)	NA

Study	Intervention Group 1	Intervention Group 2
Pennathur-2007, #2896	RFA Pneumothorax: 12 (63%) Prolonged air leak (> 5 days): 1 (5%) No procedure-related deaths	NA
Pennathur-2009, #2898	SBRT No radiation-associated adverse effects were reported Pneumothorax secondary to fiducial placement: 10 (47%) No procedure-related deaths	NA
Ricardi-2010, #3098	SBRT Late Grade 3 radiation pneumonitis: 2 (3%) Rib fracture: 1 (2%)	NA
Scorsetti-2007, #3362	SBRT Acute Grade 2 pneumonitis: 2 (5%) Late Grade 2 pneumonitis: 1 (2%)	NA
Shibamoto -2012, #4269	SBRT: NR by operability	NA
Song-2009, #3549	SBRT Grade 3 pneumonitis: 3 (9%) Partial or complete bronchial stricture: 8 (25%) Grade 5 hemoptysis: 1 (3%) No severe skin, esophageal or rib fractures were reported	NA
Stephans-2009, #3614	SBRT Grade 2 pneumonitis: 2 (2%) Grade 1 or 2 chest wall toxicity: 9 (10%)	NA
Taremi-2011, #3732	SBRT Acute Grade 3 fatigue: 1 (1%) Acute Grade 3 dyspnea: 2 (2%) Acute Grade 3 chest wall pain: 1 (1%) Late Grade 3 rib fracture: 3 (3%) Late Grade 3 dyspnea: 2 (2%) Late Grade 3 pneumonia: 1 (1%) No Grade 4 or 5 toxicities were observed	NA
Takeda-2009, #3700	SBRT No acute toxicity was observed Grade 2 pneumonitis: 1 (2%) Grade 3 pneumonitis: 2 (3%) Grade 5 bacterial pneumonia at site of Grade 3 radiation pneumonitis: 1 (2%)	SBRT NA
Turzer-2011, #3842	SBRT Grade 2 pneumonitis: 1 (3%) Grade 3 pneumonitis: 1 (3%)	NA
Vahdat-2010, #3864	SBRT NR	NA
van der Voort van Zyp 2009, #3885	SBRT Grade 3 pneumothorax: 1 (1%) Grade 3 cardiac arrhythmia: 1 (1%)	NA

Study	Intervention Group 1	Intervention Group 2
	Acute Grade 3 thoracic pain: 1 (1%) Late Grade 3 pneumonitis: 3 (4%) Late Grade 3 thoracic pain: 4 (6%) No Grade 4 or 5 toxicities were observed	
Videtic-2010, #3958	SBRT Acute Grade 3 dyspnea: 1 (4%) Late Grade 2 chest wall pain: 1 (4%) No Grade 4 or 5 toxicities were observed	NA

Appendix Table C6. Attributes of studies that address Key Question 1

ID	HC	Enroll Start	Enroll End	Design	Study Setting	Treatment Setting	Institution Setting(s)	Stage(s)	Staging Criteria	COI	Funding
Andratschke, 2011, #132	Y	12/00	03/10	RET	SI	NR	TH	I	AJCC 2002	N	G
Baumann, 2006, #271	N (24%)	XX/96	XX/03	RET	M	NR	NR	I	NR	NR	NR
Baumann, 2009, #270	N (33%)	08/03	09/05	PRO	M	NR	NR	I	NR	NR	OH
Bogart, 2009, #382	Y	12/00	07/05	PRO	NR	NR	NR	I	NR	Y	MA
Bollineni-2012, #4548	N (70%)	11/06	02/10	RET	SI	NR	TH	I	AJCC 2002	N	NR
Bradley,2003, #445	Y	XX/91	XX/01	PRO	NR	NR	NR	I	AJCC 2002	NR	NR
Burdick, 2010, #521	N (32%)	10/03	08/07	RET	SI	NR	TH	I	AJCC 2002	N	NR
Bush, 2004, #535	Yes	NR	NR	PRO	SI	NR	TH	I	NR	NR	S
Campeau, 2009, #565	Yes	01/00	12/05	RET	SI	NR	NR	I	Union Internationale Contre le Cancer	NR	NR
Coon, 2008, #803	N (39%)	01/05	01/07	RET	SI	NR	TH	I	AJCC 2002	NR	NR
Dunlap, 2010, #1032	Yes	03/05	01/08	RET	SI	NR	TH	I	AJCC 2002	NR	NR
Fritz, 2008, #1238	Yes	NR	NR	RET	SI	NR	NR	I	NR	N	NR
Graham, 2006, #1403	Yes	01/95	12/02	RET	M	NR	TH	I	NR	NR	NR
Iwata, 2010, #1747	Yes	04/03	04/07	PRO	SI	NR	TH	I	IUAC 2002	N	G
Jimenez, 2010, #1842	Yes	09/05	04/07	RET	SI	NR	TH	I	NR	N	NR
Kopek, 2009, #2040	Yes	01/00	12/07	PRO	SI	NR	TH	I	IUAC 1997	NR	MA,S,G
Mirri, 2009, #2576	N (27%)	06/03	03/07	PRO	SI	NR	TH	I	NR	NR	NR
Nakayama, 2010, #2684	N (12%)	11/01	07/08	RET	M	NR	TH	I	IUAC2002	NR	NR

C-62

ID	HC	Enroll Start	Enroll End	Design	Study Setting	Treatment Setting	Institution Setting(s)	Stage(s)	Staging Criteria	COI	Funding
Narayan, 2004, #2686	Yes	NR	NR	PRO	M	NR	TH	I	NR	NR	G
Nyman, 2006, #2750	N (20%)	09/98	03/03	RET	SI	NR	TH	I	NR	NR	NR
Olsen, 2011, #2792	N (15%)	06/04	06/09	PRO	SI	NR	TH	I	AJCC 2009	N	NR
Palma, 2011, #2843	N (68%)	01/03	03/10	PRO	SI	NR	TH	I	NR	Y	NR
Pennathur, 2007, #2896	Yes	01/02	12/05	RET	SI	NR	TH	I	NR	Y	MA,G
Pennathur, 2009, #2898	N (5%)	01/02	12/05	RET	SI	NR	TH	I	NR	NR	NR
Ricardi, 2010, #3098	N (36%)	05/03	08/07	PRO	SI	NR	TH	I	NR	N	NR
Scorsetti, 2007, #3362	N (5%)	01/04	01/06	NR	SI	NR	TH	I	NR	NR	NR
Shibamoto, 2012, #4269	Y	05/04	11/08	PRO	M	NR	TH	I	IUAC2002	N	NR
Song, 2009, #3549	Yes	06/99	05/06	RET	SI	NR	TH	I	AJCC 2002	N	G
Stephans, 2009, #3614	N (29%)	02/04	08/07	RET	SI	NR	TH	I	AJCC 2002	N	NR
Taremi, 2012, #3732	N (25%)	12/04	10/08	PRO	SI	NR	TH	I	NR	N	MA,S,G
Takeda-2009, #3700	N(18%)	12/01	05/07	RET	M	NR	TH	I	NR	N	NR
Turzer, 2011, #3842	N (26%)	09/08	04/10	RET	SI	NR	TH	I	NR	NR	NR
Vahdat, 2010, #3864	Yes	01/05	01/08	PRO	SI	NR	TH	I	NR	Y	NR
van der Voort van Zyp, 2009, #3885	N (49%)	08/05	10/07	NR	SI	NR	TH	I	NR	N	NR
Videtic, 2010, #3958	N (29%)	10/03	11/06	RET	SI	NR	TH	I	AJCC 2002	N	NR

Appendix Table C7. Description of studies that address Key Question 2

Study	Study design, enrollment numbers and lost to FU/excluded	Inclusion/exclusion criteria	Stage Distribution	Tumor/Obstruction Location & Histopathology	Patient characteristics
Chen-2012, USA, #4554	**Study design:** PRO, SAS **Patients enrolled:** 40 (100%) **Lost to FU/excluded/missing:** 0	**Inclusion criteria:** 1. Hst confirmed, primary clinical stage I NSCLC 2. Medically operable, high risk **Exclusion criteria:** Inability to safely implant fiducials for tumor tracking	Stage I: 40 (100%)	**Location:** NR **Histopathology:** Hst confirmed: 40 (100%) ACC: 19 (48%) SCC: 12 (30%) NSCLC NOS: 9 (22%)	**Age (years):** Median 76 (63-87) **Women:** 24 (60%) **Race:** Caucasian 33 (82%) **Co-morbidities:** Mean DLCO 10 (3.5-23.3 mL/min/mm Hg) Predicted mean DLCO 55% (14-128%) Predicted mean FEV1 57% (21-111%) **Current or former smoker:** 38 (95%) **Performance status:** Median ECOG 1 (0-2)
Iwata-2010, Japan, # 1747	**Study design:** NRCS, NR whether data collection was RET or PRO **Patients enrolled:** Total: 57 (100%) PBRT 80Gy: 20 (35%) PBRT 60 Gy: 37 (65%) Refusal: Total: 28 (100%) PBRT 80Gy: 10 (34%) PBRT 60 Gy: 18 (64%) **Lost to FU/excluded/missing:** None	**Inclusion criteria:** 1. Hst confirmed primary NSCLC staged IA or IB (International Union Against Cancer 2002 staging system) 2. Medically inoperable or refused surgical resection	Total: 57 (100%) Stage 1A: 27(47%) Stage 1B: 30 (57%) PBRT 80Gy: 20 (100%) Stage 1A: 6 (30%) Stage 1B: 14(70%) PBRT 60 Gy: 37 (100%) Stage 1A: 21 (57%) Stage 1B: 16 (43%)	**Location:** NR **Histopathology:** Total: 57 (100%) AC: 32 (56%) SCC: 23 (40%) Others: 2 (4%) PBRT 80Gy: 20 (100%) AC: 11 (55%) SCC: 8 (40%) Others: 1 (5%) PBRT 60 Gy: 37 (100%) AC: 21 (57%) SCC: 15 (41%) Others: 1 (3%)	**Age:** Total: 76 (48-89) PBRT 80Gy: 75 (48-87) PBRT 60 Gy: 78 (57-87) **Women:** Total: 23 (29%) PBRT 80Gy: 7 (36%) PBRT 60 Gy: 7 (19%) **Race:** NR **Co-morbidities:** Total: 28 (100%) Pulmonary: 13 (46%) CVD: 9 (32%) Severe DM: 5 (18%) Age: 2 (7%) Others: 2 (7%)

Study	Study design, enrollment numbers and lost to FU/excluded	Inclusion/exclusion criteria	Stage Distribution	Tumor/Obstruction Location & Histopathology	Patient characteristics
		3. WHO performance status ≤2 4. No history of previous LC 5. No prior chest RT or chemotherapy; **Exclusion criteria:** NR			PBRT 80Gy: 10 (100%) Pulmonary: 7 (70%) CVD: 3 (30%) Severe DM: 1 (10%) Age: 0 Others: 0 PBRT 60 Gy: 18 (100%) Pulmonary: 6 (33%) CVD: 6 (33%) Severe DM: 4 (22%) Age: 2 (11%) Others: 2 (11%) **Performance status:** NR
Lagewaard-2011, Netherlands, #2122	**Study design:** RET, SAS **Patients enrolled:** 177 (100%) **Lost to FU/excluded/missing:** 0	**Inclusion criteria:** 1. Primary clinical stage I NSCLC 2. Medically operable **Exclusion criteria:** 1. GOLD COPD class 3-4 2. FEV1 < 50% of predicted 3. DLCO < 50% of predicted 4. WHO performance status ≥ 3 5. Major comorbidity (cardiac, renal) that precludes surgery	**Stage I:** 177 (100%)	**Location:** NR **Histopathology:** Hst confirmed: 60 (33%) ACC: 20 (33%) SCC: 16 (27%) NSCLC NOS: 24 (38%) Undiagnosed: 117 (66%)	**Age (years):** 76 (50-91) **Women:** 76 (43%) **Race:** NR **Co-morbidities:** GOLD COPD No COPD: 65 (37%) Class I: 37 (21%) Class II: 75 (42%) **CCI score:** 0: 18 (10%) 1: 59 (33%) 2: 38 (22%) 3: 39 (22%) 4: 16 (9%) 5: 7 (4%) **Current or former smoker:** 168 (95%) **Performance status:** WHO < 3: 177 (100%)
Onishi-2011, Japan, #2802 (longer FU to	**Study design:** RET, SAS	**Inclusion criteria:** 1. Hst confirmed primary clinical stage I NSCLC	Stage I: 87 (100%)	**Location:** NR	**Age (years):** 74 (43-87)

Study	Study design, enrollment numbers and lost to FU/excluded	Inclusion/exclusion criteria	Stage Distribution	Tumor/Obstruction Location & Histopathology	Patient characteristics
Onishi-2007, Japan, #2803	**Patients enrolled:** 87 (100%) **Lost to FU/excluded/missing:** 0	2. Medically operable but refused surgery **Exclusion criteria:** NR		**Histopathology:** Hst confirmed: 87 (100%) ACC: 54 (62%) SCC: 25 (29%) NSCLC NOS: 8 (9%)	**Women:** 24 (28%) **Race:** NR **Co-morbidities:** Chronic lung disease: 38 (44%) **Performance status:** ECOG 0: 51 (59%) 1: 30 (34%) 2: (7%)
Shibamoto 2012, Japan, #4629	**Study design:** PRO, SAS **Patients enrolled:** Total: 180 (100%) Medically inoperable: 120 (67%) Refused surgery: 60 (33%) **Lost to FU/excluded/missing:** 0	**Inclusion criteria:** Histologically proven NSCLC stage 1 not suitable for surgery for medical or functional reasons **Exclusion criteria:** 1. Tumor > 5 cm in greatest dimension 2. WHO PS < 2 or PS 3 when not due to pulmonary disease 3. Active concurrent cancer 4. FEV1/FVC < 60% or percentage vital capacity < 75%	Stage I: 180 (100%)	**Location:** Not stated by operability **Histopathology:** Pathological confirmation: 180 (100%) Not stated by operability	**Age (years):** 77 (29-89) all cases **Women:** 57 (32%) all cases **Race:** NR **Comorbidities:** NR **Performance status:** WHO 0: 87 (48%) 1: 69 (38%) 2: 21 (12%) 3: 3 (2%) all cases
Takeda-2009, Japan, #3700	**Study design:** RET, SAS **Patients enrolled:** Total: 63 (100%) Medically inoperable: 49 (78%) Operable: 14 (22%) **Lost to FU/excluded/missing:** 0	**Inclusion criteria:** 1. Primary clinical stage I NSCLC 2. WHO performance status ≤ 2 **Exclusion criteria:** 1. Prior radiation to lung or mediastinum	Stage I: 63 (100%)	**Location:** NR **Histopathology:** Hst confirmed: 52 (82%) ACC: 35 (56%) SCC: 14: 22%) NOS: 3 (5%) Undiagnosed: 11 (18%)	**Age:** 78 (56-91) **Women:** 23 (36%) **Race:** NR **Co-morbidities:**

Study	Study design, enrollment numbers and lost to FU/excluded	Inclusion/exclusion criteria	Stage Distribution	Tumor/Obstruction Location & Histopathology	Patient characteristics
					COPD, advanced age, other illnesses: 49 (78%) **Performance status:** WHO ≤ 2: 63 (100%)

Appendix Table C8. Outcomes and interventions of studies that address Key Question 2

Study	Study Outcomes	Interventions
Chen-2012, #4554	**Study Objective:** To evaluate outcomes of SBRT in potentially operable patients with primary stage I NSCLC **Primary outcome:** NR **Definition:** NA **Secondary outcome(s):** NR **Definitions:** NA **List of outcomes:** OS, LCT **Cause of death:** Total: 12 (30%) Unrelated to lung cancer: 10 (83%) Related to lung cancer: 2 (17%) **Length of FU:** Median 44 (12-72) mos	**Intervention name:** SBRT **Vendor name:** Cyberknife (Acurray Inc., Sunnyvale, CA) **Dose/frequency/details:** Prescribed dose: 50 Gy (42-60 Gy) to the PTV 80% isodose line 3 frs Mean 7 days (5-11 days) **Technical details:** Beam energy NR **Treatment Intention:** Curative **Follow-up and Evaluation Criteria:** PET/CT scans at 3 mos intervals after SBRT Biopsy required to confirm progression
Iwata-2010, # 1747	**Study Objective:** To analyzed the safety and efficacy of high-dose proton therapy and carbon-ion therapy applied to stage I NSCLC **Primary outcome:** NR **Definition:** NA **Secondary outcome(s):** NR **Definitions:** NA **List of Outcome(s):** OS, DSS, Local control, Toxicity **Cause of death:** NR **Length of FU:** All patients observed for a minimum of 1.5 years or until death. Median duration of follow-up was 35.5 (18-66) months for living pts & 30.5 (4-66) months for all pts.	**Intervention name:** PBRT **Vendor name:** Synchrotron (Mitsubishi Electric Corporation, Kobe, Japan 3-D Rx planning system ((FOCUS-M, CMS, St. Louis, Mo and Mitsubishi Electric Corporation) **Dose/frequency/details:** PBRT 80Gy: 20 fractions, BED 10(Gy): 112 PBRT 60 Gy: 10 fractions BED 10(Gy): 96 **Technical details:** Pts were treated with 150-MeV proton beams **Treatment Intention:** NR **Follow-up and Evaluation Criteria:**

Study	Study Outcomes	Interventions
		• After Rx, pts FU at 1.5, 3, 4.5, 6, 9, and 12 months during the 1st yr, at intervals of 3 months in the 2nd yr, and at 6-month intervals in the 3rd yr. • CT, tumor marker, Brain MRI and FDG-PET were used to monitor tumor progression. • Local responses was assessed according to the modified WHO response evaluation criteria. • Toxicities were evaluated with the CTCAE version 3.0. • Medically inoperability defined as pts with poor pulmonary function (vital capacity <75% or ratio of FEV 1 to forced vital capacity <60%), a history of major CVD, severe DM, advanced age (80 years old), or other debilitating conditions that preclude surgery.
Lagerwaard-2011, #2122	**Study Objective:** To evaluate outcomes of SBRT in potentially operable patients with primary stage I NSCLC **Primary outcome:** NR **Definition:** NA **Secondary outcome(s):** NR **Definitions:** NA **List of outcomes:** OS, LCT, toxicity **Cause of death:** Total: 34 (19%) Unrelated to lung cancer: 12 (35%) Related to lung cancer: 14 (41%) Unknown: 5 (15%) **Length of FU:** Median 32 mos	**Intervention name:** SBRT **Vendor name:** NR **Dose/frequency/details:** Prescribed dose: 60 Gy to the PTV 80% isodose line BED: > 100 Gy for all fractionations 3, 5, or 8 frs 2 weeks **Technical details:** Beam energy NR **Treatment Intention:** Curative **Follow-up and Evaluation Criteria:** CT scans at 3, 6, 12 mos after SBRT FDG PET only if relapse suspected Toxicity assessed (criteria NR)
Onishi-2011, #2802 (longer FU to Onishi-2007, #2803)	**Study Objective:** To evaluate high-dose SBRT for stage I NSCLC in patients who were medically operable but refused surgery **Primary outcome:** OS, CSS, LCT, toxicity **Definition:** NR	**Intervention name:** SBRT **Vendor name:** NR **Dose/frequency/details:** Prescribed dose: 45-72 Gy at the PTV isocenter BED: Median 116 (100-141) Gy 3-10 frs

Study	Study Outcomes	Interventions
		Secondary outcome(s): NR
		Consecutive days or every other day
		Technical details: 4- and 6-MeV beam energy
		Treatment Intention: Curative
	Definitions: NA	
	List of outcomes: OS, CSS, LCT, toxicity	**Follow-up and Evaluation Criteria:** First FU at 4 weeks, then every 1-3 mos thereafter Chest CT scans every 3 mos for first year then every 4-6 mos thereafter Toxicity assessed according to CTCAE v.2.0
	Cause of death: NR	
	Length of FU: Median 55 mos	
Shibamoto -2012, #4629	**Study Objective:** To report a multi-institutional study of SBRT in inoperable and operable patients with histologically confirmed stage I NSCLC	**Intervention name:** SBRT
	Primary outcome: LC at 3-years follow-up	**Vendor name:** Novalis image-guided system (Varian Medical Systems, Palo Alto, CA) CLINAC 23EX or 21 EXS (Varian)
	Definition: Calculated from the start of SBRT	Eclipse v.7.5.14.3 (Varian) BRAINSCAN v.5.31 (BrainLAB, Feldkirchen, Germany) Pinnacle3 (Philips, Madison, WI)
	Secondary outcome(s): OS, CSS	
	Definitions: Calculated from the start of SBRT	**Dose/frequency/details:** Hypofractionated SBRT Total dose: 44-52 Gy to 90% of the isodose line of PTV in 4 frs for 9-21 days
	List of Outcome(s): OS, CSS, LCT, Toxicity	**Technical details:** 6-MV photons
	Cause of death: Dead: 65 (36%) NR by operability	**Treatment Intention:** Curative
	Length of FU: 36 months NR by operability	**Follow-up and Evaluation Criteria:** • All time intervals were calculated from the start of SBRT • CT scans of chest and upper abdomen at 2-months intervals up to 6 months, every 2-4 months thereafter • Toxicity: CTCAE v3.0 criteria during and up to 3 months after RT
Takeda-2009, #3700	**Study Objective:** To analyze clinical outcomes of SBRT for patients with stages IA and IB NSCLC	**Intervention name:** SBRT
	Primary outcome: NR	**Vendor name:** XiO treatment planning system, V.4.2 or v.4.3, CMS, St. Louis, MO Linear accelerator NR
	Definition: NA	**Dose/frequency/details:** Prescribed dose: 50 Gy to the 80% isodose line 10 Gy per fraction
	Secondary outcome(s):	

Study	Study Outcomes	Interventions
NR		5 fractions
	Definitions: NA	**Technical details:** Beam energy NR
	List of outcomes: OS, CSS, LCT, toxicity	**Treatment Intention:** Curative
	Cause of death: NR	**Follow-up and Evaluation Criteria:** • Monthly for first 6 mos, with chest X-ray • CT scans at 1 and 3 mos after SBRT, then at 3-mos intervals during first 2 years • FU interviews and CT scans at 4-6 mos intervals after 2 years • Toxicity assessed according to CTCAE v.3.0
	Length of FU: 31 (10-72) mos	

Appendix Table C9. Survival and local control outcomes of studies that address Key Question 2

Study	Survival Outcomes for Intervention Group 1	Survival Outcomes for Intervention Group 2	Local Control Outcomes for Intervention Group 1	Local Control Outcomes for Intervention Group 2	Arm
Chen-2012, #4554	SBRT Overall survival: Median ~60 mos 3-years: 75% Cancer specific survival: NR	SBRT Overall survival NA Cancer specific survival: NA	SBRT Local control:: 95% at follow-up	Local control: NA	No
Iwata-2010, # 1747	**Overall survival:** 3-years: 80% **Cancer/disease specific survival:** NR	**Overall survival:** NA **Cancer/disease specific survival:** NA	**Local control:** NR	**Local control:** NA	Yes
Lagerwaard-2011, #2122	SBRT Overall survival: Median 62 mos 1-year: 95% 3-years: 85% 5-years: 51% (only 10 pts at risk) Cancer specific survival: NR	SBRT Overall survival: NA Cancer specific survival: NA	SBRT Local control: 1-year: 98% 3-years:93%	Local control: NA	No
Onishi-2011, #2802 (longer FU to Onishi-2007, #2803)	SBRT Overall survival: 5-years: 70% (95% CI: 59-86%) Cancer specific survival: 5-years: 76% (95% CI: 66-86%)	SBRT Overall survival: NA Cancer specific survival: NA	SBRT Local control: 5-years: 87% (95% CI: 84-100%)	Local control: NA	No
Shibamoto 2012, #4629	SBRT: **Overall survival:** Median: Not reached 3-years: 74% 5-years: 70% **Cancer/disease specific survival:** NR by operability	SBRT: **Overall survival:** NA **Cancer/disease specific survival:** NA	**Local control:** NR by operability	**Local control:** NA	No
Takeda-2009, #3700	SBRT **Overall survival:** 3-years: 90% (stage IA) 3-years: 63% (stage IB) p = 0.09 3-years: 91% (operable) **Cancer/disease specific**	SBRT **Overall survival:** NA **Cancer/disease specific survival:** NA	SBRT **Local control:** 3-years: 93% (stage IA) 3-years: 96% (stage IB) p = 0.86	**Local control:** NA	No

C-72

Study	Survival Outcomes for Intervention Group 1	Survival Outcomes for Intervention Group 2	Local Control Outcomes for Intervention Group 1	Local Control Outcomes for Intervention Group 2	Arm
	survival: 3-years: 100% (stage IA) 3-years: 81% (stage IB) $p = 0.10$ 3-years: 91% (operable)				

Appendix Table C10. Miscellaneous outcomes of studies that address Key Question 2

Study	Intervention Group 1	Intervention Group 2
Chen-2012, #4554	SBRT **Lung function:** NR **Obstructive symptoms:** NR **Quality of life:** NR **Performance status:** NR **Others:** NR	SBRT **Lung function:** NA **Obstructive symptoms:** NA **Quality of life:** NA **Performance status:** NA **Others:** NA
Iwata-2010, # 1747	PBRT **Lung function:** NR **Obstructive symptoms:** NR **Quality of life:** NR **Performance status:** NR **Others:** NR	PBRT **Lung function:** NA **Obstructive symptoms:** NA **Quality of life:** NA **Performance status:** NA **Others:** NA
Lagerwaard 2011, #2122	SBRT **Lung function:** NR **Obstructive symptoms:** NR **Quality of life:** NR **Performance status:** NR **Others:** NR	SBRT **Lung function:** NA **Obstructive symptoms:** NA **Quality of life:** NA **Performance status:** NA **Others:** NA
Onishi-2011, #2802 (longer FU to	SBRT **Lung function:** NR	SBRT **Lung function:** NA

Study	Intervention Group 1	Intervention Group 2
Onishi-2007, #2803)	**Obstructive symptoms:** NR **Quality of life:** NR **Performance status:** NR **Others:** NR	**Obstructive symptoms:** NA **Quality of life:** NA **Performance status:** NA **Others:** NA
Shibamoto-2012, #4629	SBRT: **Lung function:** NR **Obstructive symptoms:** NR **Quality of life:** NR **Performance status:** NR **Others:** NR	**Lung function:** NA **Obstructive symptoms:** NA **Quality of life:** NA **Performance status:** NA **Others:** NA
Takeda-2009, #3700	SBRT **Lung function:** NR **Obstructive symptoms:** NR **Quality of life:** NR **Performance status:** NR **Others:** NR	SBRT **Lung function:** NA **Obstructive symptoms:** NA **Quality of life:** NA **Performance status:** NA **Others:** NA

Appendix Table C11. Toxicity outcomes of studies that address Key Question 2

Study	Intervention Group 1	Intervention Group 2
Chen-2012, #4554	SBRT NR	NA

Iwata-2010, # 1747	PBRT 60 Gy:
	    RP Grade 2: 4 (10.8%)
	    RP Grade 3: 0
	    Dermatitis Grade 2: 4 (10.8%)
	    Dermatitis Grade 3: 0
	    Rib fracture Grade 2: 6 (16.2%)
	    Soft Tissue Grade 2: 2 (5.4%)
	
	PBRT 80Gy:
	    RP Grade 2: 3 (15.0%)
	    RP Grade 3: 1 (5.0%)
	    Dermatitis Grade 2: 4 (20.0%)
	    Dermatitis Grade 3: 3 (15.0%)
	    Rib fracture Grade 2: 9 (45.0)
	    Soft Tissue Grade 2: 2 (10.0%)
		NA

Lagerwaard-2011, #2122	SBRT 30-day mortality: 0 (0%) Grade > 3 pneumonitis: 4 (2%) Rib fracture: 5 (3%)	NA
Onishi-2011, #2802 (longer FU to Onishi-2007, #2803)	SBRT Grade 2 pulmonary: 4 (5%) Grade 3 pulmonary: 1 (1%) Grade 3 dermatitis: 3 (3%) Grade 3 esophagitis: 1 (1%) Rib fracture: 4 (5%)	NA
Shibamoto-2012, #4269	SBRT: NR by operability	NA
Takeda-2009, #3700	SBRT No acute toxicity was observed Grade 2 pneumonitis: 1 (2%) Grade 3 pneumonitis: 2 (3%) Grade 5 bacterial pneumonia at site of Grade 3 radiation pneumonitis: 1 (2%)	SBRT NA

Appendix Table C12. Attributes of studies that address Key Question 2

ID	HC	Enroll Start	Enroll Date	Design	Study Setting	Treatment Setting	Institution Setting(s)	Stage(s)	Staging Criteria	COI	Funding
Chen-2012, #4554	Y	11/04	11/09	PRO	SI	NR	TH	I	NR	N	NR
Iwata, 2010, #1747	Yes	04/03	04/07	PRO	SI	NR	TH	I	IUAC 2002	N	G
Lagerwaard, 2011, #2122	N (66%)	04/03	12/10	RET	SI	O	TH	I	NR	Y	NR
Onishi, 2011, #2802	Yes	04/95	03/04	RET	M	NR	TH	I	NR	N	G
Shibamoto – 2012, #4269	Y	05/04	11/08	PRO	M	NR	TH	I	IUAC2002	N	NR
Takeda, 2009, #3700	N (17%)	12/01	05/07	RET	M	NR	TH, CH	I	NR	N	NR

Appendix Table C13. Description of studies that address Key Question 3

Study	Study design, enrollment numbers and lost to FU/excluded	Inclusion/Exclusion Criteria	Stage Distribution	Tumor/Obstruction Location & Histopathology	Patient Characteristics
Allison-2004, USA, #108	**Study design:** SAS, PRO **Patients enrolled:** Total: 10 (100%) **Lost to FU/excluded/missing:** None	**Inclusion criteria:** Not reported, paraphrased 1. Patients with symptomatic endobronchial recurrence 2. Non responsive to multiagent chemo and RT for initial stage III NSCLC **Exclusion criteria:** Not reported	All patients had recurrent endobronchial obstruction subsequent to stage III NSCLC	**Location:** ML: 2 (20%) UL: 3 (30%) LL: 3 (30%) MS: 2 (20%) **Histopathology:** AC: 8 (80%) SCC: 2 (20%)	**Age:** 65.9 (±8.4) 66.5 (52-77) **Women:** 2 (20%) **Race:** Not reported **Co-morbidities:** Not reported **Performance status:** Baseline KPS: 45 (±7.1) Post Rx KPS: 77 (±9.5)

Chella-2000, Italy, #654	**Study design: RCT, PRO**
	
	Patients enrolled: Total: 29 (100%)
	YAGL + BCHY: 14 (48%)
	YAGL: 15 (52%)
	
	Lost to FU/excluded/missing: None
		Inclusion criteria:
		1. NSCLC involving central airway & not eligible for further surgical, chemotherapeutic or external beam RT
		2. An expectation of life of at least 2 months
		3. A performance status score (WHO) ≤ 2
		
		Exclusion criteria: Not reported
			Not reported	**Location:**
				Trachea: 6 (21%)
				Carina & both main stems: 6 (21%)
				Carina & one main stem: 7 (24%)
				One main stem: 7 (24%)
				Lobar bronchus: 3 (10%)
				
				Histopathology:
				Total:
				  SCC: 21 (72%)
				  AC: 6 (21%)
				  LCC: 2 (7%)
				YAGL + BCHY:
				  SCC: 11 (79%)
				  AC: 2 (14%)
				  LCC: 1 (7%)
				YAGL:
				  SCC: 10 (67%)
				  AC: 4 (27%)
				  LCC: 1 (7%)
					Age:
					61 (47-76) (note this is mean with range)
					
					Women:
					6 (21%)
					
					Race: Not reported
					
					Co-morbidities: Not reported
					
					Performance status:
					Total: WHO
					  0: 3 (10%)
					  I: 11 (40%)
					  II: 15 (52%)
					YAGL + BCHY:
					  0: 1 (7%)
					  I: 4 (29%)
					  II: 9 (64%)
					YAGL:
					  0: 2 (13%)
					  I: 7 (47%)
					  II: 6 (40%)

Celebioglu-2002, Turkey, #604	**Study design:** SAS, RET **Patients enrolled:**	**Inclusion criteria:** 1. Had inoperable lung cancer, proven histologically,	Stage IIIB: 83 (87%) Stage IV: 12 (13%)	**Location:** Central: 79 (83%) Peripheral: 16 (17%)	**Age:** 60 (±7, 41-81) (note this is mean with SD & range)

Study	Study design, enrollment numbers and lost to FU/excluded	Inclusion/Exclusion Criteria	Stage Distribution	Tumor/Obstruction Location & Histopathology	Patient Characteristics
	BCHY Total: 95 (100%) **Lost to FU/excluded/missing:** Not reported	2. Had endobronchial tumor, visualized via bronchoscope, 3. Were inoperable 4. Were not subjected to standard Rx regimes because of ≥1 severe symptoms or recurrence after definitive Rx. **Exclusion criteria:** Not reported		**Histopathology:** SCC: 59 (62%) NSCC: 36 (38%)	**Women:** Female: 7 (7%) **Race:** Not reported **Co-morbidities:** Not reported **Performance status:** ECOG (baseline) 1: 14 (15%) 2: 61 (64%) 3: 17 (18%) 4: 3 (3%)
Celikoglu-2006, Turkey, #606	**Study design:** SAS, PRO **Patients enrolled:** Total: 23 (100%) No of obstructions: 28 (100%) **Lost to FU/excluded/missing:** None	**Inclusion criteria:** 1. Patients presenting with symptomatic obstruction of trachea or of a major bronchus secondary to inoperable hst cnf NSCLC 2. Near complete obstruction (quantified by ≥ 50% occlusion of at least 1 major airway) 3. Disease confined to one hemithorax and without distant metastases **Exclusion criteria:** 1. Patients requiring irradiation for palliative purposes 2. Patients with small cell carcinoma	Stage IIIA: 9 (39%) Stage IIB: 14 (61%)	**Location:** MB: 14 (48%) BI: 2 (7%) UL: 4 (14%) LL: 2 (7%) Carina, MB: 3 (10%) Trachea: 4 (14%) **Histopathology:** SCC: 19 (83%) AC: 3 (13%) SCC: 1 (4%) (poorly differentiated)	**Age:** 56.8 (±8.5, 43-78) (note this is mean with SD & range) **Women:** 3 (17%) **Race:** Not reported **Co-morbidities:** Not reported **Performance status:** Not reported
Chhajed-2006, Switzerland, #696	**Study design:** SAS, RET **Patients enrolled:** Total: 144 (100%) STNT or LASR: 52 (36%) Laser only: 13 (25%) Stent only: 13 (25%) Both: 26 (50%) **Lost to FU/excluded/missing:**	**Inclusion criteria:** 1. Central airway obstruction treated with therapeutic bronchoscopy (laser with or without stent insertion) 2. Chemotherapy 3. Eligible for radiotherapy **Exclusion criteria:** 1. Untreated central airway	Not reported	**Location:** Not reported **Histopathology:** SCC: 25 (48%) AC: 14 (27%) LCC: 4 (8%) Not specified: 9 (17%)	**Age:** 61 (mean age, SD or range) Not reported) **Women:** 14 (27%) **Race:** Not reported **Co-morbidities:** Not reported

Study	Study design, enrollment numbers and lost to FU/excluded	Inclusion/Exclusion Criteria	Stage Distribution	Tumor/Obstruction Location & Histopathology	Patient Characteristics
	Not reported	obstruction, or 2. Central airway obstruction treated with therapeutic bronchoscopy but not received chemotherapy			**Performance status:** Not reported
Guilcher-2011, France, #188	**Study design:** SAS, RET **Patients enrolled:** BCHY: 226 (100%) **Lost to FU/excluded/missing:** Not reported	**Inclusion criteria:** 1. Hst proven NSCLC, endobronchial carcinomas only, 2. Normal CT, 3. No metastases Contraindication to surgical removal and EBRT, 4. Can undergo diazepam-induced analgesia **Exclusion criteria:** 1. Visible extrabronchial extension on CT scan 2. Use of HDR brachytherapy as a boost after EBRT or to treat an endobronchial recurrence of a previously treated tumor	Tis: 60 (27%) T1: 153 (68%) T2: 9 (4%) Unknown: 4 (1%)	**Location:** Proximal: 21 (9%) Distal: 200 (89%) Unknown: 5 (2%) **Histopathology:** SCC: 217 (96%) AC: 5 (2%) Others: 4 (2%)	**Age:** 62.2 (40–84) (Note this is mean age with range **Women:** 3 (1%) **Race:** Not reported **Co-morbidities:** Not reported **Performance status:** Not reported
Jimenez-1999, Spain, #978	**Study design:** RCT, PRO **Patients enrolled:** Total: 31 (100%) PHDT: 14 YAGL: 17 **Lost to FU/excluded/missing:** Not reported	**Inclusion criteria:** 1. >18 yrs of age 2. Nonpregnant, infertile or postmenopausal females. 3. Biopsy-proven or recurrent inoperable NSCLC with totally or partially obstructive endobronchial lesions with or without extrabronchial tumor 4. Clinical evidence of airway obstruction 5. KPS ≥ 40% 6. Ability to tolerate bronchoscopic procedures 7. ≥4 weeks from the last chemotherapy cycle and ≥3 weeks from the last radiation dose	PHDT: 14 (100%) Stage I: 3 (21%) Stage II: 1 (7%) Stage III: 5 (36%) Stage IV: 3 (21%) Recurrent: 2 (14%) YAGL: 17 (100%) Stage I: 1 (6%) Stage II: 0 Stage III: 11 (65%) Stage IV: 4 (24%) Recurrent: 1 (6%)	**Location:** Total: 31 (100%) MB: 20 (65%) SB: 8 (26%) IB: 3 (10%) **Histopathology:** PHDT: 14 (100%) SCC: 13 (93%) AC: 1 (7%) Undifferentiated: 0 YAGL: 17 (100%) SCC: 12 (71%) AC: 2 (12%) Undifferentiated: 3 (18%)	**Age:** Total: 64 (±7) PHDT: 67 (Mean) YAGL: 64 (Mean) **Women:** PHDT: 0 YAGL: 0 **Race:** Not reported **Co-morbidities:** Not reported **Performance status:** Quantitative numbers not reported but stated that KPS was similar b/w groups

Study	Study design, enrollment numbers and lost to FU/excluded	Inclusion/Exclusion Criteria	Stage Distribution	Tumor/Obstruction Location & Histopathology	Patient Characteristics
		Exclusion criteria: 1. Previously undergone PHDT or YAGL resection 2. had tracheal lesions that compromised both main bronchi, brain metastasis, bone pain due to skeletal metastasis, pneumonectomy, tumors eroding or invading great vessels, haematoporphyrin hypersensitivity, leukocyte count < 2X 10^9 cells.L^{-1}, platelet count <100 x 10^9 cells L^{-1}, coagulation time ≥15 min, renal failure or liver dysfunction			
Jones-2001, USA, #1862	**Study design:** SAS, RET **Patients enrolled:** Total: 10 (100%) **Lost to FU/excluded/missing:** None	**Inclusion criteria:** 1. Patients diagnosed with stage III/IV obstructive NSCLC 2. Patients who underwent PHDT **Exclusion criteria:** Not reported	Stage III: 4 (40%) Stage IV: 6 (60%)	**Location:** Total: 17 (100%) MS: 5 (29%) Trachea: 3 (18%) LL: 4 (24%) ML: 2 (12%) UL: 1 (6%) BI: 2 (12%) **Histopathology:** AC: 7 (70%) Adenoid cystic: 1 (10%) Carcinoma: 2 (20%)	**Age:** 67 (±8.8, 48-76) (SD was calculated) **Women:** 3 (30%) **Race:** Not reported **Co-morbidities:** Not reported **Performance status:** Not reported
Langendijk-2001, Netherlands, #2144	**Study design:** RCT, PRO **Patients enrolled:** Total: 95 (100%) EBRT +BCHY: 47 (49%) EBRT: 48 (51%) **Lost to FU/excluded/missing:** 98 randomized, 3 were excluded because they did not fulfill eligibility criteria. Further, 5 patients out of 95 did not complete baseline QOL assessments and were excluded from QOL analysis.	**Inclusion criteria:** 1. Have biopsy proven NSCLC, stage I, II, III 2. Endobronchial tumor in the proximal main bronchus or lobar bronchus 3. WHO performance status 0 to 3 4. No prior or planned chemo, prior surgery, prior radiotherapy, other malignancies, pleuritis carcinomatosa, distant mets or superior vena cava syndrome.	EBRT +BCHY Stage I: 4 (9%) Stage III: 43 (91%) EBRT Stage I: 5 (10%) Stage III: 43 (90%)	**Location:** EBRT +BCHY UL: 28 (58%) ML: 4 (8%) LL: 6 (13%) MB: 9 (19%) EBRT UL: 21 (44%) ML: 4 (8%) LL: 10 (21%) MB: 13 27%) **Histopathology:** Not reported	**Age:** EBRT +BCHY: 67 (±9) EBRT: 68 (±9) **Women:** EBRT +BCHY: 9 (19%) EBRT: 8 (17%) **Race:** Not reported **Co-morbidities:** Not reported **Performance status:** Total

Study	Study design, enrollment numbers and lost to FU/excluded	Inclusion/Exclusion Criteria	Stage Distribution	Tumor/Obstruction Location & Histopathology	Patient Characteristics
		Exclusion criteria: 1. Prior Rx with Neodymium-YAG laser 2. Patients with a complete obstruction 3. Patients requiring ≥ 2 catheters			0: 23 (24%) 1: 54 (57%) 2: 13 (14%) 3: 5 (5%) EBRT +BCHY 0: 11 (23%) 1: 26 (55%) 2: 8 (17%) 3: 2 (4%) EBRT 0: 12 (25%) 1: 28 (58%) 2: 5 (10%) 3: 3 (6%)
Lencioni-2008, Multiple Countries, #2238	**Study design:** SAS, PRO **Patients enrolled:** Total: 106 (100%) NSCLC: 33 (31%) **Lost to FU/excluded/missing:** Not reported but outcomes reported for 22 patients. Unknown as to how many patients contributed to OS data.	**Inclusion criteria:** 1. Age > 18 yrs; 2. Biopsy-proven NSCLC or lung mets; 3. Patients rejected for surgery & considered unfit for RT or chemo; 4. Up to 3 tumors/lung, each 3·5 cm or smaller in greatest diameter, detected by CT; 5. Tumors located at least 1 cm from trachea, main bronchi, esophagus, aorta, aortic arch branches, main, right, or left pulmonary artery and heart; 6. Tumors accessible by percutaneous route; 7. ECOG performance status of 0, 1, or 2; 8. Platelet count >100×10^9 /L; 9. INR ≤ 1·5. **Exclusion criteria:** 1. Previous pneumonectomy; 2. Patients considered high-risk for RFA because of major comorbid medical	Stage I: 13 (39%) Recurrent: 20 (61%)	**Location:** Not reported **Histopathology:** SCC: 18 (55%) AC: 13 (29%) BC: 1 (3%) LCC: 1 (3%)	**Age:** 66.5 (11.1) 67 (29-82) **Women:** 8 (24%) **Race:** Not reported **Co-morbidities:** Not reported **Performance status:** Not reported

Study	Study design, enrollment numbers and lost to FU/excluded	Inclusion/Exclusion Criteria	Stage Distribution	Tumor/Obstruction Location & Histopathology	Patient Characteristics
		conditions 3. Tumors associated with atelectasis or obstructive pneumonitis; 4. Renal failure needing hemo or peritoneal dialysis; 5. Active clinically serious infection; 6. History of organ allograft; substance abuse or any medical, psychological, or social conditions that might interfere with the patients participation in the study or assessment of the study findings			

Moghissi-1999, UK, #2591	**Study design:** RCT, PRO
	
	Patients enrolled:
	Total: 75 (100%)
	EBRT: 38 (51%)
	EBHT: 37 (49%)
	
	Lost to FU/excluded/missing:
	16 excluded
		Inclusion criteria:
		1. No previous thoracic RT
		2. Partial obstruction of trachea or partial or complete obstruction of bronchus or a lobar bronchus
		3. Microscopically confirmed NSCLC
		4. Locally too advanced for surgical resection or radical RT.
		
		Exclusion criteria:
		Not reported
			Not reported	**Location:**
				EBRT:
				  Trachea: 1 (3%)
				  MB: 22 (53%)
				  Others: 15(39%)
				EBHT:
				  Trachea: 1 (3%)
				  MB: 21 (57%)
				  Others: 1 (41%)
				
				Histopathology:
				Not reported
					Age:
					EBRT: 72
					EBHT: 71
					(Note these are median age)
					
					Women:
					EBRT: 15 (39%)
					EBHT: 13 (35%)
					
					Race:
					Not reported
					
					Co-morbidities:
					Not reported
					
					Performance status:
					EBRT (WHO PS):
					  0: 3 (8%)
					  1: 16 (42%)
					  2: 14 (37%)
					  3: 5 (13%)
					EBHT (WHO PS):
					  0: 2 (1%)
					  1: 16 (43%)
					  2: 14 (38%)
					  3: 5 (14%)

Muto-2000, Italy, #2665	**Study design:** SAS, PRO **Patients enrolled:** Total: 320 (100%) BCHY (10 Gy): 84 (26%)	**Inclusion criteria:** 1. Histological proven NSCLC 2. Stage IIIA-IIIB 3. KPS > 60 4. Life expectancy > 6	Not reported	**Location:** Not reported **Histopathology:** Not reported	**Age:** Not reported **Women:** Not reported

Study	Study design, enrollment numbers and lost to FU/excluded	Inclusion/Exclusion Criteria	Stage Distribution	Tumor/Obstruction Location & Histopathology	Patient Characteristics
	BCHY (14Gy) + EBRT: 47 (15%) BCHY (15Gy, 1cm) + EBRT: 50 16%) BCHY (15Gy, 0.5 cm) + EBRT: 139 (43%) **Lost to FU/excluded/missing:** LTFU: 40 (13%) Evaluable patients: BCHY (10 Gy): 78 (28%) BCHY (14Gy) + EBRT: 46 (16%) BCHY (15Gy, 1cm) + EBRT: 36 (13%) BCHY (15Gy, 0.5 cm) + EBRT: 120 (43%)	months 5. Presence of cough and/or dyspnea, hemoptysis, obstr pneumonia 6. No chemo before or after RT **Exclusion criteria:** Not reported			**Race:** Not reported **Co-morbidities:** Not reported **Performance status:** Not reported
Mallick-2006, India, #2417	**Study design:** PRO, RCT **Patients enrolled:** Total: 45 (100%) EBRT + BCHY-16Gy: 15 (33.3%) EBRT + BCHY-10Gy: 15 (33.3%) BCHY-15Gy: 15 (33.4%) **Lost to FU/excluded/missing:** None	**Inclusion criteria:** 1. Previously untreated, inoperable, locally advanced NSCLC patients. 2. Endoscopically proven endobronchial disease with ≥ 1 symptom (dyspnea, cough, hemoptysis or obstructive pneumonia) 3. KPS score between 60 to 80 **Exclusion criteria:** 1. Previously Rx patients 2. Those with mets who would require primary chemo.	Stage III: 45 (100%)	**Location:** EBRT+BCHY-16Gy: 15 MB: 6 (40%) LB: 9 (60%) EBRT+BCHY-10Gy: 15 MB: 6 (40%) LB: 9 (60%) BCHY-15Gy: 15 MB: 8 (53%) LB: 7 (47%) **Histopathology:** EBRT+BCHY-16Gy: 15 SCC: 13 (87%) AC: 1 (7%) LCC: 1 (7%) EBRT+BCHY-10Gy: 15 SCC: 13 (87%) AC: 2 (13 %) BCHY-15Gy: 15 SCC: 14 (93%) AC: 1 (7%)	**Age:** Total: 64.5 (35-75) EBRT+BCHY-16Gy: 68.9 (45-75) EBRT+BCHY-10Gy: 63.1 (46-70) BCHY-15Gy: 61.5 (35-70) (Age is in mean) **Women:** Total: 2 (4%) EBRT+BCHY-16Gy: 0 EBRT+BCHY-10Gy: 1 (7%) BCHY-15Gy: 1 (7%) **Race:** Not reported **Co-morbidities:** Not reported **Performance status:** Not reported
Petera-2001, Czech Republic, #2914	**Study design:** SAS, PRO **Patients enrolled:** Total: 67 (100%) BCHY (Cur): 20 (30%) BCHY (Pall): 21 (31%)	**Inclusion criteria:** BCHY (Cur): 1. Inoperable LC with WHO PS 0 to 2 2. Without wt loss >10% in previous 6 months	BCHY (Cur): Stage II: 2 (10%) Stage III: 16 (80%) Stage IV: 1 (5%) Other: 1 (5%) BCHY (Pall):	**Location:** BCHY (Cur): MS: 6 (30%) Lobar bronchus: 9 (45%) > 1 location: 5 (25%) BCHY (Pall): MS: 5 (24%)	**Age:** BCHY (Cur): 59 (46-75) BCHY (Pall): 63 (49-83) (Note: This is mean with range) **Women:**

C-84

Study	Study design, enrollment numbers and lost to FU/excluded	Inclusion/Exclusion Criteria	Stage Distribution	Tumor/Obstruction Location & Histopathology	Patient Characteristics
	Lost to FU/excluded/missing: BCHY (Pall): 1 (1%)	BCHY (Pall): 1. Advanced disease 2. Poor performance status 3. With wt loss >10% in previous 6 months **Exclusion criteria:** Not reported	Stage III: 16 (76%) Stage IV: 3 (14%) Other: 2 (10%)	Lobar bronchus: 11 (52%) > 1 location: 5 (24%) **Histopathology:** BCHY (Cur): SC: 18 (90%) AC: 1 (5%) NSCLC unspec: 1 (5%) BCHY (Pall): SC: 19 (90%) AC: 1 (5%) NSCLC unspec: 1 (5%)	BCHY (Cur): 0 (0%) BCHY (Pall): 3 (14%) **Race:** Not reported **Co-morbidities:** Not reported **Performance status:** Not reported
Stout-2000, UK, #3640	**Study design:** RCT, PRO **Patients enrolled:** Total: 108 (100%) BCHY: 49 (49%) EBRT: 50 (51%) **Lost to FU/excluded/missing:** 9 (8%) excluded- relapsed after surgery	**Inclusion criteria:** 1. Thoracic symptoms limited to cough, hemoptysis or breathlessness 2. fit to undergo therapeutic bronchoscopy or fractionated EBRT (WHO PS 0 to 2) 3. no clinical evidence of malignant disease beyond thorax 4. histologically confirmed NSCLC medically operable **Exclusion criteria:** Not reported	Not reported	**Location:** Not reported **Histopathology:** SCC: 81 (82%)	**Age:** 68 (40-84) Note this is mean) **Women:** 20 (20%) **Race:** Not reported **Co-morbidities:** Not reported **Performance status:** WHO BCHY: 2: 8 (16%) 3: 3 (6%) NR: 32 (78%) EBRT: 2: 13 (27%) 3: 4 (8%) NR: 32 (65%)
van Boxem-1999, Netherlands, #427	**Study design:** NRC, RET **Patients enrolled:** Total: 31 (100%) YAGL: 14 (45%) ECAU: 17 (55%)	**Inclusion criteria:** 1. Patients had centrally located inoperable NSCLC and underwent bronchoscopic Rx because of dyspnea due to tracheobronchial obstruction caused by	**YAGL** Stage IV: 6 (43%) Stage IIIB: 6(43%) Stage IIIA: 2 (14%) **ECAU** Stage IV: 6 (35%) Stage IIIB: 10 (59%)	**Location:** YAGL Trachea: 3 (21%) Bronchi: 11 (79%) **ECAU** Trachea: 3 (18%) Bronchi: 14 (82%)	**Age:** YAGL: 61 (37-88) ECAU:62 (47-79) **Women:** YAGL: 3 (21%) ECAU: 7 (41%)

Study	Study design, enrollment numbers and lost to FU/excluded	Inclusion/Exclusion Criteria	Stage Distribution	Tumor/Obstruction Location & Histopathology	Patient Characteristics
	Lost to FU/excluded/missing: Total: 0 YAGL: 0 ECAU: 0	intraluminal tumor **Exclusion criteria:** Not reported	Stage IIIA: 1 (6%)	**Histopathology:** **YAGL** AC: 1 (7%) SCC: 10 (71%) LCC: 3 (21%) **ECAU** AC: 5 (29%) SCC: 4 (24%) LCC: 8 (47%)	**Race:** YAGL: Not reported ECAU: Not reported **Co-morbidities:** YAGL: Not reported ECAU: Not reported **Performance status:** YAGL: Not reported ECAU: Not reported
Vucicevic-1999, Yugoslavia, #4010	**Study design:** SAS, RET **Patients enrolled:** Total: 39 (100%) **Lost to FU/excluded/missing:** Not reported	**Inclusion criteria:** 1. Inoperable, occlusive histologically confirmed stage IIIB NSCLC **Exclusion criteria:** Not reported	Stage III: 39 (100%)	**Location:** Not reported **Histopathology:** AC: 2 (5%) SCC: 37 (95%)	**Age:** 60.6 (42-75) **Women:** 2 (5%) **Race:** Not reported **Co-morbidities:** Not reported **Performance status:** KPS: Range was 70-100%
Weinberg-2010, USA, #4066	**Study design:** SAS, RET **Patients enrolled:** Total: 9 (100%) **Lost to FU/excluded/missing:** None	**Inclusion criteria:** 1. Patients received PHDT & HDR BCHY for endobronchial tumors **Exclusion criteria:** Not reported	I/II: 1 (11%) II: 1 (11%) III: 6 (67%) IV: 1 (11%)	**Location:** UL: 7 (29%) LL: 4 (17%) ML: 1 (4%) MS: 5 (21%) Bl: 2 (8%) Trachea: 1 (4%) Lymph node: 2 (8%) Hilum: 1 (4%) Lingual: 1 (4%) **Histopathology:** SCC: 9 (100%)	**Age:** (52-73) **Women:** 1 (11%) **Race:** Not reported **Co-morbidities:** Not reported **Performance status:** Not reported

Appendix Table C14. Outcomes and interventions of studies that address Key Question 3

Study	Study Outcomes	Interventions
Allison-2004, #108	**Study Objective:** Authors reported in a case series fashion outcomes of 10 patients with symptomatic endobronchial	**Intervention name:** Stenting plus HDR brachytherapy

Study	Study Outcomes	Interventions
	recurrence who underwent 2 simultaneous interventions: stenting and HDR brachytherapy **Primary outcome:** Not reported **Definition:** NA **Secondary outcome(s):** Not reported **Definitions:** NA **List of Outcome(s):** Local control, OS **Cause of death:** Progression of LC: 10 (100%) **Length of FU:** Not reported	**Vendor name:** Self-expanding metallic stent (Nitinol/Ultraflex, Boston Scientific Co., Natick, MA) **Dose/frequency/details:** 6 Gy was delivered to 0.5-cm depth via a Nucletron HDR for brachytherapy. Two additional HDR Rx were delivered at weekly intervals for a total dose of 18 Gy. **Technical details:** Flexible bronchoscope was used to place stent and simultaneously an HDR catheter was introduced. **Treatment Intention:** Palliative **Follow-up and Evaluation Criteria:** • Patients underwent bronchoscopy at each HDR and FU bronchoscope 1 & 3 months after the last HDR Rx, as well as when clinically indicated. • Biopsy was taken 1 or 3 months after the last HDR Rx. • All patients were FU to progression or death
Chella-2000, #654	**Study Objective:** To compare the efficacy of the combined Nd-YAG laser: HDR brachytherapy versus bronchial debulking with Nd-YAG laser alone in a prospective randomized study treatment. **Primary outcome:** Disease progression free period **Definition:** Not reported **Secondary outcome(s):** Not reported **Definitions:** NA **List of Outcome(s):** Further endoscopic Rxs, median survival, PFT, blood gas analysis, Speiser's index **Cause of death:** Dead: 18 (62%) 　Local progression: 13 (72%) 　Distant mets: 5 (28%) **Length of FU:** Median FU: 17.8 months (9–35)	**Intervention name:** Laser and HDR brachytherapy **Vendor name:** Rigid bronchoscope (Wolf or Effer –Dumon) Catheter for BCHY (Nucletron) **Dose/frequency/details:** YAGL: Energy of 25–45 W, using pulses up to 1.2 s, was used for a mean total amount of 1850 J (range 1400–2200 J) BCHY: HDR brachytherapy 15–18 days after Nd-YAG laser debulking. High radioactive Iridium-192 source (10 Ci), prescribed dose was 5 Gy at 0.5 cm, with a total exposition time variable from 10 to 15 min. Rx was repeated 3 times every 7 days for a total dose of 15 Gy. **Technical details:** None **Treatment Intention:** Not reported **Follow-up and Evaluation Criteria:** • Pulmonary function tests; arterial blood gas assessment; chest radiograph; fiberoptic bronchoscopy at baseline, 14 days after the laser debulking and from 30 to 45 days after HDR brachytherapy • A radiological (chest film and CT scan) and endoscopic followup

Study	Study Outcomes	Interventions
		performed every 2 months.
		• Airway obstruction grade was calculated according to Speiser's obstruction score method
		• Intraluminal radiotherapy associated morbidity was assessed according to Gollins's scoring system
Celebioglu-2002, #604	**Study Objective:** To compare the palliation improvement pre- and post-radiotherapy.	**Intervention name:** HDR brachytherapy
	Primary outcome: Not reported **Definition:** NA	**Vendor name:** 3D planning unit (Nucletron Plato) HDR unit (Nucletron)
	Secondary outcome(s): Not reported **Definitions:** NA	**Dose/frequency/details:** Total Rx length: 4–8 cm Total Rx time: 10–16 min. Brachytherapy delivered at weeks 1, 2 and 3 at 7.5 Gy per fraction or at weeks 1 and 2 at 10 Gy per fraction. In poor performance status patient's two fractions were preferred.
	List of Outcome(s): Symptom control, toxicity	
	Cause of death: Not reported	**Technical details:** Bronchoscopy under local anesthesia, used opaque dummy wire for fluoroscopic verification
	Length of FU: Surviving patients FU for a minimum of 3 months with a mean of 7.5±5.4 months	**Treatment Intention:** Palliative
		Follow-up and Evaluation Criteria: • All patients eval at 6th wk and at the 3rd month of Rx • Speiser's scoring index for scoring endobronchial obstruction • Performance status - ECOG scale
Celikoglu-2006, #606	**Study Objective:** To study the effectiveness, safety, and feasibility of initial debulking by intratumoral chemotherapy with cisplatin followed by irradiation in the treatment of obstructive inoperable NSCLC.	**Intervention name:** Intratumoral cisplatin followed by radiation
	Primary outcome: Not reported **Definition:** NA	**Vendor name:** Not reported
	Secondary outcome(s): Not reported **Definitions:** NA	**Dose/frequency/details:** Intratumoral chemotherapy was performed under LA through a flexible fiber optic bronchoscope Chemotherapy: Injection of up to 40 mg cisplatin (approx. 2 mg cisplatin per cubic centimeter of the tumor) at each Rx session. Cisplatin given every week, for 3 weeks (on days 1, 8, 15 and 22).
	List of Outcome(s): % obstruction, mean survival	

Study	Study Outcomes	Interventions

	Cause of death: Not reported
	
	Length of FU: Not reported
		Radiation: At 3–7 days after the last session of intratumoral chemotherapy 60 Gy in 24 fractions (2.5 Gy per fraction)
		
		Technical details: None
		
		Treatment Intention:
		Curative
		
		Follow-up and Evaluation Criteria:
		• In the absence of a bronchial residual tumor 1 month after irradiation, the patient's condition was assessed at 3-monthly intervals by clinical findings, chest X-ray film, and bronchoscopy.
		• Survival period was measured from the first intratumoral session day.
		• Criteria for efficacy of debulking:
		    Good response: >50% ↑ in diameter of the airway's lumen
		    Moderate response: 25—50% ↑ in diameter of the lumen
		    Small response: <25% ↑ in diameter of the lumen

Chhajed-2006, #696	**Study Objective:** In patients with advanced NSCLC treated with chemotherapy, we compared survival in patients with treated central airway obstruction to those who did not have central airway obstruction. **Primary outcome:** Not reported **Definition:** NA **Secondary outcome(s):** Not reported **Definitions:** NA **List of Outcome(s):** Survival, toxicity **Cause of death:** Not reported **Length of FU:** Not reported	**Intervention name:** Therapeutic bronchoscopy (laser and/or stent insertion) Patients received chemotherapy (with or without external beam radiation) prior or after or both time periods after therapeutic bronchoscopy (laser and/or stent insertion) **Vendor name:** Rigid bronchoscopy (Efer-Dumon; Karl Storz Optics; Tuttlingen, Germany) Laser ablation (Smart 1064 DW; Deka Medical Electronic Associates; Calenzano, Italy) **Dose/frequency/details:** NA **Technical details:** Rigid bronchoscopy under general anesthesia Laser ablation using either rigid or flexible bronchoscope **Treatment Intention:** Not clearly stated **Follow-up and Evaluation Criteria:** Survival calculated from the date of administration of chemotherapy or therapeutic bronchoscopy, whichever was earlier.
Guilcher-2011, #188	**Study Objective:** To assess retrospectively the efficacy and tolerance of HDR brachytherapy alone in the Rx of patients with	**Intervention name:** HDR-brachytherapy

Study	Study Outcomes	Interventions
	endobronchial tumors that cannot be removed surgically or benefit from EBRT	**Vendor name:** Not reported
	Primary outcome: Not reported **Definition:** NA	**Dose/frequency/details:** Total dose: <30 Gy: 160 (71%); ≥30 Gy: 66 (29%) Fractions: ≤5: 106 (47%); > 5: 120 (53%) Dose/fraction: ≤5: 148 (65%); > 5: 78 (35%)
	Secondary outcome(s): Not reported **Definitions:** NA	**Technical details:** Tumor located by bronchoscopy. ≥ 1 catheters were implanted next to the lesion via the working channel of the bronchoscope. Target volume was drawn with a 1-to 2-cm safety margin. The dose was prescribed to be delivered at 1 cm from an Iridium-192 source.
	List of Outcome(s): OS, CSS, Local Control, Toxicity	
	Cause of death: Total dead: 128 (57%) LC: 57 (45%) Intercurrent disease: 45 (35%) Rx toxicity: 13 (10%) Other cancers: 12 (9%) Unknown cause: 1 (1%)	**Treatment Intention:** Not reported **Follow-up and Evaluation Criteria:** • FU varied according to the center but usually included bronchoscopy and chest CT scan every 6 months. • Speiser and Spratling scale to assess radiation bronchitis
	Length of FU: 30.4 months (9-116) (note this is mean with range)	
Jimenez-1999, #978	**Study Objective:** To conduct a prospective RCT in order to assess the effectiveness and safety of photodynamic therapy versus laser resection in 31 patients with partial or complete tracheobronchial obstruction due to inoperable NSCLC.	**Intervention name:** PHDT YAGL **Vendor name:** Photofrin; Lederle, Vancouver, Canada
	Primary outcome: Not reported **Definition:** NA	**Dose/frequency/details:** PHDT: Tumors were irradiated (630-nm light) via a flexible fibreoptic bronchoscope 40-50 h after IV 2 mg/kg DHE. 2nd irradiation done if parts of tumor failed to show signs of necrosis 96-120 h after 1st irradiation. Max of 3 doses of DHE at 1-month intervals and up to 6 laser photoradiations, with max of 2 photoradiations/ session. YAGL: Rigid bronchoscope, general anesthesia, performed using 15-80 W pulses and a pulse duration of 0.5-1.5 s. Sessions repeated every 2-4 days until it was considered that further application would not give additional benefits.
	Secondary outcome(s): Not reported **Definitions:** NA	
	List of Outcome(s): Survival, toxicity, response rate, time to Rx failure	
	Cause of death: Total dead: 23 (74.2%) Progression of malignancy PHDT: 7 (50%) YAGL: 12 (71%) Probably related to Rx: PHDT: 1 (7%) YAGL: 0	**Technical details:** None

Study	Study Outcomes	Interventions
	Death from hemoptysis and presumed progression of the disease PHDT: 1 (7%) YAGL: 1 (6%) Unknown reasons: 3 (10%) **Length of FU:** Protocol specified all patients to be followed for 24 months.	**Treatment Intention:** Palliation **Follow-up and Evaluation Criteria:** Control bronchoscopy after either PDT or Nd-YAG laser resection was performed 1 week after PDT, every month for 3 months and at 6 and 12 months (and at 18 months, if possible) thereafter. A
Jones-2001, #1862	**Study Objective:** To summarize early experience with PHDT in the palliation of symptoms in patients with terminal lung cancer and obstructing endobronchial lesions. **Primary outcome:** Not reported **Definition:** NA **Secondary outcome(s):** Not reported **Definitions:** NA **List of Outcome(s):** Survival, symptoms **Cause of death:** Not reported **Length of FU:** Not reported	**Intervention name:** PHDT **Vendor name:** Coherent Lambda plus Argon Laser (Santa Clara, CA) **Dose/frequency/details:** Porfirmer sodium (2.0 mg/kg) given 48 hours prior to laser, 630 nm wavelength, average light delivered per session (200 J/cm) **Technical details:** Flexible bronchoscope was used **Treatment Intention:** Palliation **Follow-up and Evaluation Criteria:** Not reported
Langendijk-2001, #2144	**Study Objective:** To test the hypothesis that the addition of endobronchial BCHY to EBRT provides higher levels of palliation of dyspnea and other respiratory symptoms and improvement of QOL in patients with NSCLC with endobronchial tumor **Primary outcome:** Response rate of dyspnea **Definition: Response was defined as** • Baseline score 'moderate or severe', with improvement to 'mild' or 'nil' on at least 2 consecutive assessments in the first 3 months after the end of RT=improvement • Baseline score 'mild', with improvement to 'nil' on at least 2 consecutive assessments in the first 3 months after the end of RT= improvement • Baseline score 'mild', with 'mild' on at least 2 consecutive assessments in the first 3 months after the end of RT= control • Baseline score 'nil', with 'nil' on at least 2 consecutive assessments in the first 3 months after the end of RT = prevention	**Intervention name:** BCHY **Vendor name:** For BCHY: HDR-microselectron (Nucletron, Leersum, The Netherlands) **Dose/frequency/details:** Palliative schedule: 3 Gy/fraction (4 times a week) up to a total dose of 30 Gy (100%) without correction for lung tissue density. Radical schedule: 2.25 Gy/fraction (4 times a week) to a total dose of 45 Gy followed by a boost up to 60 Gy using fraction doses of 2.5 Gy (four times a week). Correction was made for lung tissue density (0.3). BCHY: Under LA, Iridium 1^{92} stepping source, using a stepping size of 2.5 or 5 mm Palliative: 23% (11 of 48) in EBRT; 19% (9 of 47) in EBRT+BCHY Radical: 77% (37 of 48) in EBRT; 81% (38 of 47) in EBRT+BCHY **Technical details:** Note that both palliative & radical RT based on severity of disease and

Study	Study Outcomes	Interventions
	Secondary outcome(s): Re-expansion of atelectasis, survival and complications **Definitions:** Not reported **List of Outcome(s):** QOL and other respiratory symptoms were evaluated on exploratory basis **Cause of death:** EBRT +BCHY: Total: 44/48 (92%) Local progression: 12 (26%) Massive hemoptysis: 7 (15%) Mets: 16 (34%) Local progression + mets: 1 (2%) Intercurrent disease: 1 (2%) Unknown: 6(13%) EBRT: Total: 40/47 (85%) Local progression: 17 (35%) Massive hemoptysis: 6 (13%) Mets: 11(23%) Local progression + mets: 2 (4%) Intercurrent disease: 4 (8%) Unknown: 1(2%)	performance status was given to both Rx arms. **Treatment Intention:** • Note that both palliative & radical RT based on severity of disease and performance status was given to both Rx arms. • Palliative RT: Patients with WHO performance status 3, supraclavicular lymph node mets and/or distant mets with symptoms related to intrathoracic tumor • Radical RT: Patients with stage I or II disease with a tumor diameter > 4 cm or stage IIIa and stage IIIb disease without supraclavicular lymph node mets and a WHO performance ≤2 **Follow-up and Evaluation Criteria:** • QOL and RS were assessed before the start of RT and subsequently 2 weeks, 6 weeks and 3, 6 and 12 months after end of RT • Dutch version of the EORTC QLQ-C30 (version 1.0) and the lung cancer module QLQ-LC13 were used to measure QOL
	Length of FU: Not reported	
Lencioni-2008, #2238	**Study Objective:** To assess the feasibility, safety, & effectiveness of percutaneous CT-guided RFA in the Rx of NSCLC & pulmonary mets. **Primary outcome:** Technical success, safety (Rx-related complications & changes in pulmonary function), and confirmed CR of the target tumors **Definition:** Technical success defined as correct placement of the ablation device into all target tumors with completion of the planned ablation protocol—i.e, maintenance of the target temperature of 90°C for the required time according to tumor size. Treatment-related complications were those occurring within 30 days from treatment. Complications were assessed on a per-procedure basis and defined as follows. Minor: Those resulting in no sequel or needing nominal treatment or a short hospital stay for observation. Major: Those resulting in readmission to the hospital for Rx, extended an unplanned increase in the level of care, extended	**Intervention name:** RFA **Vendor name:** RITA Medical Systems Model 1500 and Model 1500X (AngioDynamics, Queensbury, NY) **Dose/frequency/details:** Time spent achieving target temperature of 90 degree Celsius. **Technical details:** Not reported **Treatment Intention:** Not reported **Follow-up and Evaluation Criteria:** • OS: Time from the beginning of Rx to last FU visit or death from any cause was used. • CSS: Time from the beginning of Rx to last FU visit or cancer related death was used. • FU visits scheduled 1 & 3 months after Rx & then at 3-months intervals for up to 2 years.

Study	Study Outcomes	Interventions
		• Physical examination; radiological imaging for tumor assessment, including CT, KPS, PFT, FACT-L, SF-12, adverse events.
	hospitalization, permanent adverse sequel, or death.	
	Secondary outcome(s): OS, CSS, QOL **Definitions:** Not reported	
	List of Outcome(s): NA	
	Cause of death: Reported but cannot be discerned	
	Length of FU: Mean 15 months (1-30)	
Moghissi-1999, #2591	**Study Objective:** To compare the efficacy and adverse effects of the two Rx in terms of palliation of breathlessness, cough, hemoptysis, chest pain, stridor, resp function, performance status, QOL, days of inpatient management and survival.	**Intervention name:** EBRT EBHT (Brachytherapy, Cryotherapy, Laser)
		Vendor name: Not reported
	Primary outcome: Not reported **Definition:** NA	**Dose/frequency/details:** EBRT: 17 Gy in 2 fractions (n=12) EBHT: 13 Gy (n=13)
	Secondary outcome(s): Not reported **Definitions:** NA	**Technical details:** Not reported
	List of Outcome(s): Survival, Obstructive symptoms, PS	**Treatment Intention:** Palliative
	Cause of death: Not reported	**Follow-up and Evaluation Criteria:** • Patients assessed before Rx, at time of randomization, then 4 weeks, 2, 4 & 6 months thereafter
	Length of FU: NA	• QOL: Rotterdam Symptoms checklist and patient diary
Muto-2000, #2665	**Study Objective:** To demonstrate that a fractionated HDR BCHY is tolerable for patients with advanced NSCLC and improves symptoms	**Intervention name:** EBRT HDR BCHY
		Vendor name: Not reported
	Primary outcome: Not reported **Definition:** NA	**Dose/frequency/details:** EBRT: 15 MV linear accelerator, daily dose 2 Gy, delivered 60 Gy to tumor bed and 50 Gy to mediastinum.
	Secondary outcome(s): Not reported **Definitions:** NA	BCHY (10 Gy): 10 GY in single fraction BCHY (14Gy) + EBRT: 14 Gy (2 fractions of 7 Gy)
	List of Outcome(s): Survival, toxicity	

Study	Study Outcomes	Interventions
	Cause of death: Not reported **Length of FU:** 5-36 months	BCHY (15Gy, 1cm) + EBRT: 15 Gy (3 fractions of 5Gy each) (1 cm from central axis) BCHY (15Gy, 0.5 cm) + EBRT: 15 Gy (3 fractions of 5Gy each) (0.5 cm from central axis) **Technical details:** None **Treatment Intention:** Palliative **Follow-up and Evaluation Criteria:** Chest x-ray after 1-3 months from last HDR BCHY Bronchoscopy & CT scan after 6 months
Mallick-2006, #2417	**Study Objective:** To compare the subjective and objective responses to 3 Rxs for endobronchial palliation, response duration, QOL and complications in stage III NSCLC. **Primary outcome:** Not reported **Definition:** NA **Secondary outcome(s):** Not reported **Definitions:** NA **List of Outcome(s):** Symptom and obstruction score, duration of symptoms, QOL, complications **Cause of death:** Not reported **Length of FU:** 6 months (2-17)	**Intervention name:** Brachytherapy External beam radiation **Vendor name:** BCHY (Treatment planning done with Nucletron PLATO treatment) **Dose/frequency/details:** i. EBRT-30 Gy in 10 fractions+ BCHY-16Gy in 2 fractions; ii. EBRT-30 Gy in10 fractions+ BCHY-10Gy single fraction; iii. BCHY-15Gy single fraction **Technical details:** EBRT: Megavoltage photon beam of Co^{60} or a 6-MV linear accelerator **Treatment Intention:** Palliative **Follow-up and Evaluation Criteria:** • Symptoms were scored before Rx and at monthly intervals after Rx completion. Chest X-ray was done at monthly intervals. QOL assessments (EORTC QLQ-C30 and LC 13 version) were done before and at end of 1 months after Rx. • Speiser Score for Symptom and Obstruction • Toxicity: RTOG morbidity scoring criteria
Petera-2001, #2914	**Study Objective:** To report the effect of combination therapy (teletherapy + brachytherapy) given as curative & palliative on symptomatic response, tumor response, survival rate and complications (paraphrased)	**Intervention name:** Teletherapy + BCHY **Vendor name:** HDR loading system (Gammamed, MDS, Nordion, Hahn, Germany)

Study	Study Outcomes	Interventions
	Primary outcome: Not reported **Definition:** NA **Secondary outcome(s): Not reported** **Definitions:** NA **List of Outcome(s):** Survival, symptoms **Cause of death: Not reported** **Length of FU:** Median FU of living patients: BCHY (Cur): 304 days (92-638) BCHY (Pall): 274 days (212-881) Calculated from the first BCHY Rx.	**Dose/frequency/details:** BCHY (Cur): BCHY dose was 3X5 Gy, teletherapy dose was 50 Gy in 25 fractions to the mediastinum and 60Gy in 30 fractions to the primary tumor. BCHY (Pall): BCHY dose was 3X7.5 Gy, mean dose from EBRT was 42.3 Gy (10-56). **Technical details:** None **Treatment Intention:** Curative and palliative **Follow-up and Evaluation Criteria:** Symptom evaluation: Scoring system by Speiser & Spralling Bronchoscopy & chest X-ray 6 weeks after compulsion of RT.
Stout-2000, #3640	**Study Objective:** To evaluate the clinical and QOL of patients receiving BCHY and EBRT as a primary palliative Rx in advanced lung cancer. **Primary outcome: Not reported** **Definition:** NA **Secondary outcome(s): Not reported** **Definitions:** NA **List of Outcome(s):** Symptoms (clinician & patient assessment), survival, QOL (Hospital Anxiety and Depression Scale) **Cause of death:** Not reported **Length of FU:** Not reported. Patients followed up till dead.	**Intervention name:** BCHY EBRT **Vendor name:** BCHY: HDR-microselectron **Dose/frequency/details:** BCHY: 15 Gy dose, flexible bronchoscope EBRT: 8 exposures over 10-12 days- max s/c dose of 30Gy **Technical details:** None **Treatment Intention:** Palliative **Follow-up and Evaluation Criteria:** • Positive symptom: If symptom absent at baseline and absent at follow-up assessment OR if symptom is graded mild at baseline and graded mild OR absent at follow-up assessment OR if symptom is graded moderate or severe at baseline and graded mild or absent at follow-up assessment. • Global palliation: Each negative symptom endpoint was assigned a score of 0 and a positive endpoint 1, giving a range of scores 0 to 9. A total score of 0 to 4 was poor palliation and 5 to 9 good palliation. • Baseline & 4, 8, 16, 26, 38 and 52 weeks and every 3 months afterwards. • Acute Rx side effects: those that occurred within 4-8 weeks of Rx.
van Boxem-	**Study Objective:** To evaluate the cost-effectiveness of YAGL and	**Intervention name:**

Study	Study Outcomes	Interventions
1999, #427	ECAU for palliation in patients with symptomatic endoluminal obstruction due to NSCLC	YAGL ECAU
	Primary outcome: Not reported **Definition:** NA	**Vendor name:** YAGL: Sharplan Lasers, Allendale, NJ ECAU: Valleylab; Boulder, CO
	Secondary outcome(s): Not reported **Definitions:** NA	**Dose/frequency/details:** Coagulation with both interventions was performed using power settings up to 55 W YAGL: 1.1 ±0.3 session per patient ECAU: 1.2 ±0.4 session per patient
	List of Outcome(s): Improvement of symptoms, complication rate, mean survival	**Technical details:** Flexible and rigid bronchoscopes were used in most cases.
	Cause of death: Not reported	**Treatment Intention:** YAGL: Palliative ECAU: Palliative
	Length of FU: Not reported	**Follow-up and Evaluation Criteria:** • Planned FU times Not reported • Calculated from time after therapy ends **Note:** Dyspnea improvement was evaluated as yes or no by 2 authors
Vucicevic-1999, #4010	**Study Objective:** To assess the results of HDR BCHY in combination with EBRT in NSCLC patients	**Intervention name:** EBRT plus HDR BCHY
	Primary outcome: Not reported **Definition:** NA	**Vendor name:** Not reported
	Secondary outcome(s): Not reported **Definitions:** NA	**Dose/frequency/details:** HDR BCHY: Mean dose of 2100 cGy in 3 fractions (1 fraction per week) EBRT: High energy photo beam (6 or 10 MV) up to a total dose of 3000-4500 cGY in 10-22 fractions/ 5 fractions per week.
	List of Outcome(s): Survival, symptoms, toxicity	**Technical details:** None
	Cause of death: Not reported	**Treatment Intention:** Palliative
	Length of FU: Average FU: 7 months (2-19)	**Follow-up and Evaluation Criteria:** Bronchoscopy & chest X-ray 1-3 months after BCHY Rx. OS was calculated by Kaplan Meier from the time of completion

Study	Study Outcomes	Interventions
Weinberg-2010, #4066	**Study Objective:** To review the outcomes of combined PHDT + HDR-BCHY for patients with symptomatic obstruction from endobronchial NSCLC **Primary outcome:** Not reported **Definition:** NA **Secondary outcome(s):** Not reported **Definitions:** NA **List of Outcome(s):** Survival, toxicity **Cause of death:** Not reported **Length of FU:** Not reported	**Intervention name:** HDR-BCHY Chemotherapy PHDT **Vendor name:** Not reported **Dose/frequency/details:** BCHY: Flexible bronchoscope, 500 Gy delivered to 0.5cm depth via a nucletron remote after loading HDR unit. 2 additional HDR Rx delivered at weekly intervals for a total dose of 15 Gy in 3 fractions. PHDT: 2 mg/kg photoforin 48 hrs prior to given Rx. 630 nm light to a dose of 200 J/cm^2 **Technical details:** None **Treatment Intention:** Palliative **Follow-up and Evaluation Criteria:** All patients had a routine monthly bronchoscopy for first 3 months and then every 3-6 months as indicated

Appendix Table C15. Survival and local control outcomes of studies that address Key Question 3

Study	Survival Outcomes for Intervention Group 1	Survival Outcomes for Intervention Group 2	Local Control Outcomes for Intervention Group 1	Local Control Outcomes for Intervention Group 2	Arm
Allison-2004, #108	**Overall survival:** 10.3 months (±4.1) (calculated) **Cancer/disease specific survival:** Not reported	**Overall survival:** NA **Cancer/disease specific survival:** NA	**Local control:** 100 %. No patient had local recurrence till they all died. However, mean or median FU time not reported.	**Local control:** NA	No
Chella-2000, #654	YAGL + BCHY **Overall survival:** Median survival: 10.3 months (method Not reported) **Cancer/disease specific survival:** Not reported	YAGL **Overall survival:** Median survival: 7.4 months (method Not reported) **Cancer/disease specific survival:** Not reported	YAGL + BCHY **Local control:** Not reported	YAGL **Local control:** Not reported	No
Celebioglu-2002, #604	**Overall survival:** Not reported **Cancer/disease specific survival:** Not reported	**Overall survival:** NA **Cancer/disease specific survival:** NA	**Local control:** Not reported	**Local control:** NA	No
Celikoglu-2006, #606	**Overall survival:** Not reported **Cancer/disease specific survival:** Not reported	**Overall survival:** NA **Cancer/disease specific survival:** NA	**Local control:** Not reported	**Local control:** Not reported	No
Chhajed-2006, #696	STNT or LASR: **Overall survival:** Median survival : 8.4 months (4.8-17.1), 3-months survival: 90% 6-months survival: 71% 12-months survival: 40% **Cancer/disease specific survival:** Not reported	**Overall survival:** NA **Cancer/disease specific survival:** NA	**Local control:** 9 patients had tumor growth. Thus local control was 87% (at unspecified time, assumption at the time of study closeout, average FU period not given)	**Local control:** NA	Yes
Guilcher-2011, #188	**Overall survival:** Median survival: 28.6 months 2 yr: 57% 5 yr: 29% **Cancer/disease specific survival:** 2 yr: 81% 5 yr: 56%	**Overall survival:** NA **Cancer/disease specific survival:** NA	**Local control:** G3data	**Local control:** NA	No

Study	Survival Outcomes for Intervention Group 1	Survival Outcomes for Intervention Group 2	Local Control Outcomes for Intervention Group 1	Local Control Outcomes for Intervention Group 2	Arm
Jimenez-1999, #978	PHDT: Overall survival: Median survival: 265 days Cancer/disease specific survival: Not reported	YAGL: Overall survival: Median survival 95 days (p=0.007) Cancer/disease specific survival: Not reported	PHDT: Local control: Not reported	YAGL: Local control: Not reported	No
Jones-2001, #1862	Overall survival: Mean survival: From diagnosis: 10.5 months Post PHDT Rx: 5.5 months Cancer/disease specific survival: Not reported	Overall survival: NA Cancer/disease specific survival: NA	Local control: Not reported	Local control: NA	No
Langendijk-2001, #2144	EBRT +BCHY: Overall survival: Median survival: 7.0 months (95%CI: 5.3 to 8.9) Cancer/disease specific survival: Not reported	EBRT: Overall survival: Median survival: 8.5 months (95%CI: 5.4 to 11.6) Cancer/disease specific survival: Not reported	EBRT +BCHY: Local control: Not reported	EBRT: Local control: Not reported	No
Lencioni-2008, #2238	Overall survival: 1 yr: 70% (95% CI: 51 to 83) 2 yr: 48% (95% CI: 30 to 65) Cancer/disease specific survival: 1 yr: 92% (95% CI: 78–98) 2 yr: 73% (95% CI: 54–86)	Overall survival: NA Cancer/disease specific survival: NA	Local control: Not reported	Local control: NA	Yes
Moghissi-1999, #2591	EBRT: Overall survival: Median survival: 182 days 1 yr survival: 26% Cancer/disease specific survival: Not reported	EBHT: Overall survival: Median survival: 150 days 1 yr survival: 29% Cancer/disease specific survival: Not reported	Local control: Not reported	Local control: Not reported	No
Muto-2000, Italy, #2665	Overall survival: Mean survival from diagnosis: 11.1 months Mean survival from last HDR BCHY Rx: 9.7 months Cancer/disease specific survival: Not reported	Overall survival: NA Cancer/disease specific survival: NA	Local control: Not reported	Local control: NA	No
Mallick-2006, #2417	Overall survival: Not reported Cancer/disease specific survival: Not reported	Overall survival: Not reported	Local control: Not reported	Local control: Not reported	No
Petera-2001, #2914	Overall survival: Median survival (from diagnosis)	Overall survival: NA	Local control: Not reported	Local control: NA	Yes

Study	Survival Outcomes for Intervention Group 1	Survival Outcomes for Intervention Group 2	Local Control Outcomes for Intervention Group 1	Local Control Outcomes for Intervention Group 2	Arm
	BCHY (Cur): 365 days (92-670) BCHY (Pall): 242 days (30-881) Median survival (1st BCHY Rx) BCHY (Cur): 245 days (1-396) BCHY (Pall): 242 days (1-850) **Cancer/disease specific survival:** Not reported	**Cancer/disease specific survival:** Not reported			
Stout-2000, #3640	BCHY: **Overall survival:** Median: 250 days 1 yr: 22% 2 yr: 2% **Cancer/disease specific survival:** Not reported	EBRT: **Overall survival:** Median: 287 days (p=0.042) 1 yr: 38% 2 yr: 10% **Cancer/disease specific survival:** Not reported	**Local control:** Not reported	**Local control:** Not reported	No
van Boxem-1999, #427	**Overall survival:** YAGL: 8.0 ± 2.5 m **Cancer/disease specific survival:** Not reported	**Overall survival:** ECAU: 11.5 ± 3.5 m **Cancer/disease specific survival:** Not reported	**Local control:** Not reported	**Local control:** Not reported	No
Vucicevic-1999, #4010	**Overall survival:** G3 data Fig 5 page 380 **Cancer/disease specific survival:** Not reported	**Overall survival:** NA **Cancer/disease specific survival:** NA	**Local control:** Not reported	**Local control:** NA	No
Weinberg-2010, #4066	**Overall survival:** Consult TR Page 54 table 2 **Cancer/disease specific survival:** Not reported	**Overall survival:** NA **Cancer/disease specific survival:** NA	**Local control:** Not reported	**Local control:** NA	No

Appendix Table C16. Miscellaneous outcomes of studies that address Key Question 3

Study	Intervention Group 1	Intervention Group 2
Allison-2004, #108	**Lung function:** Not reported	**Lung function:** NA
	Obstructive symptoms: Not reported	**Obstructive symptoms:** NA
	Quality of life: Not reported	**Quality of life:** NA
	Performance status: Not reported Baseline KPS: 45 (±7.1) Post Rx KPS: 77 (±9.5) Diff: p<0.001 using Wilcoxan rank sum	**Performance status:** NA
	Others: Not reported	**Others:** NA
Chella-2000, #654	YAGL + BCHY **Lung function:** FEV_1 (L): 　　Pre: 1.43 (±0.6) 　　Post: 2.32 (±0.4) FEV_1 (%): 　　Pre: 53.2 (±11.2) 　　Post: 65.4 (±12.1)	YAGL **Lung function:** FEV_1 (L): 　　Pre: 1.35 (±0.7) 　　Post: 2.16 (±0.6) FEV_1 (%): 　　Pre: 52.4 (±10.7) 　　Post: 63.4 (±12.3)
	Obstructive symptoms: Speiser's index: 　　Pre: 6.9 (±0.7) 　　Post: 2.7 (±0.9)	**Obstructive symptoms:** Speiser's index: 　　Pre: 6.4 (±0.7) 　　Post: 3.0 (±0.8)
	Quality of life: Not reported	**Quality of life:** Not reported
	Performance status: Not reported	**Performance status:** Not reported
	Others: Not reported	**Others:** Not reported
Celebioglu-2002, #604	**Lung function:** Not reported	**Lung function:** NA
	Obstructive symptoms: BCHY Dyspnea: 　　Pre: 2 　　Post: 0 (<0.05) Cough: 　　Pre: 2 　　Post: 1 (<0.05) Hemoptysis: 　　Pre: 2 　　Post: 1 (<0.05) Pneumonitis: 　　Pre: 2 　　Post: 1 (<0.05) BOI:	**Obstructive symptoms:** NA

Study	Intervention Group 1	Intervention Group 2
	Pre: 6 Post: 4 (<0.05) **Quality of life:** NA **Performance status:** NA **Others:** NA	**Quality of life:** NA **Performance status:** NA **Others:** NA
Celikoglu-2006, #606	**Lung function:** Not reported **Obstructive symptoms:** Reported as % obstruction without any detail Pre Rx: 86.8 %±15.2 (for 28 obstructive sites) Post Rx: 36.0 %± 31.1 (for 28 obstructive sites) Obstruction improvement Good: 11 (48%) Moderate: 8 (35%) Small: 4(17%) **Quality of life:** Not reported **Performance status:** Not reported **Others:** Not reported	**Lung function:** NA **Obstructive symptoms:** NA **Quality of life:** NA **Performance status:** NA **Others:** NA
Chhajed-2006, #696	**Lung function:** Not reported **Obstructive symptoms:** Not reported **Quality of life:** Not reported **Performance status:** Not reported **Others:** Not reported	**Lung function:** NA **Obstructive symptoms:** NA **Quality of life:** NA **Performance status:** NA **Others:** NA
Guilcher-2011, #188	**Lung function:** Not reported **Obstructive symptoms:** Not reported **Quality of life:** Not reported **Performance status:** Not reported **Others:** Not reported	**Lung function:** NA **Obstructive symptoms:** NA **Quality of life:** NA **Performance status:** NA **Others:** NA
Jimenez-1999, #978	**Lung function:** Not reported **Obstructive symptoms:** Amelioration of symptoms was similar in both the groups. Quantitative data not reported. **Quality of life:** Not reported	**Lung function:** Not reported **Obstructive symptoms:** Amelioration of symptoms was similar in both the groups. Quantitative data not reported. **Quality of life:** Not reported

Study	Intervention Group 1	Intervention Group 2
Jones-2001, #1862	**Performance status:** Not reported **Others:** Not reported **Lung function:** Not reported **Obstructive symptoms:** Not reported **Quality of life:** Not reported **Performance status:** Not reported **Others:** Improvement I in subjective symptoms of obstruction: 9 (90%) Acute hemoptysis resolved: 7 (70%)	**Performance status:** Not reported **Others:** Not reported **Lung function:** NA **Obstructive symptoms:** NA **Quality of life:** NA **Performance status:** NA **Others:** NA
Langendjik-2001, #2144	**Lung function:** NA **Obstructive symptoms:** EBRT +BCHY: % Response Dyspnea: 18/39 (46%) Cough: 24% Hemoptysis: 86% Chest pain: 80% Pain in arm/shoulder: 74% Dyspnea symptom score (all patients): 2 wks: -5.4 6 wks: -3.9 3 months: 5.7 6 months: 15.0 12 months: 2.2 Dyspnea symptom score (patients with tumor in main bronchus): 2 wks: -22.6 6 wks: -10.8 3 months: -6.8 **Quality of life:** Not reported **Performance status:** Not reported	**Lung function:** NA **Obstructive symptoms:** EBRT: % Response Dyspnea: 16/43 (37%) (p=0.29) Cough: 38% (NSS) Hemoptysis: 82% (NSS) Chest pain: 67% (NSS) Pain in arm/shoulder: 69% (NSS) (Note: numerator and denominator unknown and not advisable to calculate as patients may have been omitted and assumptions may give false results) Dyspnea symptom score (all patients): 2 wks: 7.4 (Δ-12.9) 6 wks: 8.9 (Δ-12.8) (p=0.02) (note: unclear about p value) 3 months: 10.8 (Δ-5.1) 6 months: 10.6 (Δ4.3) 12 months: 15.2 (Δ-13.0) Dyspnea symptom score (patients with tumor in main bronchus): 2 wks: 12.4 (Δ-35.0) 6 wks: 17.8 (Δ-28.6) 3 months: 24.8 (Δ-31.6) **Quality of life:** Not reported **Performance status:** Not reported

Study	Intervention Group 1	Intervention Group 2
	Others: None	**Others:** None
Lencioni-2008, #2238	**Lung function:** (n=22) FEV, L 0 months: 1·9 (±0·9) 1 months: 1·7 (±1·1) 3 months: 1·7 (±0·9) 6 months: 1·6 (±0·9) 12 months: 1·5 (±0·7) FEV, % predicted 0 months: 68·8 (±26·9) 1 months: 65·3 (±24·6) 3 months: 71·0 (±27·2) 6 months: 62·5 (±18·5) 12 months: 63·4 (±20·7) **Obstructive symptoms:** Not reported **Quality of life:** FACT-G 0 months: 80·5 (±11·2) 12 months: 82·2 (±11·1) LCS 0 months: 22·5 (±3·9) 12 months: 23·6 (±3·1) TOI 0 months: 64·2 (±10·6) 12 months: 67·5 (±8·0) PCS 0 months: 44·4 (±10·8) 12 months: 46·0 (±10·2) MCS 0 months: 47·6 (±9·6) 12 months: 49·6 (±10·3) **Performance status:** Not reported	**Lung function:** NA **Obstructive symptoms:** NA **Quality of life:** NA **Performance status:** NA **Others:** NA
Moghissi-1999, #2591	**Others:** None EBRT: **Lung function:** Relief of breathlessness: 32% **Obstructive symptoms:** Not reported **Quality of life:** Not reported **Performance status:**	EBHT: **Lung function:** Relief of breathlessness: 28% **Obstructive symptoms:** Not reported **Quality of life:** Not reported **Performance status:**

Study	Intervention Group 1	Intervention Group 2
	WHO PS: 14%	WHO PS: 38% (difference 24%; 95%CI: 8 to 56)
	Others: Palliation of major thoracic symptoms: 27%	**Others:** Palliation of major thoracic symptoms: 22%
Muto-2000, Italy, #2665	**Lung function:** Not reported	**Lung function:** NA
	Obstructive symptoms:	**Obstructive symptoms:** NA

Obstructive symptoms:

Dyspnea:
BCHY (10 Gy):
    Pre: 90 %
    Post: 20 %
BCHY (14Gy) + EBRT:
    Pre: 87 %
    Post: 15%
BCHY (15Gy, 1cm) + EBRT:
    Pre: 88 %
    Post: 10 %
BCHY (15Gy, 0.5 cm) + EBRT:
    Pre: 85 %
    Post: 5 %

Cough:
BCHY (10 Gy):
    Pre: 92 %
    Post: 42 %
BCHY (14Gy) + EBRT:
    Pre: 96 %
    Post: 28 %
BCHY (15Gy, 1cm) + EBRT:
    Pre: 90 %
    Post: 12 %
BCHY (15Gy, 0.5 cm) + EBRT:
    Pre: 91 %
    Post: 11 %

Hemoptysis:
BCHY (10 Gy):
    Pre: 10 %
    Post: 0 %
BCHY (14Gy) + EBRT:
    Pre: 7 %
    Post: 1 %
BCHY (15Gy, 1cm) + EBRT:
    Pre: 8 %
    Post: 1 %
BCHY (15Gy, 0.5 cm) + EBRT:
    Pre: 12 %
    Post: 0 %

Quality of life:

Quality of life:

Study	Intervention Group 1	Intervention Group 2
	Performance status: Not reported	NA
	Performance status: Not reported	**Performance status:** NA
	Others: None	**Others:** NA
Mallick-2006, #2417	**Lung function:** Not reported	**Lung function:** Not reported
	Obstructive symptoms: Obstructive pneumonia (% incidence) EBRT+BCHY-16Gy: Pre: 9 (60%) Post: 9 (100%) (NSS) EBRT+BCHY-10Gy: Pre: 10 (67%) Post: 7 (70%) (NSS) Obstructive pneumonia (median time to relapse in months) EBRT+BCHY-16Gy: 4 EBRT+BCHY-10Gy: 5 Obstructive pneumonia (median time to progression in months) EBRT+BCHY-16Gy: 7 EBRT+BCHY-10Gy: 7	**Obstructive symptoms:** Obstructive pneumonia (% incidence) BCHY-15Gy: Pre: 10 (67) Post: 8 (80) (NSS) Obstructive pneumonia (median time to relapse in months) BCHY-15Gy: 6 (NSS) Obstructive pneumonia (median time to progression in months) BCHY-15Gy: 6 (NSS)
	Quality of life: QLQ-C3 (Global Health status): EBRT+BCHY-16Gy: Pre: 37 Post: 75 (↑103%) EBRT+BCHY-10Gy: Pre: 35 Post: 63 (↑80%) QLQ-C3 (Physical Functioning): EBRT+BCHY-16Gy: Pre: 71 Post: 90 (↑27%) EBRT+BCHY-10Gy: Pre: 74 Post: 85 (↑15%) QLQ-LC13 (Symptom Scale: Dyspnea) EBRT+BCHY-16Gy: Pre: 33 Post: 4 (↓88%) EBRT+BCHY-10Gy: Pre: 25 Post: 13(↓48%) QLQ-LC13 (Symptom Scale: Cough)	**Quality of life:** QLQ-C3 (Global Health status): BCHY-15Gy: Pre: 34 Post: 62 (↑82%) QLQ-C3 (Physical Functioning): BCHY-15Gy: Pre: 56 Post: 78 (↑39%) QLQ-LC13 (Symptom Scale: Dyspnea) BCHY-15Gy: Pre: 33 Post: 13 (↓61%) QLQ-LC13 (Symptom Scale: Cough)

Study	Intervention Group 1	Intervention Group 2

	QLQ-LC13 (Symptom Scale: Cough)
	EBRT+BCHY-16Gy:
	    Pre: 67
	    Post: 40 (↓40%)
	EBRT+BCHY-10Gy:
	    Pre: 65
	    Post: 36 (↓45%)
	
	QLQ-LC13 (Symptom Scale: Hemoptysis)
	EBRT+BCHY-16Gy:
	    Pre: 20
	    Post: 0 (↓100%)
	EBRT+BCHY-10Gy:
	    Pre: 47
	    Post: 9 (↓81%)
	
	Performance status:
	Not reported
	
	Others:
	Dyspnea (% incidence)
	EBRT+BCHY-16Gy:
	    Pre: 15 (100)
	    Post: 14 (93) (NSS)
	EBRT+BCHY-10Gy:
	    Pre: 13 (87)
	    Post: 12 (92) (NSS)
	Dyspnea (median time to relapse in months)
	EBRT+BCHY-16Gy: 4
	EBRT+BCHY-10Gy: 5
	Dyspnea (median time to progression in months)
	EBRT+BCHY-16Gy: 7
	EBRT+BCHY-10Gy: 7
	Cough (% incidence)
	EBRT+BCHY-16Gy:
	    Pre: 15 (100)
	    Post: 12 (80) (NSS)
	EBRT+BCHY-10Gy:
	    Pre: 15 (100)
	    Post: 13 (87) (NSS)
	Cough (median time to relapse in months)
	EBRT+BCHY-16Gy: 4
	EBRT+BCHY-10Gy: 7
	Cough (median time to progression in months)
	EBRT+BCHY-16Gy: 7
	EBRT+BCHY-10Gy: not reached
	Hemoptysis (% incidence)
	EBRT+BCHY-16Gy:
	    Pre: 9 (60)
		BCHY-15Gy:
		    Pre: 56
		    Post: 22 (↓61%)
		
		QLQ-LC13 (Symptom Scale: Hemoptysis)
		BCHY-15Gy:
		    Pre: 27
		    Post: 9 (↓67%)
		
		Performance status:
		Not reported
		
		Others:
		Dyspnea (% incidence)
		BCHY-15Gy:
		    Pre: 15 (100)
		    Post: 13 (87) (NSS)
		
		Dyspnea (median time to relapse in months)
		BCHY-15Gy: 6 (NSS)
		
		Dyspnea (median time to progression in months)
		BCHY-15Gy: 6 (NSS)
		
		Cough (% incidence)
		BCHY-15Gy:
		    Pre: 15 (100)
		    Post: 13 (87) (NSS)
		
		Cough (median time to relapse in months)
		BCHY-15Gy: 4 (NSS)
		
		Cough (median time to progression in months)
		BCHY-15Gy: not reached (NSS)
		
		Hemoptysis (% incidence)
		BCHY-15Gy:
		    Pre: 12 (80)
		    Post: 10 (82) (NSS)

Study	Intervention Group 1	Intervention Group 2
	Post: 9 (100) (NSS) EBRT+BCHY-10Gy: Pre: 13 (87) Post 13 (100) (NSS) Hemoptysis (median time to relapse in months) EBRT+BCHY-16Gy: 8 EBRT+BCHY-10Gy: not reached Hemoptysis (median time to progression in months) EBRT+BCHY-16Gy: 11 EBRT+BCHY-10Gy: not reached	Hemoptysis (median time to relapse in months) BCHY-15Gy: 5 (p=0.01) Hemoptysis (median time to progression in months) BCHY-15Gy: 6 (p=0.01)
Petera-2001, #2914	**Lung function:** Not reported **Obstructive symptoms:** BCHY (Cur): Improvement in dyspnea: 11 (61%) Cough: 7 (44%) Hemoptysis: 4 (67%) BCHY (Pall): Improvement in dyspnea: 14 (74%) Cough: 12 (70%) Hemoptysis: 5 (71%) **Quality of life:** Not reported **Performance status:** Not reported **Others:** None	**Lung function:** NA **Obstructive symptoms:** NA **Quality of life:** NA **Performance status:** NA **Others:** None
Stout-2000, #3640	**Lung function:** Not reported BCHY: **Obstructive symptoms:** (% of +ve symptom endpoints) 4 weeks: Cough: 59% (n=41) Hemoptysis: 85% (n=41) Breathlessness : 78% (n=41) 8 weeks: Cough: 50% (n=46) Hemoptysis: 78% (n=46) Breathlessness: 59% (n=46) **Quality of life:** Not reported **Performance status:** Not reported	**Lung function:** Not reported EBRT: **Obstructive symptoms:** (% of +ve symptom endpoints) 4 weeks: Cough: 59% (n=29) Hemoptysis: 90% (n=29) Breathlessness : 66% (n=29) 8 weeks: Cough: 67% (n=46) Hemoptysis: 89% (n=46) Breathlessness: 78% (n=46) **Quality of life:** Not reported **Performance status:** Not reported

Study	Intervention Group 1	Intervention Group 2
	Others: (Global palliation) BCHY: 76%	**Others:** EBRT: 91% (0.09)
van Boxem-1999, #427	**Lung function:** Not reported	**Lung function:** Not reported
	Obstructive symptoms: YAGL: 10 (71%) (on a yes no dichotomous scale as rated by study authors)	**Obstructive symptoms:** ECAU: 13 (76%)
	Quality of life: Not reported	**Quality of life:** Not reported
	Performance status: Not reported	**Performance status:** Not reported
	Others: Not reported	**Others:** Not reported
Vucicevic-1999, #4010	**Lung function:** Not reported	**Lung function:** NA
	Obstructive symptoms: BCHY + EBRT: Dyspnea: Pre: 26/39 (67%) Post: 3/39 (8%) Cough: Pre: 35/39 (90%) Post: 8/39 (21%) Hemoptysis Pre: 22/39 (56%) Post: 1/39 (3%) Massive hemoptysis Pre: 6/39 (15%) Post: 0/39 (0%)	**Obstructive symptoms:** NA
	Quality of life: Not reported	**Quality of life:** NA
	Performance status: Not reported	**Performance status:** NA
	Others: None	**Others:** None
Weinberg-2010, #4066	**Lung function:** Not reported	**Lung function:** NA
	Obstructive symptoms: Not reported	**Obstructive symptoms:** NA
	Quality of life: Not reported	**Quality of life:** NA
	Performance status:	**Performance status:**

Study	Intervention Group 1	Intervention Group 2
	Not reported	NA
	Others:	**Others:**
	None	NA

Appendix Table C17. Toxicity outcomes of studies that address Key Question 3

Study	Intervention Group 1	Intervention Group 2
Allison-2004, #108	Not reported	NA
Chella-2000, #654	YAGL + BCHY: Death due to hemoptysis: 1 (7%) (12 months after Rx)	YAGL Not reported
Celebioglu-2002, #604	BCHY: Hemoptysis requiring hospitalization: 1 (1%) Pneumothorax: 0 Fistula: 0 Cardiovascular problems: 0	NA
Celikoglu-2006, #606	Not reported	NA
Chhajed-2006, #696	STNT + LASR Stent migration: 3 (6%) Mucous plugging of the airway stent: 2 (4%) Moderate-to-severe bleeding during bronchoscopy: 1 (2%) Death within 24 h of the procedure: 1 (2%)	NA

Guilcher-2011, #188	Respiratory insufficiency during HDR BCHY: 2 (1%)
	Grade III mucositis: 2 (1%)
	Grade II radiation bronchitis: 28 (12%)
	Pneumothorax: 3 (1%)
	Bronchial stenosis: 21 (9%)
	Necrosis of bronchial wall: 7 (3%)
	Hemoptysis: 15 (7%)
	Death due to complication: 13 (6%)
	    Death due to hemoptysis: 10 (4%)
	    Death due to necrosis: 2 (1%)
	    Death due to radiation stenosis: 1 (0.4%)
		NA

Jimenez-1999, #978	PHDT Death from hemoptysis and presumed progression of the disease: 1(7%)	YAGL Death from hemoptysis and presumed progression of the disease: 1 6%)
Jones-2001, #1862	Not reported	NA
Langendjik-2001, #2144	EBRT +BCHY: Death due to massive hemoptysis: 7(15%) Broncho-esophageal fistula: 1 (2%)	BCHY: Death due to massive hemoptysis: 6(13%)
Lencioni-2008, #2238	40 procedures were done in NSCLC patients and there were 5 large or symptomatic pneumothorax needing drainage as a major complication.	
Moghissi-1999, #2591	Not reported	Not reported

Muto-2000, Italy, #2665	Grade 2 Radiation Bronchitis:
	    BCHY (10 Gy): 13/78 (17%)
	    BCHY (14Gy) + EBRT: 4/46 (9%)
	    BCHY (15Gy, 1cm) + EBRT: 0/36 (0%)
	    BCHY (15Gy, 0.5 cm) + EBRT: 3/120 (3%)
	Grade 3 Radiation Bronchitis:
	    BCHY (10 Gy): 17/78 (22%)
	    BCHY (14Gy) + EBRT: 3/46 (7%)	

Study	Intervention Group 1	Intervention Group 2

	BCHY (15Gy, 1cm) + EBRT: 3/36 (8%)
	BCHY (15Gy, 0.5 cm) + EBRT: 5/120 (4%)
	Grade 4 Radiation Bronchitis:
	  BCHY (10 Gy): 12/78 (15%)
	  BCHY (14Gy) + EBRT: 3/46 (7%)
	  BCHY (15Gy, 1cm) + EBRT: 3/36 (8%)
	  BCHY (15Gy, 0.5 cm) + EBRT: 5/120 (4%)
	Fatal hemoptysis:
	  BCHY (10 Gy): 2/78 (3%)
	  BCHY (14Gy) + EBRT: 3/46 (7%)
	  BCHY (15Gy, 1cm) + EBRT: 2/36 (6%)
	  BCHY (15Gy, 0.5 cm) + EBRT: 3/120 (3%)
	Broncho esophageal fistulas:
	  BCHY (10 Gy): 1/78 (1%)
	  BCHY (14Gy) + EBRT: 1/46 (2%)
	  BCHY (15Gy, 1cm) + EBRT: 1/36 (3%)
	  BCHY (15Gy, 0.5 cm) + EBRT: 0 (0%)	

Mallick-2006, #2417	No grade II-grade IV acute complications occurred	No grade II-grade IV acute complications occurred 1 patient died due to fatal hemoptysis at 7 months
Petera-2001, #2914	Not discernible	NA
Stout-2000, #3640	BCHY: Fatal hemoptysis: 4 (8%)	EBRT: Fatal hemoptysis: 3 (6%)
Study	Intervention Group 1	Intervention Group 2
van Boxem-1999, #427	YAGL: Hypotension: 1 (7%)	ECAU: Hemoptysis/respiratory failure: 1 (6%)

Vucicevic-1999, #4010	Acute
	  Esophagitis: 3/39 (8%)
	  Cardiac arrhythmia: 1/39 (3%)
	Chronic
	  Pulmonary fibrosis: 4/39 (10%)
	  Esophageal stricture: 1/39 (3%)
	  Fistulae: 1/39 (3%)
	  Massive hemoptysis: 1/30 (3%)
		NA

Weinberg-2010, #4066	Bronchial contraction: 5/9 (56%) Occlusion from bronchial contraction: 2/9 (22%) Photosensitivity: 2/9 (22%)	NA

C-112

Appendix Table C18. Study attributes - Key Question 3

Study	HC	Enroll Start	Enroll End	Time	Study Setting	Treatment Setting	Institution Setting(s)	Stage(s):	Staging Criteria:	COI	Funding
Allison-2004,	Yes	NR	NR	PRO	SI	O	TH	Recurrence	NR	No	NR
Celebioglu-2002,	Yes	05/97	03/99	RET	SI	I	TH	Stage 3, Stage 4, Recurrence	Int. Staging System of Lung Cancer	NR	NR
Celikoglu-2006,	Yes	NR	NR	PRO	SI	O	TH	Stage 3	AJCC	NR	NR
Chella-2000,	Yes	Dec-95	Dec-98	PRO	SI	O	TH	NR	NR	NR	NR
Chhajed-2006,	No	NR	NR	RET	SI	NR	TH	NR	NR	No	NR
Guilcher-2011,	No	1991	2004	RET	M	NR	Other : Unable to make judgment	NR	NR	No	NR
Jimenez-1999,	Yes	NR	NR	PRO	SI	NR	Other : Hospital	Stage 1, Stage 2, Stage 3, Stage 4, Recurrence	NR	NR	Manufacturer
Jones-2001,	Yes	08/1998	12/2000	RET	SI	I	TH	Stage 3, Stage 4	NR	NR	NR
Langendijk-2001,	Yes	NR	NR	PRO	M	NR	TH	Stage 1, Stage 3	UICC 1992	No	Professional Society
Lencioni-2008,	Yes	07/2001	12/2005	PRO	M	NR	TH	Stage 1, Recurrence	NR	No	Manufacturer
Mallick- 2006, # 2417	Yes	05/2003	02/2005	PRO	SI	O	TH	Stage 3	NR	No	Not supported
Moghissi-1999,	Yes	05/1993	11/1996	PRO	MI	O	CH, CC	NR	NR	NR	NR
Muto-2000,	Yes	01/1992	07/1997	PRO	SI	NR	TH	Stage 3	NR	NR	NR
Petera-2001,	No	12/1996	04/1999	NR	SI	NR	TH	Stage 2, Stage 3, Stage 4	NR	NR	NR
Stout-2000,	Yes	07/1989	07/1993	PRO	M	O	CH	NR	NR	NR	NR
van Boxem-1999,	Yes	01/94	12/96	RET	SI	I	TH	Stage 3, Stage 4	NR	NR	NR
Vucicenic-1999,	Yes	01/1996	12/1997	RET	SI	NR	TH	Stage 3	NR	NR	NR
Weinberg-2010,	Yes	1/2001	8/2008	NR	SI	NR	TH	Stage 1, Stage 2, Stage 3, Stage 4	NR	NR	NR

Appendix Table C19. Carey and Boden assessment tool for Key Questions 1 and 2

ID	KQ	Clearly Defined Question	Well-described study population	Well-described intervention	Use of Validated Outcome Measures	Appropriate Statistical Analysis	Well-Described Results	Discussion/Conclusions Supported by Data	Funding/Sponsor Source Acknowledged
Andratschke, 2011	KQ1	Y	Y	Y	Y	U	Y	U	Y
Baumann, 2006	KQ1	N	Y	Y	Y	Y	Y	Y	N
Baumann, 2009	KQ1	Y	Y	Y	Y	Y	Y	Y	Y
Bogart, 2010	KQ1	Y	N	N	Y	Y	Y	Y	Y
Bollineni, 2012	KQ1	Y	Y	N	Y	Y	Y	U	Y
Bradley, 2003	KQ1	Y	Y	Y	Y	Y	Y	Y	N
Burdick, 2010	KQ1	Y	Y	Y	Y	Y	Y	Y	N
Bush, 2004	KQ1	Y	Y	Y	Y	Y	Y	Y	Y
Campeau, 2009	KQ1	Y	Y	Y	Y	Y	Y	Y	N
Chen, 2012	KQ2	Y	Y	N	Y	Y	N	U	N
Coon, 2008	KQ1	Y	Y	Y	Y	N	Y	Y	N
Dunlap, 2010	KQ1	Y	Y	Y	Y	Y	Y	Y	N
Fritz, 2008	KQ1	Y	Y	Y	Y	Y	Y	Y	N
Graham, 2006	KQ1	Y	Y	Y	Y	Y	Y	Y	N
Iwata, 2010	KQ1/2	Y	Y	Y	Y	Y	Y	Y	Y
Jimenez, 2010	KQ1	Y	Y	Y	Y	Y	N	U	N
Kopek, 2009	KQ1	Y	Y	Y	Y	Y	Y	Y	Y
Mirri, 2009	KQ1	Y	N	Y	Y	U	N	U	N
Nakayama, 2010	KQ1	Y	Y	N	Y	Y	N	U	N
Narayan, 2004	KQ1	Y	N	Y	Y	Y	N	U	Y

ID	KQ	Clearly Defined Question	Well-described study population	Well-described intervention	Use of Validated Outcome Measures	Appropriate Statistical Analysis	Well-Described Results	Discussion/Conclusions Supported by Data	Funding/Sponsor Source Acknowledged
Nyman, 2006	KQ1	Y	Y	Y	Y	Y	Y	Y	N
Olsen, 2011	KQ1	Y	N	Y	Y	Y	Y	U	N
Palma, 2011	KQ1	Y	N	Y	Y	Y	Y	U	Y
Pennathur, 2007	KQ1	Y	Y	Y	Y	Y	Y	Y	Y
Pennathur, 2009	KQ1	Y	Y	Y	Y	Y	Y	Y	N
Ricardi, 2010	KQ1	Y	Y	Y	Y	Y	Y	N	N
Scorsetti, 2007	KQ1	N	Y	Y	Y	Y	Y	Y	N
Shibamoto, 2012	KQ1/2	Y	Y	Y	Y	Y	Y	Y	Y
Song, 2009	KQ1	Y	Y	Y	Y	Y	Y	Y	Y
Stephans, 2009	KQ1	Y	Y	Y	Y	Y	Y	Y	Y
Takeda, 2009	KQ1/2	Y	Y	Y	Y	Y	Y	Y	N
Taremi, 2011	KQ1	Y	N	Y	Y	Y	Y	Y	Y
Turzer, 2011	KQ1	Y	Y	Y	Y	Y	Y	Y	N
Vahdat, 2010	KQ1	Y	N	Y	Y	Y	N	N	N
van der Voort van Zyp, 2009	KQ1	Y	N	Y	Y	Y	Y	Y	N
Videtic, 2010	KQ1	Y	Y	Y	Y	Y	Y	Y	N
Lagerwaard, 2011	KQ2	Y	Y	N	Y	Y	Y	Y	N

ID	KQ	Clearly Defined Question	Well-described study population	Well-described intervention	Use of Validated Outcome Measures	Appropriate Statistical Analysis	Well-Described Results	Discussion/Conclusions Supported by Data	Funding/Sponsor Source Acknowledged
Onishi, 2011	KQ2	Y	Y	Y	Y	Y	Y	Y	Y

Appendix Table C20. Carey and Boden assessment tool for Key Question 3

ID	KQ	Clearly Defined Question	Well-described study population	Well-described intervention	Use of Validated Outcome Measures	Appropriate Statistical Analysis	Well-Described Results	Discussion/Conclusions Supported by Data	Funding/Sponsor Source Acknowledged
Allison, 2004	3	Y	Y	Y	Y	N	Y	Y	N
Chhajed, 2006	3	N	N	N	Y	Y	N	N	N
Lencioni, 2008	3	Y	Y	Y	N	N	Y	N	Y

Abbreviations Used in This Appendix

Abbreviation	Definition
3DRT	Three dimensional radiation therapy
AC	Adenocarcinoma
ACE-27	Adult Co-Morbidity Evaluation-27 scoring system
BAC	Bronchoalveolar carcinoma
BED	Biologically Effective Dose
BI	Bronchus intermedius
BOI	Bronchial abstraction index
CAD	Coronary Artery Disease
CCI	Charlson Comorbidity Index
CGE	Cobalt Gray equivalent
CHF	Congestive Heart Failure
CI	Confidence interval
COPD	Chronic Obstructive Pulmonary Disease
CPD	Chronic Pulmonary Disease
CSS	Cancer-specific survival
CT	Computed Tomography
CTC	Common Toxicity Criteria
CTCAE	Common Terminology Criteria for Adverse Events
CVD	Cardiovascular disease
CWP	Chest Wall Pain
DLCO	Diffusion Lung Capacity for Carbon Monoxide
DM	Diabetes mellitus
CSS	Disease-specific survival
ECOG	Eastern Cooperative Oncology Group
EORTC	European Organization for Research and Treatment of Cancer
FACT-G	Functional Assessment of Cancer Therapy- General
FDG	Fluorodeoxyglucose
FEV	Forced expiratory volume
FRS	Fractions
FU	Followup
GTV	Gross tumor volume
GY	Gray
HC	Histopathology confirmation
HDR	High-dose-rate
Hst	Histologically
IGRT	Image-Guided Radiotherapy
IMRT	Intensity-modulated radiotherapy
INR	International Normalized Ratio
KFI	Kaplan-Feinstein index
KPS	Karnofsky performance status
LB	Lobar bronchus
LC	Lung cancer
LCC	Large cell carcinoma
LCS	Lung Cancer Subscale
LCT	Local control
LENT-SOMA	Late Effects Normal Tissue Task Force -Subjective, Objective, Management, Analytic *scales*
LL	Lower lobe
MB	Main bronchus
MCS	Mental Component Summary
MeV	Million electron volts
MI	Myocardial Infarction
ML	Middle lobe
mos	Months

MS	Main stem
N	Number
NA	Not applicable
NCI	National Cancer Institute
NOS	Not otherwise specified Non-Small Cell Lung Cancer
NR	Not reported
NSCC	Non squamous cell lung cancer
NSCLC	Non-small cell lung cancer
NSS	Not statistically significant
OMC	Other Medical Comorbidities
OS	Overall Survival
PCS	Physical Component Summary
PET	Positron Emission Tomography
PHDT	Photodynamic therapy
PFS	Progression-free survival
PRO	Prospective
PS	Performance status
Pts	Patients
PTV	Planning target volume
PVD	Peripheral Vascular Disease
QLQ	Quality of life Questionnaire
QOL	Quality of life
RECIST	Response Evaluation Criteria in Solid Tumors
RET	Retrospective
RFA	Radio-frequency ablation
RT	Radiation Therapy
RTOG	Radiation Therapy Oncology Group
Rx	Treatment
SAS	Single arm study
SB	Superior bronchus
SBRT	Stereotactic body radiotherapy
SCC	Squamous cell carcinoma
SCS	Simplified comorbidity score
SWOG	Southwest Oncology Group
TOI	Trial Outcome Index
UICC	Union Internationale Contre le Cancer
UL	Upper lobe
UNSCLC	Unclassified Non-Small Cell Lung Cancer
WHO	World Health Organization
YAGL	Yttrium aluminum garnet laser